MEDICAL ETHICS

THIRD EDITION

ALASTAIR CAMPBELL

GRANT GILLETT

GARETH JONES

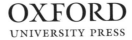

OXFORD

UNIVERSITY PRESS

OXFORD
UNIVERSITY PRESS

253 Normanby Road, South Melbourne, Victoria 3205, Australia

Oxford University Press is a department of the University of Oxford. It
furthers the University's objective of excellence in research, scholarship, and
education by publishing worldwide in

Oxford New York

Athens Auckland Bangkok Bogotá Buenos Aires Cape Town Chennai
Dar es Salaam Delhi Florence Hong Kong Istanbul Karachi Kolkata
Kuala Lumpur Madrid Melbourne Mexico City Mumbai Nairobi Paris
Port Moresby São Paulo Shanghai Singapore Taipei Tokyo Toronto Warsaw

with associated companies in Berlin Ibadan

OXFORD is a trade mark of Oxford University Press in the UK and in certain
other countries

ISBN 0 19 558445 7

Text designed by Patrick Cannon
Cover designed by Deb Snibson, Modern Art Production Group
Typeset by Solo
Printed through Bookpac Production Services, Singapore

Contents

The Authors

Alastair Campbell is Professor of Ethics in Medicine at the University of Bristol. His academic career began at the University of Edinburgh in the Department of Christian Ethics and Practical Theology, and he spent six years as Director of the Bioethics Research Centre in the Dunedin School of Medicine, University of Otago. He was founding editor of the *Journal of Medical Ethics*.

Grant Gillett is a professor of medical ethics at the University of Otago. He is also a practising neurosurgeon. He qualified in medicine at the Auckland Medical School in New Zealand, and also completed a Masters degree in psychology. For some years, while completing his own studies, he was a lecturer in physiological psychology. He trained as a neurosurgeon and worked at the Radcliffe Infirmary in Oxford. He then gained a D Phil in philosophy at Oxford University and became a fellow at Magdalen College in 1985. In 1988 he moved to the University of Otago. He is the author of *Representation, Meaning and Thought* (1992), *Reasonable Care* (1989), and is a co-author of *The Discursive Mind* (1994). His latest book is *The Mind and its Discontents* (1999). He has also edited several books, and published widely in the areas of philosophy and medical ethics.

Gareth Jones has been Professor and Head of the Department of Anatomy and Structural Biology at the University of Otago since 1983. Prior to that he held appointments at University College London, and at the University of Western Australia. He has had a close association with the Bioethics Centre at the University of Otago since its inception, and has had periods as its Acting Director. He has published widely both in neurobiology and bioethics, and his latest book is *Speaking for the Dead: Cadavers in Biology and Medicine* (2000).

Preface

This book is intended as a practical introduction to the ethical questions doctors and other health care professionals can be expected to encounter in their practice. The original edition was released in 1992 as *Practical Medical Ethics*, with the second edition, *Medical Ethics*, appearing in 1997. The current edition builds on the last edition, and has taken on more of a United Kingdom emphasis, to reflect its popularity there. There are new chapters on organ transplantation (including xenotransplantation and stem cells), and innovative and unorthodox treatments. In addition, changes have been made to a number of other chapters to include discussion of autopsies, the use of biopsies from surgical operations, brain death, and up-dated discussions to take account of the plethora of developments in cloning and the human genome project.

We envisage this book, like its predecessors, to be of immediate relevance to health care professionals and to the users of health services. Since we start from the premise that medical ethics is embedded in the dilemmas of everyday practice, we consider that our argument should return repeatedly to specific cases, following critical reflection on our own views and the views of others. Our aim has thus been to integrate theoretical discussion with its practical application.

Although we have a health professional readership in mind, especially medical students and medical practitioners at all stages of their careers, we do not believe that medical ethics is a domain restricted to doctors. Our intention is to inform a broad section of society, and therefore it is our hope to attract a wide readership from outside the medical profession. Nevertheless, in the first instance, we have written this book with that profession in mind, since we believe that each health care profession has particular challenges to meet and particular blind spots to overcome. As with its predecessors, we would like to see this volume emerge as a basic textbook on medical ethics for any medical curriculum that has ethics as a serious component.

The emphasis on the basic biomedical sciences has increased in this edition, a reflection of the flurry of activity in that realm. While we do not want this emphasis to predominate, we also realise that these sciences inform clinical practice to an increasing degree. Consequently, those starting out on a medical career and therefore having to reflect on ethical issues in medicine, will have to contend more and more with the considerable range of delicate issues raised by this burgeoning area.

As in previous editions, each chapter presents a range of ethical views, drawn from both traditional philosophical responses and the most recent of contemporary responses. The case studies and examples that illustrate theoretical discussion are suitable both for private study and for use in group discussions.

While we leave it to readers to make up their own minds on the many contentious issues in medical ethics, we have not refrained, at times, from offering our own conclusions, backed by the arguments that have led us to them. Such an approach gives readers something to react to, by providing a launching pad for formulating their own approaches to the numerous dilemmas facing them.

This book is the result of a team effort. Since the authors come from different theoretical backgrounds and professional perspectives, we have worked hard to express ourselves consistently, in both linguistic style and ethical approach. Our aim has been to produce a unified work that reads as though it emanates from one author. We have deliberately provided no indication of who has written which chapters. In this edition we return to the three authors of the first edition. While all three of us were originally at the University of Otago in Dunedin, New Zealand, Alastair Campbell has been at the University of Bristol, England since the publication of the second edition. Consequently, we have aimed to broaden the perspective somewhat to take account of the United Kingdom situation, and to down play what was originally a strong New Zealand emphasis. We hope that the result will be of assistance to readers in a wide variety of cultural contexts. We would like to take this opportunity to thank Max Charlesworth for his contribution to the second edition, and for the breadth of perspective he brought to our thinking in many aspects of medical ethics.

We wish to record our thanks to Dr Kerry Galvin, who has assisted in major ways with the editing and collating of the material and preparing the typescript, and without whom this edition may not have seen the light of day. We also wish to thanks Cindy Towns for her assistance in the early stages.

Gareth Jones, on behalf of the authors
Department of Anatomy and Structural Biology
University of Otago
November 2000

PART I

Foundations

1
Theories of Medical Ethics

Introduction

Medical ethics is an applied branch of ethics or moral philosophy. It attempts to unravel the rights and wrongs of different areas of health care practice in the light of philosophical analysis.

> Dr A has a daring theory about leukemia. If he is right, he will save his patients from a burdensome course of treatment because his theory concerns the use of vitamins and diet rather than standard courses of chemotherapy. If he is wrong, the patient stands to die of a potentially treatable disease. The doctor knows that most patients would be quite alarmed if he told them they had leukemia. He does not want them 'hiving off' to other doctors and/or asking a lot of awkward questions about conventional treatment, so he tells them they have some blood cells that are a little disordered in their growth and need extra vitamins and careful watching. He does not tell them that some people would regard their disease as malignant, nor does he explain the risks to their health that might result from his singular approach to the disease. After a few months it becomes apparent that his approach is not working. He admits that he is wrong and goes back to administering conventional treatment.

Many of us realise that this doctor has not acted correctly, but when we come to analyse just what is wrong and how one should act in such situations, that realisation alone is not enough. It is here that applied moral philosophy makes its contribution.

Some Historical Background

Ethics itself has a long history. In the fourth century BC, Socrates related ethics to personal morality and character when he asked, 'What sort of person ought one to be?' The subject of ethics is best thought of as the critical scrutiny of moral thought and practice. For instance, we think it is wrong to kill, as a matter of moral law, but an ethicist would want to know why we think this, whether it is always wrong to kill, and how we justify our conviction of its wrongness in different cases. An ethicist might, for instance, ask us to imagine that someone was about to kill our child: would we think it wrong to kill the potential murderer if that were the only way to save the child? Or he might ask a deep question such as 'So what is bad about human death?' (In some traditions, including that to which Socrates himself subscribed, death is regarded as entry into paradise, or at least as a passage to a higher state of being.)

Plato answered the ethical question 'What sort of person ought one to be?' by stating that a good person was one who, in his mind, attended to and was guided by the 'form' of the good. This was a divine and eternal reality only imperfectly seen in everyday human existence but supremely disclosed by the calm contemplations of wise men. We, however, recognise that great thoughts do not always mean good deeds, and that morality is essentially to do with our attitudes, behaviour, and relations to one another.

Aristotle offered a more pragmatic analysis than Plato's, according to which 'forms' were modes of being found in the creatures around us, and the form of human excellence was that which best suited rational social animals (or mortal beings). For Aristotle, the qualities that make us human were shown in our thinking, our associations with each other, and our functions as members of the natural order. Aquinas and some of the Christian Moralists have grafted onto Aristotle's theory the doctrine that the ideal of human function is the way we are meant to be because it represents the design of our Creator. This, like the Aristotelian tradition, allows us to examine what counts as human excellence or well-being in an attempt to discover how we should act. Aristotle's view is, however, consistent with an underlying theory about human nature and its origins, including an evolutionary one. In fact, Aristotle and Hippocrates, the medical teacher credited with the first ethical codes in medicine, shared a methodology that began with observations of the actual world in which they lived, rather than beginning with theories about life, the universe, and everything.

The leap from Aristotle to David Hume takes us to a further naturalistic theory, but for Hume the form that constitutes right living is taken to be exemplified by decent, clear-thinking eighteenth-century gentlemen. Such people acted on the basis of their moral *sentiments*, having regard for norms with a broader basis than their own good opinions of themselves. However, it was clear to Hume that morals, depending as they do on the sentiments of decent people, were essentially a matter of emotion. When we translate this into terms suited to medical ethics, we get the image of decent, kind medical persons with sound opinions. Such doctors would do what they felt was best for their patients but perhaps not what they would prefer, not because they were ill-intentioned but only because the patients might not understand or share their point of view in a given situation. The problem is that the basis for our assessments can vary from sensitive and informed consideration for another person's feelings to 'paternalism', a rather arrogant assumption that one knows best.

Paternalistic doctors make decisions for others on the basis of their own values, which others may not share. Such doctors, if misguided, can be positively harmful to their patients. Imagine, for instance, an enthusiastic young cardiologist who believes that everyone with chest pain should have a cardiac catheter investigation. In pursuing this policy she may have little regard for the patient's wishes regarding intervention for heart disease, or for properly informing the patient about the risks and benefits of the test being contemplated (indeed, she may not have thought those out properly for herself). This approach ignores what we might regard as proper ethical constraints on medical practice because it tends to equate the right decision with what the doctor feels to be right for the patient. The difficulty with a focus on the doctor's character and the soundness of his or her sentiments is that it can divert our attention from the fact that it is the patient's interests that have always (since Hippocrates at least) been paramount in medical ethics. However, we ought not to abandon the attempt to find a moral guide in our own being, provided only that we are attuned to and care about the needs and well-being of others and do not merely follow our own inclinations.

Codes of Conduct

A more contemporary version of the ethical question has shifted from character to conduct and asks: 'What should a person do?' Or, in the matter of health care ethics, 'What should a health professional do?'

The most forthright answer is contained in Kantian theories: a person should do his duty. In fact this is a degenerate version of Kant's answer, which was that one should act in such a way that, in a community whose members all acted that way, one would order one's life according to reason and the lives of all would be enhanced. To be sure, he saw the more general imperative as generating a series of specific duties, and it is these that have been picked up in the post-Kantian strands of medical ethics. Kantian ethics focuses on rights and duties, and tends to stress the absolute and complementary nature of the two. Thus, we are told that patients have a right to life or a right to information. We are also told by some that doctors should always save life and always preserve confidences. Some of these rights and duties emerge when one tries to draw up practical guidelines for regulating the conduct of the diverse members of a community, but they seldom emerge as absolutes. Such a conception of rights can be attacked as a purely social creation, but this does not square with the idea that we believe all human beings ought to be treated in decent ways, and that therefore any society has an obligation to respect what we might call human rights. However, it remains a mystery from where the relevant rights originate, when we try to give them a more fundamental basis than societal arrangements (a basis such as statutory law), or when they are discussed in an area like patient care, where the law does not comment in detail.

A further danger is that talk of rights can seem to close a moral issue. The statement that we have a right to free speech or a right to freedom of worship appears to be definitive, even if it is not enough to clinch an argument. Indeed the extent to which these rights justify our actions might be subject to fierce debate when we consider things like pornography, or the ritual abuse of children. The recognition of a right or duty might serve as a point at which to begin a moral discussion, but it rarely helps to resolve a genuine moral problem.

The great weakness of Kantian theories is that one can easily conjure up situations where rights and duties conflict. Consider the following situation.

> Agnes, an elderly lady with severe dementia, in fact almost vegetative, is in a rest home. She suffers a fractured neck of a femur, then a stroke and pneumonia. As she is dying, a priest visits her to administer the final absolution. He requests that her nasogastric tube be removed while he gives her the wafer, and this is done. Just as he is finishing, the nurse returns and reinserts the tube because it is time for the patient's afternoon feed and it is the nurse's duty not to hasten her death. Ten minutes later Agnes dies.

We all realise that something has gone wrong here, and that it can probably be attributed to a case of unswerving adherence to absolute duty. The problem is that it is difficult to see what we should put in the place of duty, even if we get a clue to the fact that we need more than just a list of duties when we have to resolve a conflict between them. For instance, we consider that a health professional is justified in waiving the absolute duty of confidentiality if he or she learns that a male patient is systematically abusing his infant children. So how do we decide what is the right thing to do in these cases? Our conceptions of duty cannot help because they merely prescribe specific types of conduct and do not tell us of any deeper values that can be used to resolve conflicts between them.

In order to produce an overarching theory, we could regard duties as no more than relatively stable rules devised within a more general moral system that takes account of the overall good resulting from a situation. This moral system pays close attention to the *effects* or *consequences* of what we do, applying in a special way to those in medical practice. But where does such a system originate from and what is its underlying rationale? Such questions have produced an answer that has formed the basis of another major strand of thinking in medical ethics.

Utilitarian Theories

A utilitarian approach rests on the premise that the right thing to do is to create the greatest good for the greatest number. It therefore focuses not on our actions and their accord with our conceptions of duty but on the consequences of those actions. This system generates an obligation to do our best to increase happiness and diminish suffering so as to secure net overall benefit for everybody concerned. This is a very congenial aim for most health care workers, who tend to see their profession as involved in benefiting humankind in ways to do with health. However, things are not quite that simple because utilitarianism has problems of its own (Gillett 1996).

The first we might call, after Roald Dahl, the 'Congratulations Mrs Schicklegruber' problem. This problem has to do with calculating the value of the various possible outcomes of one's actions. It is illustrated by the Austrian doctor who struggles to help a woman give birth to a live baby and then turns to her at the end and says, 'Congratulations, Mrs Schicklegruber, you have a fine son'. The problem is that so many of the consequences of what we do are not obvious to us at the time we have to do something. With clinical interventions the calculations may seem to be easy. However, people differ greatly in their perceptions of what is of value and thus, even in health care, it might not be possible to gauge the net benefits. Even if there is some agreed conception of what, in general, is a good outcome, it soon becomes apparent that the sums are going to be hideously difficult in all but the simplest cases. The things we must compare include not only quantitative differences in outcome—for instance, survival for one year versus three—but also qualitative differences. Health care ethics has to consider the value of one person having an operation for glue ear versus another person having a varicose vein operation; or a short life with cancer versus a longer life in which one might feel unwell and be disabled in certain ways. We might try to sidestep the problem of 'third-person' or absolute values by relating outcomes to the preferences of those affected by them. But as micro-economists are sceptical not only about *inter*-personal comparisons of preference and value but also about *intra*-personal preference rankings, the idea of a useful arithmetic guide to benefit arising from preferences looks not only bleak but hopeless.

A second problem is what we might call the 'Brave New World' problem. It suggests that we have intuitions about goodness and preference that make purely preference-based utilitarianism very suspect. If we lived in Huxley's *Brave New World*, we would probably prefer a life of convenient and shallow hedonistic pleasures to any struggle with the uncertainties of 'normal', uncontrolled, and sometimes unpleasant human existence. But most of us regard the fact that one would have been conditioned to enjoy the standard Brave New World contented life from before birth as a morally odious feature of such a life.

But if it is morally odious, that is not because it goes against our preferences. In a similar vein, if electrodes were implanted in a man's brain so that stimulating them caused him great pleasure (which he preferred to anything else whatsoever), he might perform a socially useful function for a considerable part of his waking life, with the obtaining of such stimulation his sole reward. But we have to ask ourselves whether this balding human organism, whose sole enjoyment is having his brain electrically stimulated, is living what anyone ought to call a good life, even though he might prefer it.

As if this were not enough, we also have the 'Christians and lions' problem. Imagine that we have a small minority of Christians within a bloodthirsty populace that enjoys seeing people torn apart by lions. When we do the sums, the happiness of the bloodthirsty majority is much more substantial than the misery of the victims. It emerges that, from a utilitarian viewpoint, we should just throw the Christians to the lions because morality demands it. Morality demands it because it would increase the net happiness in the situation and therefore be of overall benefit to our community. A similar neglect of the claims of individuals because of a wider benefit motivates a utilitarian argument for punishing the innocent. If punishment decreases crime, and we want to achieve that good end, we should make sure we find a criminal for every serious crime, so that the social mythology becomes 'You always get caught'. If this should result in killing or punishing a few innocent victims, it could still be morally justified by the net deterrent effect and consequent security and contentment in society. Of course, it would have to be a closely guarded secret that some of the convictions were rigged. As a matter of social policy, this view cannot be right. Anyone prepared to justify on moral grounds the execution of the innocent is not worth talking to about ethics because that person has a corrupt mind (Anscombe 1981).

To bring these objectives home to roost in a health care setting we can consider the child abuse paradox. If a child is being abused at a very young age then we can draw three fairly safe conclusions:

1   the parents are unhappy with the child; it is crying or whatever;
2   the child is having a miserable life; and
3   the child will probably grow up to be an abuser and perpetuate the misery.

It could be argued that, if the child is young enough, it has no formed preferences about the future and therefore could be painlessly euthanised (put to death) without any suffering. Hence, the right way to manage child abuse is to kill the child and either reform or sterilise the parents. However, most of us do not regard this as a good resolution to the problem. In fact, it seems as wrong as breaking a promise to a dying person or doing a vaginal examination on a woman under general anaesthetic when she has explicitly requested that it not be done. But why are these two things wrong if they don't cause any harm to those involved? Most would answer that they are wrong because they indicate a lack of moral sensitivity and integrity, and a lack of appreciation of what really matters in relationships between people.

Some of the problems with utilitarianism or consequentialism in general can be avoided by adopting *rule utilitarianism* and arguing that a society or individual should formulate rules that take into account what is most likely to be of benefit, all things considered, and then sticking by the rules as if they were duties (Hare 1991). The difficulty with this theory is that it is hard to decide whether it is a kind of utilitarianism or a kind of rights and duties theory. It could even be considered to be a virtue theory in which the relevant rights, duties, and virtues are not blind to the normal consequences of human actions, and a society that acted in accordance with fair and caring rules in their dealings with each other would compromise virtuous people.

In the text that follows we often discuss the consequences of decisions, but that does not mean we espouse consequentialism. Failure to take a careful view of consequences in planning actions would be a silly policy. In addition, the upright moral agent will recognise that means and ends are inseparable. To achieve a particular end, actions have to be performed in certain ways and certain attitudes have to be exhibited. This forms part of the moral assessment of both the action itself and the kind of agent a person is. Traditionally, moral theorists who are interested in what kind of character a person has, have been called virtue ethicists.

Virtue Ethics

The problems evident with codes of conduct, the over-use of 'rights', and social values such as utilitarian benefit have forced us to reconsider the question of personal character. We have focused on the qualities of moral sensitivity and integrity, and now must ask what it is to be a person of sensitivity and integrity. We might suggest that it is to be a 'person of sound character'. This claim brings us close to what is called *virtue theory*, and is reminiscent of Hume's person of sound sentiment. According to virtue theory, it is character that is the focus of moral concern, and someone who shows virtues, such as kindness, generosity, respect for others, honesty, and compassion, will be the model of moral conduct.

This appears to bring us full circle in that it suggests that medical ethics rests on the opinions and judgment of health care workers. However, this is too vague, and in any case even the most vitriolic critics of doctors would accept, as we have, that most health care professionals are decent people acting as best they can according to their own lights. We will, therefore, have to spell out how a decent person ought to act in day-to-day health care. We need to devise a conception of virtuous practice that does not suggest that a doctor or nurse can dictate what ought to happen to other people. An experienced health care worker's opinions are, of course, somewhat special as they are informed by and based on scientific knowledge and long acquaintance with clinical problems. The health care professional's experience will be an invaluable asset in weighing up the pros and cons and the likely outcomes of a given situation. In fact, we might moderate the professional clinician's view of what ought to happen by arguing that the good clinician will always listen to the patient, and try to do what is in the patient's best interests, even if their values differ. But such judgments are prone to error and so we must seek less subjective grounds for action. We should, however, realise that virtues such as caring, concern for others, appreciation of their predicament, and the ability to communicate clearly and effectively to a person under a great deal of stress, are the heart and soul of good clinical judgment. Before we eventually return to virtue-related theories of moral judgment and their importance in health care settings, we will canvass other sources of guidance for ethical conduct.

A Professional Ethic

We are not totally bereft of guidance in seeking a foundation for medical ethics because the Hippocratic Oath, despite its archaic terms of reference, is fairly demanding in its requirements on health care practice. It has historically been owned by doctors but, in fact, has also served as a founding document for the codes of other health care professions. We can, therefore, say that health care ethics has a Hippocratic ethos. Hippocrates' code begins with a rather forceful statement about duties belonging to a special group. This special group was to be given dangerous knowledge, and therefore, had to swear to use it only for good. Although the loyalty that individual professionals are urged to show to their colleagues can lead to gross distortions in health care practice, we must remember that the context of the Oath was one in which a number of practitioners were going about doing things to people, allegedly for the betterment of their health but without any training or regulation of their practices. As is the way with experts, one continually strikes the 'who will guard the guardians problem'. What is more, if we accept that health care should benefit the patient, a fundamental feature of ethical practice is a growing body of knowledge about what will protect and enhance health. Thus, there is a sound basis for individuals to make a commitment to an accredited and well-trained group of professionals if they presume to deliver health care. With this commitment in place, we can go on to establish a notion of professional integrity so that certain duties and standards apply to what we do.

The first concern of the Hippocratic Oath was, it seems, to set apart those individuals prepared to submit to the discipline and standards of medicine.

While these have changed a great deal since the days of Hippocrates, the Oath reminds us that the *sine qua non* of the ethical analysis of a problem in medicine must be to ask whether the individuals concerned have acted in accordance with adequate standards of health care practice. If they have not done that, they have failed at the starting gate. It is under this head that we place those who do not see their patients when they should, who see and treat patients while in an impaired state, or who neglect to act with due care and attention in their professional conduct. In modern health care practice, the standards are both clinical and scientific.

In the New Zealand setting a concept that avoids the gendered language of the ancient oath is one that says we should treat our colleagues as *whānau*. *Whānau* is a Māori term referring to the family to which one belongs, and whose honour is an important part of one's life. Once this is in clear focus, it also becomes clear that one is jealous of the honour of one's *whānau*, but also concerned that family honour has a sound basis. Thus, the concept strikes the right balance between criticism and correction, and concerned solidarity that ought to prevail in a health care profession.

A second provision of the Hippocratic Oath is that one ought to act in the best interests of patients, or for their benefit, or 'to keep them from harm and injustice'. Thus, we have a duty to determine what the welfare of the patient requires us to do, and to do it in such a way as to maximise the chances of the patient getting the best possible outcome in terms of his or her life and purposes. This introduces something that is implicit in the phrase 'best interests', but is never stated explicitly in the Oath: one ought to find out what the patient actually wants. It is quite legitimate for a patient to say, 'Well, thank you doctor, I realise that I have got a cancer in my liver but, rather than having all those tests and operations, I would just as soon go home and end my life in peace.' The final arbiter of the patient's best interests is, almost always, the patient. The doctor must always discuss and respect the patient's perspective on the problem, just as the captain of a ship will always discuss major decisions with the owner of that vessel.

Respect For Persons

This feature of good health care is implicit in a broadly Aristotelian approach to ethics and is of vital importance to patients and their well-being. Respect for the patient as a person is also something that emerges from a Kantian approach to ethics and to our relations with one another. Being individuals, patients have their own opinions and aims in life, which require them to act intelligently in most of the things they do. But in order to act intelligently, patients must (a) be given information, and (b) be allowed to make up their own minds. It is incumbent therefore on the professional to inform his or her patients about their disease and its management, and to allow them to make those significant choices required where the disease affects the course of their life and career. There is no single right way to manage a health problem in any but the simplest of conditions (surgeons tend to act as if there is because they like things to be simple, but the evidence on which they base their firm opinions often does not bear the weight of the opinion that rests upon it). Some people have problems that require careful and sensitive handling if their best interests are to be served. For this reason doctors, and health care professionals in general, must abandon paternalistic attitudes and include their patients as participants in their health care decisions; that is what respect for people involves. We could say that the best model of the doctor–patient relationship is one of cooperative partnership in facing a serious life problem.

We should note that this moral consideration assumes what we would properly call autonomy, and not mere wilfulness. It therefore implies a respectful and broadly rational dialogue between doctor and patient, in order to combine the patient's values and the doctor's expertise to produce benefit. For this to happen, the patient and the doctor must be prepared to listen to each other, think about what is being said, and be responsible about their respective roles. This is facilitated only in a climate of openness and trust.

A Worthwhile Life

Regarding people first and foremost as persons, and not just as biological entities, has the added implication that there may be situations in which the patient's autonomy and the doctor's beneficence may point away from preserving life.

People have their own identities, experiences of life, and ability to act on things around them. These capacities are basic to formulating a person's own values and exercising autonomy. However, even though they are not merely biological, the functioning of such capacities depends on biological integrity and they can be destroyed, for instance, by a devastating injury to the brain. This means that the special moral concern we normally have for a person may not apply to what is no more than a living human body. The idea that there can be kinds of life that a reasonable human being will not find worth living is often used to drive a wedge between the sanctity of life and the quality of life. We discuss some of the specific issues arising from this in later chapters but, for the present, we note that our medical assessments of benefit should take careful account of what will actually give the patient an acceptable quality of life.

This does not mean that we can decide that certain persons are substandard and ought to be disposed of; nor does it mean that we deny treatment to human beings who are less fit than their fellows; nor that we apportion health care on the basis of merit. The concept of a life worth living merely implies that human beings can quite reasonably and with sound moral judgment decide that certain kinds of life and their prolongation are of no benefit to themselves or anyone else. The admission that such a judgment is possible does not mean that we must take certain actions, such as mercy killing, in those circumstances. But it does mean that sometimes a patient's evaluation of outcomes will lead to a reasonable decision not to undertake certain kinds of treatment, even those considered by some doctors to be 'life-saving'.

Some Principles

We can now articulate some broad principles allowing us to undertake the ethical analysis of a problem in medicine (Beauchamp & Childress 1989). This may be approached in terms of basic questions to be asked in situations of uncertainty, and cannot be regarded as a set of self-sufficient guides for the good clinician.

Non-maleficence/beneficence

Which situations are possibly harmful to patients? For instance, if we find that there is a doctor who regularly turns up to see patients in a semi-inebriated state, it is only going to be a matter of time before an error of judgment leads to a serious outcome for one of the unfortunate patients dependent upon the doctor for care. Steps must be taken to ensure that this does not happen (*primum non nocere*).

The other side of this coin is a notion of substantial benefit. We could define this as an outcome that now or in the future would be regarded by the patient as worthwhile. Note that this is patient-centred, and not professional-centred, although it may take account of the expert knowledge of the health care professional. Agnes, in our earlier example, suffered the indignity of the insertion of a nasogastric tube ten minutes before her death. This had no chance of meeting any needs that she, then or in the future, would have been glad to have been met; therefore the tube was not ethically justified. We should always gear our medical practice to producing substantial benefit. An informed patient is able to insist upon it, and it should always be the basis on which we judge treatment.

Autonomy

At what point in the situation is the patient's status as a person, with the power to decide and act in his or her own best interests, threatened? Here we can imagine a situation involving a disturbed young man, perhaps with a psychiatric problem, who is incapable of acting rationally or of taking reasonable care of himself. We incur an obligation to attempt to remove this threat to his autonomy as a thinking being and to restore him to normal function. But only *that* is our responsibility; it is not our role to strip him of his status as a person and force him into a pattern of behaviour that we might more easily cope with. There should be no mandate in the care of a disturbed patient to downgrade his or her status permanently. For this reason, a periodic review of our justification for treating a patient as incompetent is ethically demanded of any professional or team of professionals who act to override that patient's autonomy. This also implies that we cannot undertake any so-called therapeutic measures that will cause a patient to become permanently incapable of functioning as a participant in human society with some degree of control over his or her own life.

Of course, some patients have permanently lost the capacity for autonomous decision-making, and choices must be made for them. Because of the importance of autonomy, however, we are bound to act in such a situation as we think the patient would have wanted. A doctor may justify a decision by saying, 'Well, that is what I would want if it were me' or, even better, may validate his or her own judgment by getting an independent but concerned perspective from someone else, such as a relative or friend of the patient, or perhaps a nurse or social worker.

> Beatrice has a lump in her breast. The surgeon advising her does not tell her that the lump is possibly a cancer and he 'jollies her along' with reassurances that 'everything will be fine'. He mentions, but does not explain in any depth, the fact that she will need a breast operation. She, predictably, decides not to have the operation or attend follow-up because the prospect of it alarms her. At no stage is she clearly told about the risks she is running, and the possible outcome she is facing.

This doctor is ethically at fault because he is not treating Beatrice as a responsible person. He is thereby pre-empting her ability to make significant decisions about her own life. Autonomy, information, and respect all go together to form the crux of current ethical views of the professional–patient relationship as a partnership of intelligent equals.

Professional Integrity

What is the impact of what one does in a given situation on the practice and profession of health care? This ethical question is not just a matter of protectionism for a set of closed professions but is, in fact, an important concern for any society that wants to have good health care. Health care is not just an instant transaction but is, as we have noted, a growing body of expertise and shared skills. Since the time of Hippocrates it has depended and still depends on respectful and collegial relations between health care workers. These are, in fact, vital to good standards of practice in any unit or institution. For instance, we might find that a certain senior nurse cannot bear criticism or subject his ideas to analysis in any kind of review. He may, as far as one can tell, be a very good clinician but there is something wrong with his practice because it lacks an essential element of humility and answerability for what he is doing. In the long term he might cease to treat his patients according to the best standards of nursing practice and they might well suffer because of it. To forestall this eventuality, we must detect and remedy the distorted relations that have developed so that his practice is assured of a scrutiny beyond his own impressions of it. We will expand on this in our discussion of the healing ethos.

Justice

Are we discriminating unfairly in the availability and kind of medical care we offer? This could arise if, for example, two people with equal and telling needs for a certain treatment were handled differently on the basis of wealth or race. It does not mean that we will provide a compulsory and uniform standard of medical care for everyone, but rather that we will accept a certain responsibility to treat people, within certain limits, in a fair way. It seems undeniable that a caring society will aim to make a decent minimum of medical care available to all its members.

Above and beyond this distribution of resources that a society sees fit to make available for medical care, there might be forms of treatment that are discretionary and available only to those prepared to sacrifice some other good. For such inequity to be just, we need to explore what we consider to be a justified and equitable level of health care, and remain committed to providing it in some principled way. If we care for people regardless of their worth, the basis of this should probably be need.

The problem with principles such as the four outlined is exactly the problem that we found with rights and duties: they sometimes conflict. In this case, there needs to be an underlying value or ethos. This 'bedrock' of our moral perception would seem to be the Aristotelian realisation that we are all reasoning and social beings who have in common certain biological and psychological needs and vulnerabilities, and that, on the basis of the commitments and relationships that bind us together, we should care for one another.

Filling Out the Picture

Several thinkers have recently caused us to reconsider the theoretical framework within which we examine issues in health care ethics. We may identify critical and postmodern theory, feminist ethics, and ethics of care as particularly relevant here.

Critical and postmodern theory both focus on the institutional and cultural practices that disempower certain individuals or types of individuals. The lack of power and the abuses that result from it can make concepts like autonomy seem peculiarly naive. Such a stance is highly relevant to health care ethics because there is such an inherent imbalance of power between the medical profession, other health care professions, and patients. The doctor has traditionally had a socially validated place as the highest level of authority on health care questions and therefore the doctor is often seen as the most powerful person in the health care setting. This results in patients being dependent and relatively silenced in health care interactions, and also sometimes in other health care professionals being disempowered. The power imbalance, we might say, permeates the system to disempower those in the less dominant positions, especially the person receiving care.

When there was very limited knowledge of health science, the experts were autocratic and made decisions because they were entrusted with that role even though they often did not have a firm foundation for the judgments they made. This did not change as the system increasingly benefited from the growth of bio-medical knowledge. Medical judgments, scientifically informed, remain expert and inaccessible to uneducated or lay people, although when the problem is explained most patients can understand what is happening. The tendency to create expert or privileged knowledge confirms the power of those who know, and we add to the traditional structural power within the system a new expert power based on the successes of biomedical science.

Unfortunately the distance created between the professional and the patient can lead to ignorance, by the professional, of the real situation and real needs of the person he or she is trying to help. The privileges that result from being part of a wealthy, powerful, and morally validated profession can also blind professionals to the real predicaments being undergone by their patients and clients.

It is at this point that feminist ethics and the ethics of care are sharply relevant. Feminist ethics looks closely at the kinds of moral phenomena that occur when one group is oppressed by another. The dominance of men in social and political life has been all too evident before and during the growth of modern health care. Women, as an oppressed group, notice this dominance in many ways and have had to adjust to roles that perpetually embody the assumption that the woman will be the helper, the second tier of activity and importance, and of less consequence than the man in a mixed situation. Women's voices are often unheard in literature about science, medical advances, higher management, and so on. Concepts like invisibility, silence, and disempowerment reveal different aspects of this experience. They allow us to come to an appreciation of the lived experience of somebody who feels lessened in a given context and point out how common that experience is in health care settings. The phenomenon is not hard to find: the obstetric patient who loses control of her pregnancy and labour because she is submitted to an obstetric protocol carried out by experts; the surgical patient who agrees to an operation because he feels it is expected of him; the patient who cannot tell her doctor about being abused because she is afraid that the delicate balance she is keeping in her life between loneliness, the care of her children, some kind of companionship, and an appearance of normality will be upset. In each case the language of autonomy, beneficence, and justice may hide needs, fears, and loss of self-worth. To act ethically in such a situation is to see beyond duties, rights, and choices and to begin to discover a different world whose challenges must be met by a delicate balance of attentive and critical understanding, professionalism, and care.

The ethics of care focuses on the moral perceptions, dispositions, and thoughts that arise from the actual business of caring for people. It has grown up in nursing ethics, where the problems of power hierarchies, the role of women, and the actual experiences of tending to people's needs have combined to yield a very different perspective on the clinical situation from that traditionally found in books of medical ethics. In some ways it is a virtue theory, which emphasises the moral importance and insights of lived experience in the development of a caring character. It is also like virtue theory in that it privileges the judgment of those who have actually been involved in the morally challenging situations under discussion, and struggled to cope with the experiences they found there.

What it has added is not a mere substitution of the concept of care for concepts like autonomy and beneficence, but rather a sensitive appreciation of practical needs, caring responses to those needs, and the wisdom resulting from such encounters. This is a crucial ingredient in practical health care ethics because it enables judgment, negotiation, responsiveness, and understanding to moderate rules, principles, and codes and to take due account of consequences. We could say it is like the fluid that makes a set of dry ingredients into a cake. Care is flexible and fluid; it binds individuals together and brings the complex demands of a moral situation into a conversation that can produce a good response. The practice of care is educative and character-changing, and issues in a set of virtues, such as the ability to detect vulnerability and insecurity, the ability to notice and read silences, the ability to moderate one's actions so as not to dominate or override the views of others, the ability to see ourselves as others see us, and the ability to appreciate the felt but unspoken needs of those with whom one is dealing. These are vital additions and transformations in our understanding of health care ethics.

The importance of what is not said between a patient and doctor is thrown into sharp relief by a postmodern emphasis on power and position in discourse. The patient does not say certain things either because he or she cannot, or because there is no space for them to be said. A person cannot speak about some aspects of his or her life in some settings because those things seem shameful. We should also notice the authority of the expert or legitimated knowledge that is the preserve of medicine in particular, and health care in general. The effect of these things is to make the patient reluctant to talk about things where he or she feels that the doctor will disapprove. It is an ethos of care that allows these silences to be opened up and things that hide within them to be voiced. It is, therefore, part of our calling as members of a caring profession to be sensitive to the points at which this needs to happen, and to make space for things to be said that would otherwise never be heard.

An Illustration

We could illustrate and apply these basic principles by returning to the case of Dr A, the eccentric oncologist, with which we began this chapter. The principles, in effect, identify the ethical features of the case and the more general lessons that it has to teach. They highlight the facets of the case that caring practice will need to address.

First, Dr A submitted his patients to a real risk of harm, which contravenes our standards of health care practice. Second, his actions contravened the *autonomy* of his patients in that he did not explain the situation to them. If he had, he might have been able to claim that he was allowing the patients to define their own *best interests*, and been justified to some extent if any of them opted for a trial of the 'treatment' he offered in preference to the unpleasant chemotherapy that is standard for their problem. He cannot claim this mitigation because he neither told them of the risks they were running, nor gave them any indication that there were alternative ways of dealing with the problem. It is indefensible to act in such a way without telling patients, and therefore the profession would be ethically bound to attempt to offset the harm that was being done.

In a case like this, some would argue that professional etiquette, which comprises the rules of thumb that preserve and protect collegial relations within the profession, prevents one from interfering with the practice of a colleague. However, etiquette must give way to ethics when a doctor's conduct poses a serious threat to patient welfare and the practice of good medicine. We are not treating our colleague as *whānau* if we let that colleague endanger the honour of the family without seeking to correct the error of his ways.

This case is hypothetical and one can imagine additional features that would have made the doctor's unethical behaviour even more dangerous. He could, for instance, have obstructed his patients' access to normal advice and care by colleagues who did not agree with his hypothesis. This would contravene by positive commission, and not just omission, the principle that one should do no harm. He could have proclaimed his theory, unsupported and dubious as it was, to those receiving training under his supervision. This would have prejudiced the future practice of medicine by those he influenced. He could have refused to submit to any review of his results so that the harm caused by his views would remain undetected and uncorrected. This, again, would have contravened the idea of a collegial profession. That principle and *primum non nocere* would both be threatened if he systematically distorted his data so that the real preventable harm befalling his patients continued and could not be revealed.

Quite apart from what *he* could have done, there are a number of ways in which others might have compounded and worsened his errors. His colleagues could have allowed him to treat their patients without warning those patients or informing them of the truth about their disease, and so colluded in his offences against the patients' best interests and autonomy. Similar ethical criticisms would apply if his colleagues let his scientific deceptions go unchallenged, so that his trial of treatment was able to continue long after its tragic results had become evident; or if they refused to confront him or discipline him when it did become evident that basic ethical matters touching the medical care of his patients were being neglected under the influence of his prejudices. They could have allowed him to 'experiment on' only those patients dependent upon the institution for their care, so that patients were treated differentially according to factors such as socio-economic status or ability to pay. This would violate the principle of justice in health care. Any of these unethical modes of behaviour would have made the situation even worse.

The overarching concern in this case is medical hubris. The doctor made a decision, and his colleagues allowed him to act on it. The thoughts, wishes, and vulnerabilities of his patients are clouded in silence. We get no sense that he really understood them or tried to listen to their stories even if his demeanour was caring and concerned. His theory dominated his mind and practice and blinded him to the lived tragedies with which he had to deal. This in itself is damning, even if all else could be justified. The failure of care and understanding is a defect that, if not rectified, renders his acts totally misguided and potentially dangerous. It is far more important than the legal requirements that interact with our codes of medical ethics.

Summary and Conclusions

There are certain foundations on which we can build an outline of medical ethics. First, our practice ought to be in accord with a *techne* (skilled form of knowledge) or art whose aim is to confer substantial benefit on suffering human beings. This *techne* is governed by an ethic that is committed to restoring and repairing, as far as possible, the form and function of a human being. Any health care worker should be able to assure patients, with sincerity and integrity, that the care they will receive is at least as good as (and perhaps better than) that defined by the accepted standards of contemporary medical practice.

Second, we must always treat our patients as people, involving them in those significant decisions about their care that will affect their lives and well-being. That is why our conception of substantial benefit is and should remain patient-centred, and the patient should be able to regard the doctor as a partner and an experienced guide on the journey that is their illness. We must be particularly strict about any violation of this principle.

Third, we must safeguard the continuity and standards of medicine and other health care professions, taking care to ensure that what is done and taught is consistent with an ongoing enterprise in service of those people who suffer. Any health care professional should regard themselves as part of a family enterprise where the standards must be kept high, and we should work together with understanding and integrity. Only by zealous attention to this aspect of our ethical responsibilities can we be sure that what will be offered to patients by our successors will be as good as, if not better than, the treatment we are now empowered to offer them.

Fourth, we must practise health care in the light of our patients' needs without being influenced or prejudiced by factors that have nothing to do with their diseases. Thus, we must act with justice and impartiality, ensuring that our care is given in a spirit of compassion and a desire to benefit, rather than being distorted by any other motive or interest.

With these principles in hand and, one would hope, a genuine sensitivity to the people and situations we encounter, we are equipped to address the ethical problems of modern health care in the spirit of Hippocrates. Our conclusions should be informed by an awareness of health care and its inherent power imbalances, and they should reflect the insights emerging from hands-on caring for people who suffer. In the following chapters we look in detail at the general principles outlined here, relating them to a series of issues in such a way as to try to give the reader an insight into the ethical challenges of contemporary health care practice.

2
The Healing Ethos

Introduction

What is it that makes a person into a medical practitioner? In one way the answer may seem obvious: it is the learning process spread over six or more years that inculcates the required basic knowledge and skills to qualify for professional registration. However, this is really too simple a view. Like all professional education, medical training is more than just the passing on of knowledge and the teaching of skills. It is also the transmission of a whole set of attitudes that the profession has acquired over many years, attitudes passed on in many subtle ways by more experienced practitioners as they instruct the novice doctors under their tutelage.

This set of attitudes may be described as the *ethos* of medicine. The transmission of this ethos begins as soon as the student of anatomy learns to dissect a human cadaver clinically and to put aside those feelings of revulsion that most people would naturally feel when asked to perform such a task (see Chapter 4). A kind of emotional hardening has to take place, an attitude that marks out the medical student as a member of a group with privileged access to the bodies of others, in life and in death. The student must quickly learn ways of coping not only with cadavers, but with the pain, distress, and mutilation associated with serious disease and injury. Yet, paradoxically, those who learn to distance themselves from their emotions in order to be clinically competent doctors will not necessarily be good ones. The healing ethos combines this necessary detachment with a genuine concern for the individual patient, an attitude requiring a degree of empathy and emotional closeness. Only when the medical ethos includes a profound respect for the individuality of each patient will it serve the true purpose of medicine—the health of the patient. Ethos and ethics are not always the same thing, and what has become accepted practice must be open to continual ethical scrutiny to ensure that the needs of the patient are truly served.

In this chapter, we survey the ethical features of professional relationships in medicine by first considering the general features of the relationship between doctors and patients, and then focusing more specifically on informed consent, confidentiality, and truth-telling. In a final section, we consider relationships between colleagues both within and outside the medical profession as these affect the welfare of patients.

The Doctor–Patient Relationship

'He [the physician] would be like God, saviour equally of slaves, of paupers, of rich men, of princes, and to all a brother . . . for we are all brothers.' This quotation from the ancient 'Hymn of Serapion', addressed to the god of healing, Asclepius, illustrates the powerfully religious origins of medicine. In the ancient world all healers were seen as sharing in the power of God or the gods to overcome evil. Medicine was an ancient craft, and in the West, traced its origins to the school of Hippocrates (fifth century BC), in which brotherly allegiance, respect for the gods, and commitment to the welfare of all patients were seen to be wholly interdependent. In this regard a sentence from the *Precepts* of Hippocrates is often quoted: 'Where there is love of man there is also love of the art.'

How relevant are these ancient perceptions of doctoring to the modern practice of medicine? It is obvious that medicine is now more commonly seen to be associated with science than with religion. For example, Pellegrino and Thomasma in *A Philosophical Basis of Medical Practice* (1981) describe medicine as 'the most scientific of the humanities and the most humane of the sciences'. In a largely secular society, patients and doctors alike are inclined to see the gods as irrelevant to both the science and the art of medicine. Nevertheless, the doctor is often still invested with a godlike authority, and faith in the doctor's ability to diagnose correctly and to prescribe effective treatment can be seen as an important component in the healing process. There is still a power associated with medicine that seems to derive partly from the highly specialised nature of the knowledge required to practise it, and partly from people's need to find some force that will protect them from disease and death.

An assessment of the ethical implications of this trust in the power of medicine requires a careful look at the character of the relationship provided in the modern practice of medicine. There is still a danger that, despite (or perhaps even because of) the rise of medical science, the autonomy of patients will be ignored and the paternalistic attitude—'doctor knows best'—will be used to control the situation. Leo Tolstoy has a vivid description of this attitude in his 1886 story *The Death of Ivan Ilyich*:

> The whole procedure followed the lines he expected it would; everything was as it always is. There was the usual period in the waiting-room, and the important manner assumed by the doctor . . . and the weighty look which implied, You just leave it all to us, and we'll arrange matters—we know all about it and can see to it in exactly the same way as we would for any other man [Tolstoy 1960, p. 126].

A different model of the medical relationship is required to ensure that patients are treated in a way that respects their individuality and their capacity to make judgments for themselves. With this aim in view, the term 'client' is sometimes substituted for 'patient', and it is argued that the medical relationship is really a form of 'contract' to be fully negotiated by the practitioner and the client. Similarly, the contractual nature of the relationship can be conveyed by substituting 'consumer' for 'patient'. This approach does have some advantages over the old paternalistic model. It may prevent doctors from acting in what they consider to be the 'best interests' of the patient without establishing whether this is in fact what the patient would choose (Veatch 1981). It can also help the patient to think through the implications of treatment, to take responsibility for the health care decisions that are made, to know what to expect from the doctor, and to take action when the contractual obligations have not been honoured.

However, the contractual model has a number of problems. First, the substitution of 'client' for 'patient' is a semantic change of little significance. The term itself does not necessarily convey an equal relationship (the Latin root—*cliens*—signifies a person under the protection or patronage of a superior). The use of 'client' in law and social work is no guarantee that these professions act less paternalistically than do doctors. 'Patient' is a more accurate description of the recipient of medical treatment and care, since it means simply 'the person who is suffering'.

Second, the use of 'consumer' in health care transactions can be very misleading because it ignores the inevitable vulnerability of the patient in most situations of illness. It is relatively rare for a person to be in a position to negotiate appropriate treatment, as one would negotiate a business contract or decide on the purchase of consumer goods in a supermarket or appliance store. The technicalities of medical diagnosis and treatment are such that patients are heavily dependent on the interpretation of the medical practitioner to understand the options properly. In addition, illness often has a disabling effect on one's capacity to judge between options, to view the situation objectively and to pay attention to all the detail provided. The principle *caveat emptor* (let the buyer beware) is a safeguard people can observe when, for example, they are considering the purchase of 'bargain price' goods. But, such a prudent regard for one's own interests is not possible in many medical encounters. There has to be confidence in the goodwill, competence, and commitment of the doctor in the light of these uncertainties. We often need to seek help, with only the moral trustworthiness of the provider of care to rely on.

For these reasons it has been suggested that 'covenant' is a more appropriate term than 'contract' for the health care relationship (Campbell 1984; May 1983). The advantage of this change in terminology is that it offers a different approach to the medical relationship. Although covenant is closely related to contract, it contains a greater sense of personal commitment, which transcends a careful calculation of individual advantage. The covenant relationship is open-ended, a promise to show active concern for the welfare of the other. Thus, it seems to be a more accurate reflection of the sense of professional dedication that most health professionals bring to their work. It implies that respect for the patient as a person is more important to the doctor than a constant striving for status, income, and power. Such a view does justice to the religious or humanistic convictions of those who choose medicine out of a sense of vocation and a desire to help those in need.

There are, of course, dangers in the covenant model and it becomes a question of whether these are better risks to accept than the risks of the contractual emphasis. The obvious difficulty is that it may put the doctor in an elevated moral position that seems to suggest some superiority over other professions and occupations and over patients (who are not expected to have an equal covenantal commitment to their doctors). The result can be an over-idealistic portrayal of medical work that obscures the obvious advantages to the practitioner in both social and economic terms. Conversely, the notion of commitment can result in exploitation of the practitioner, with nothing expected from the patient or society in terms of an active involvement in the promotion of individual or social health. The doctor becomes a 'lone ranger' battling the forces of disability and disease single-handedly. The result can be an over-involved style of practice that fails to encourage the patient to be an active participant in his or her own recovery, and can lead to sacrifice of the practitioner's own personal and family life. Moreover, an emphasis on the moral trustworthiness of the practitioner can be used to justify the kind of paternalistic attitude that sees no need to enlist the patient fully as a partner in the medical relationship. 'You can trust us' can be used as an evasion of proper scrutiny of what actually takes place.

A solution to these difficulties, however, can be found by insisting that one of the professional obligations of the doctor is commitment to an open, truthful, and fully cooperative relationship with patients.

Information and Consent

Consider the following case.

A general practitioner is aware that some of the symptoms being presented to her are suggestive of carcinoma of the urinary tract, but obviously this cannot be confirmed or discounted without further tests. What should she say to the patient, in referring him for investigation? Should she mention cancer as a possibility at this stage, or is this creating unnecessary alarm?

In the past, it would have been argued that the best interests of the patient would not be served by sharing with him, at this stage, the medical possibilities. The traditional beneficent approach was to reassure the patient that there was probably nothing to worry about—'just a few tests to check things out'. The problem with this approach is that it creates a relationship between practitioner and patient that is hard to change at a later stage, if things turn out as the practitioner fears. Moreover it denies a fundamental value within the professional relationship as we have been describing it—the value of honesty or truthfulness.

An open and straightforward sharing of the available information and the steps that are necessary to advance the investigation creates instead a cooperative relationship in which the patient is prepared for a later discussion of treatment options, if this is required. If the doctor 'babies' the patient at the outset, it is difficult to change the encounter to a more adult footing later in the process. The doctor in this case could first say something like this: 'I'd like to arrange for you to have some tests to find out what's causing the pain and bleeding. It could be something quite simple and easily remedied, or it could be a more serious problem, in which case we shall want to do something about it as soon as we can.' This statement leaves the patient free to ask further and more detailed questions if he wishes. The doctor has not specifically mentioned cancer as a possibility, but she has left it open for this to be explained if the patient follows through with further questions. When the full information is available from the test results, this opening discussion has prepared the way for a full sharing of the information now available. At this stage the treatment options are discussed with the patient as a partner in the decision-making process and fully informed of the options open to him.

How much information is required in order to ensure that a patient is genuinely consenting to treatment after a careful consideration of the options? The General Medical Council of Britain has described the fundamental right to adequate information as follows:

> Patients have a right to information about their condition and the treatment options available to them. The amount of information you give each patient will vary, according to factors such as the nature of the condition, the complexity of the treatment, the risks associated with the treatment or procedure, and the patient's own wishes [General Medical Council 1999].

The following statement, which was included in a Code of Health and Disability Services Consumers' Rights prepared by the New Zealand Health and Disability Commissioner, provides a useful general criterion: 'Every consumer has the right to the information that a reasonable consumer, in that consumer's circumstances, would expect to receive.'

This is really a double criterion: first, the circumstances of the individual patient or 'consumer' are a relevant factor; second, in order for an 'informed decision' to be made there must be an assessment of what any *reasonable* person would wish to know in the circumstances. Beginning with the second criterion, we cannot expect people to make a reasoned decision if they are not in full possession of the relevant facts. They need to know the benefits of the various treatments that could be offered, and the corresponding risks (including side effects). They must be told who will be carrying out the treatment and how soon it will be available, and they need to be informed of the likely consequences of not having any treatment. These are the minimum requirements for any discussion of treatment options.

Knowledge of the particular patient is used to guide the doctor about how best to convey what can be quite technical and, at times, alarming information. The aim must be to enable the patient to participate in a choice that reflects his or her own values, aims, and aspirations rather than those of the doctor. A patient who then says: 'What do you recommend, doctor?' is expressing a wish to rely on expert advice. This is a perfectly reasonable request, but in this situation the practitioner must be doubly sure that the patient understands what the nature of that advice is. Relying on expert advice does not relieve the patient of responsibility for the decision. For this reason, it is now being suggested that the phrase 'informed consent' should be replaced by some alternative phrase like 'informed choice' or 'informed request', emphasising the patient's primary role in the process.

In practice, many difficulties will be encountered in trying to achieve informed consent—or 'informed choice'. Because the partnership between patient and doctor will always be an unequal one, it is rarely a totally independent choice by the patient. Only a medically trained person can appreciate the uncertainties and complexities of many treatment options, however much of an effort is made to convey some of these to the patient; and inevitably a doctor will have preferences, which may well differ in emphasis from those of some of his or her colleagues. Thus, however much we struggle to exclude bias, it has to be said honestly that the choice the patient makes will often be dependent upon the particular practitioner who describes the options. A doctor who puts faith in one particular form of chemotherapy for cancer, for example, is likely to present it in such a way that his patients see it as the best option. (This is a variation of the well-known phenomenon that patients of Freudian or of Jungian analysts always seem to dream the 'right' kind of dreams for their respective analyst's theories!)

A practical solution to undue influence in the obtaining of consent can be found only by encouraging patients to make themselves better informed. Increasingly patients are themselves taking the initiative by seeking out information about their condition and the treatment options from the world wide web. They will often seek advice about treatments promoted on the web and request an explanation of why some are not being offered to them as options. Some doctors find this increased knowledge in patients alarming and a challenge to their authority. But, in fact, it can only be for the good that patients are better informed and are taking more responsibility for finding solutions to their medical problems. The role of the doctor in these circumstances is to act as a trustworthy resource to the patient, based on the doctor's specialist knowledge of the issues. The doctor can help the patient evaluate the information they have discovered and can place it in the context of a full understanding of the patient's specific condition. In this way the sense of partnership between doctor and patient can be enhanced rather than diminished. Far from making the medical profession redundant, the information explosion of our times makes it ever more important that doctors are truthful, objective, and scholarly interpreters of the confusing array of information now available to patients.

In the final analysis, therefore, there will always remain an element in the doctor–patient relationship that depends upon the trustworthiness and integrity of the doctor. No ethical or legal requirements for informed consent will be effective without the willingness of those with the knowledge and power to be constantly critical of their own practice and always open to a perception of the needs of individual patients. The covenantal relationship cannot be replaced by some cast-iron contract that will infallibly protect the rights of patients. Moreover, there are many situations in which the capacity of the patient to decide is either impaired or totally absent, and in these circumstances the doctor (in conference with the family) must be trusted to make appropriate decisions on behalf of the patient. Thus, although the old paternalistic attitude in which patients were kept in virtual ignorance must be rejected, there will be many situations in which the capacity of the *doctor* to make the right treatment choices is still the most important factor. An emphasis on consent, where appropriate and possible, does not remove the need for a profession that will act 'for the patient's good' (Pellegrino & Thomasma 1988).

Confidentiality

A doctor has two homosexual men as patients, each of whom consults him regularly with symptoms possibly suggestive of the onset of AIDS. One patient agrees to have a blood test and proves to be HIV antibody positive. He begs the doctor not to inform his partner, fearing that this will mean the end of their relationship. The partner adamantly refuses to have a test, saying that he doesn't want to know if he ever does get AIDS, and that in any case he 'knows how to be careful'. The doctor is also aware that this patient has a number of casual sexual relationships, of both a homosexual and a heterosexual nature. Should he inform him that his partner is HIV positive to warn him of the dangers to himself and his other contacts, or must he respect the confidentiality of the information, and hope that 'careful' means no possibility of transmission of the virus?

This case illustrates the complexity of the notion of confidentiality in the medical relationship. There are circumstances in which a doctor's obligation to respect the confidentiality of the information gained about a patient seems to be in direct conflict with one's duties to other patients or to the wider society. How is the dilemma to be resolved?

We must first consider why confidentiality is regarded as so important in health care relationships. The provision of medical care always involves an invasion of privacy. Without access to the patient's body and to a wide range of personal information about the patient, it is not possible either to achieve an adequate diagnosis or to provide appropriate treatment. This privileged access, however, is justified only because it is to the patient's benefit, and it is only obtained (except in an emergency) if the patient consents to it. Thus, the information gained in the medical consultation, although contained in records that are the property of either an individual practitioner or a health institution, should normally be used only for purposes the patient authorises. Any other use of the information represents an invasion of the privacy of the patient and a breach of the trust that made the patient willing to consult the practitioner in the first place. In other words, confidentiality constitutes an essential element in the therapeutic relationship, and must be regarded as integral to the 'sacred trust' described in the Oath of Hippocrates.

Does this mean that confidentiality is an absolute that can never be outweighed by other moral considerations? Until recently it was viewed in this light, rather on a par with the secrets of the confessional. To take this view commits us to a totally individualistic outlook on medical care. Doctors clearly have some obligations to those around the individual patient, even though the patient is usually given prime consideration. In circumstances where active harm to others will be caused, the obligation to confidentiality cannot be an absolute. The problem is defining what constitutes 'active harm'. It is already well established that when a patient is rendered unfit to drive by a medical condition, this information must be passed on to the appropriate authorities if the patient refuses to do it on their own behalf (Cole 1987; General Medical Council 2000). Equally, health professionals have an obligation to breach confidentiality, when only by so doing can a child be protected from sexual abuse or physical harm. Sometimes, however, the risk to others is less clearly predictable. The Tarasoff case in the USA (California Supreme Court 1976) found a psychologist and his employers negligent in their failure to inform the girlfriend of a psychiatric patient that he was threatening to kill her—a threat he did in fact carry out (see Chapter 10). This seems to extend, far beyond any immediately predictable dangers, the duty to breach confidentiality in an effort to protect others.

What of the homosexual man, in the case above, who was in danger of unknowingly spreading the AIDS virus widely among his sexual partners? This example is complicated by his explicit statement that he did not wish to know if he was HIV positive. But the requirement to protect others does still apply, and would have to influence the doctor's decision in this case. In simpler cases, where a bisexual infected man is concealing his condition from his female partner, the guideline has now been established that confidentiality can be breached to warn the unaware partner of the risk she is exposed to, if the infected person refuses to pass on the information (see Chapter 9). This guideline might be extended to cover the doctor's obligation to provide some added protection for the unknown partners of his promiscuous patient. The decision is a very hard one since, in order to achieve this somewhat uncertain objective, the doctor would be obliged to override the expressed wishes of *both* of the patients for whom he has direct responsibility.

In most everyday clinical situations, however, the requirement for confidentiality is much more straightforward. It can be understood as an explicit recognition of the respect a doctor shows for every patient as an individual. To respect the privacy of the information is to respect patients themselves, and thus to justify the trust that is placed in the doctor as a person of discretion and sensitivity. Unfortunately, both the content of some medical records and the manner in which they are handled, often represent a betrayal of that basic trust. (Access to records for research purposes raises different issues, which are discussed in Chapter 13.) In a hospital setting especially, notes on patients can be much too readily accessed by individuals who have no direct clinical involvement with the patient, and therefore no right to the personal details contained in the record. Moreover, notes can contain highly subjective and prejudicial comments on patients. If such comments are discovered by the patient, the whole basis of the relationship is undermined.

> A young woman patient had presented herself frequently at the surgery of a general practitioner complaining of tiredness and persistent headaches. She had been referred for several specialist consultations, but no reason for her symptoms had been established. On one occasion she had turned up at a casualty department in a severe panic and with hyperventilation tetany, and was discharged with an appointment for a psychiatric consultation at the outpatient clinic. She did not keep this appointment, but returned to her general practitioner for further advice. During that consultation an interruption gave her an opportunity to look at her case file on the doctor's desk. Written in large letters in the front of the file was the following comment: 'Beware, hysterical and manipulative, determined to be unwell.' The patient lodged a complaint against the doctor, and was left with a sense of being humiliated and degraded by the medical profession as a whole.

Whatever the correct assessment of this patient's condition, the doctor showed a total lack of understanding as to the nature of confidential medical notes, using them as a cloak for interprofessional communication or as an *aide-mémoire* for himself. Notes should always be written in the form of a record of objectively established findings that have been—or will be—shared with the patient, with an appropriate interpretation of the technical details. (Rights of access to one's own medical record have now been established in the United Kingdom by the *Access to Health Records Act 1990*). The shared status of clinical notes reinforces the basic ethical notion that confidentiality aims primarily to enable an open and safe relationship between doctor and patient.

In addition to the moral obligation to maintain confidentiality and to show respect for patients in one's record-keeping and communication with colleagues, practitioners must operate within the legal constraints of privacy legislation. In the United Kingdom, the adoption of the *European Convention on Human Rights* within the *Human Rights Act 2000* has established a set of basic rights, including a right to privacy. Similar legislation is already in force elsewhere. For example, in New Zealand, the Privacy Commissioner issued a *Health Information Privacy Code* that has the force of law (Privacy Commissioner 1994). The code lays down rules relating to all health information about identifiable individuals. Its rules govern the collection, secure storage, access to, use of, and disclosure of all such information. Although the code is complex in some respects, its basic approach is very straightforward: the individual concerned should know that the information is being collected and why. We should also note that special provisions relate to the collection, storage, and transmission of electronic data. In the United Kingdom the confidentiality of all computerised records is now protected by the *Data Protection Act 1988*, which came into force in March 2000. The security of such records is of paramount importance in the medical context.

Some doctors may feel that legal codes of this kind represent an interference with their clinical autonomy. But, in reality, such legislation reinforces the profession's commitment to patient confidentiality and provides solutions to the dilemmas of exceptional disclosure of information that are very similar to those already accepted by the professional codes of ethics. The fundamental principle must be respect for the privacy of the individual patient, and breach of this privacy must have clear ethical justification.

Truthfulness

Throughout this chapter we have been stressing the special character of the relationship between patient and doctor, a relationship that seeks to make the patient a partner in the healing endeavour but recognises the inequality created by the sick person's vulnerability and sense of dependence. In order to avoid the paternalism of the past, the interaction between patient and doctor must be characterised by truthfulness on the part of the doctor (but equally by the patient, who cannot be helped if he or she acts in a deceptive or manipulative way). Truthfulness describes much more than simply the passing on of accurate information. It is expressed in an attitude towards the other person that seeks to create open and mutually respectful communication (Bok 1980; Higgs 1985). It is possible to avoid lying to a person and yet disregard truthfulness by concealing facts or creating false impressions. For example, it was common in the recent past to avoid, wherever possible, the use of the word 'cancer'. Instead, 'wart' or 'growth' might be used, and any diagnosed malignancy would simply not be mentioned unless the patient asked directly about it. Such subterfuges are now uncommon, largely because the more open attitudes towards cancer have made them ineffective. However, there remains a considerable hesitation to communicate a bad prognosis to a patient, while at the same time the family may be 'let into the secret'. It is obvious that such devices create a relationship with patients that is deficient in truthfulness, even if no direct lies are told. The argument that this is 'kinder' to patients does not appear to be supported by the facts, since surveys have shown that the vast majority of people would prefer to be told directly what their chances of survival are, rather than being left worrying about the true nature of their condition and unable to trust those around them to be honest with them.

Are there no situations in which concealment is the preferable moral choice? The so-called 'therapeutic privilege' has been found in at least one legal case to exempt doctors from passing on information when in their judgment it would be therapeutically counterindicated. There are some clinical situations in which the condition of the patient is so fragile that a full disclosure of all known facts would be overwhelming for them at that time. For example, a person in a critical condition after a road accident might ask about the survival of other family members. A temporary concealment of the full facts might be indicated to save the psychological trauma of hearing that someone had died or was also critically ill. The same argument is often used to justify a certain vagueness about the extent of a person's own burns or internal injuries during the critical phase. It should be noted, however, that these are exceptional circumstances that cannot justify a policy of concealment of bad prognoses from patients, on the false assumption that it will always jeopardise their chances of recovery. Truthfulness is not the bald communication of facts: it is the kind of sensitivity to individual need that knows there is a time to speak and a time to remain silent.

Collegial Relationships

We must consider finally how relationships between colleagues should be managed in order to serve the primary end of medicine—the health of the patient. 'My colleagues will be my brothers', declares the Hippocratic Oath. This ancient atmosphere of brotherly loyalty lingers on in medicine despite the total change in social circumstances since the Oath was formulated two and a half millennia ago. The 'band of brothers' who followed the Oath of Hippocrates constituted virtually a priestly group within ancient society, and they were bound together by a semi-mystical religious allegiance to Asclepius, the god of healing. Today the medical profession consists of men and women of widely differing religious beliefs, whose common allegiance is to a code of ethics that transcends national boundaries and specific religious affiliations—the Geneva Convention Code of Medical Ethics, set out in the Appendix of this book. The fundamental principle of the code is: 'The health of my patient will be my first consideration.'

Thus the doctor's first loyalty is not to colleagues but to patients. This does not mean, however, that loyalty to colleagues is of no importance. Members of the public often suspect that professions look after their own members to the detriment of patients or clients or, in the famous phrase of George Bernard Shaw (borrowed from Adam Smith), that 'all professions are conspiracies against the laity'. This suspicion is sometimes well founded. Disciplinary and complaints procedures are often painfully slow and not easy for the ordinary member of the public to understand (see Chapter 15 for a fuller discussion of this problem).

Although loyalty within a profession can sometimes work to the disadvantage of patients, especially when it leads to the covering up of the incompetence or impairment of colleagues, it is certainly more than merely a self-serving and protective device. Critics of loyalty to colleagues overlook the fact that the most dangerous practitioner is the 'loner' who attempts to work in isolation from colleagues in the field, and without reference to those who have different expertise either within the medical disciplines or in other professional fields. The provision of health care is demanding, both emotionally and intellectually. In order to work in the best interests of patients, every practitioner must learn to share the decision-making process with others, to consider alternative diagnoses and treatment, and to find correction or support when the decisions are especially difficult and uncertain.

To clarify the point further, we must distinguish between etiquette and ethics in collegial relationships. The rules of medical etiquette have tended to create a medical hierarchy in which each consultant is king of their own kingdom and therefore not subject to 'interference' by colleagues, even those of equal rank. In addition, this approach has tended to guard medical territory very carefully, and has resisted encroachment by other disciplines. Great emphasis has been placed on the clinical autonomy of the individual practitioner, and to challenge this autonomy has been seen as, at best, discourteous and, at worst, positively dangerous to the patients for whom the practitioner holds ultimate responsibility.

Although it is important that the judgment and experience of a skilled professional be respected and not be subject to ill-informed outside interference, it does not follow that the totally independent professional is the best safeguard of the patient's interests. On the contrary, the complexity of health care interventions demands that the needs of the patient be viewed from a whole range of different perspectives, and in many instances the viewpoint of the nurse or the social worker can provide a much needed corrective to an overly narrow medical view. We therefore agree with Hampton that 'clinical freedom is dead'.

> Clinical freedom is dead, and no-one need regret its passing. Clinical freedom was the right—some seemed to believe the divine right—of doctors to do whatever in their opinion was best for patients. In the days when investigation was non-existent and treatment as harmless as it was ineffective, the doctor's opinion was all that there was, but now opinion is not good enough [Hampton 1983, p. 1237].

The ideal relationship between colleagues, within the medical profession and between health care professionals generally, is a mutual one of both support and honest criticism. The modern professional expects to be accountable, both to colleagues and to the public that grants the profession the privilege of self-regulation. This entails both regular peer review of one's practice and the willingness to review decisions in an interdisciplinary context. The health of patients is often jeopardised by professional imperialism or interprofessional rivalry. Conversely, when a case conference approach is adopted, with free communication between staff of different grades and varying professions, the needs of the patient are much more likely to be perceived and appropriately met.

Recent changes to the organisation of the Health Service in the United Kingdom have created new structures to ensure that the mechanisms of peer review and for achieving quality care cannot be viewed as optional extras, but become a fundamental contractual responsibility of all institutions that provide health care. These new responsibilities have been described as 'clinical governance' and the mechanisms for ensuring it takes place are currently being instituted (Department of Health 1999). Time will tell whether the new phrase 'clinical governance' is merely a political buzzword or whether there will be a real change in the ethical scrutiny of patient care and in the support available to colleagues who are failing to act in their patients' best interests.

Conclusion

In this chapter we have sought to describe a 'healing ethos' that will do justice to the range and complexity of modern health care interventions. We have stressed the need for a relationship between patients and doctors that respects the personal nature of the relationship as well as its grounding in the knowledge and skill of the trained professional. We do not believe that patients will be appropriately helped unless their autonomy is fully respected, and this entails improving their capacity for making choices by the provision of full information, and honouring their trust in the profession by maintaining high standards of confidentiality and truthfulness.

The healing ethos is one that must also recognise the vulnerability and inevitable dependency of those who are critically ill and for whom recovery may not be an option. There is an ethics of care that is as important as the ethics of cure (Campbell 1998), and death need not always be viewed as a medical failure. It is an impoverished medical relationship that can operate only within a scenario of successful outcomes. The professional relationship described in this chapter is designed to assist both patient and doctor through all the vicissitudes of illness, or in the words of a traditional medical saying: 'To cure sometimes, to relieve often, to comfort always'.

3
Health Care Ethics in Diverse Cultures

Cultural Tensions in Health Care

We have outlined some of the major ideas that have shaped contemporary health care ethics. It is worth noting that most of these ideas arise from the Western cultural traditions of Greece, Rome, and Christendom. Dominant within this tradition has been recent Anglo-American writing based in British moral philosophy. There has, until recently, been a paucity of writing from other cultural traditions and a neglect of critical or 'postmodern' views in the discussion of ethical issues. This has led to a version of the liberal ideal of a society of free, economically independent, and competing individuals becoming the conceptual framework for medical ethics. The liberal emphasis on personal autonomy and rational egoism in ethics does not necessarily imply that there is no place for altruism or communitarian values, but it does tend to give these a fairly minor role in ethical discussions. So dominant has the liberal discourse been that, in the recent attempt to address the multicultural situation, the traditional principles of autonomy, beneficence, non-maleficence, and justice almost invariably form the background to discussion (Serour 1994; Steinberg 1994). However, for many (and particularly for women) the individualistic type of liberalism often prevalent within Western medical ethics presents an unrealistic caricature of the human condition. A system of ethics based on it becomes a castle of sand, rather than an insightful and reflective discipline (Warren 1992).

In addition, there has been criticism of Western medicine over the problem posed by combining cultural and social norms with the medical technology developed by the West (Hoffmaster 1994). The complaint is often made that Western, middle-class values, espoused and enunciated by a relatively wealthy, secular, and educated elite, are being sold to technologically dependent nations, without any attempt to adapt to their cultural norms. This is seen by some as a perpetuation of colonial practices that have led to the discounting of traditional insights into the human condition. However, some of the norms dominant in certain cultural settings seem intrinsically abusive or discriminatory, for instance, against women or against whole groups of people.

Some of these societal norms have immediate relevance to bioethics. The prominence given to female circumcision in recent debates forces us to ask whether bioethics can condemn a practice regarded by some as central to the identity and integrity of their culture. A further example is the widespread conviction among Japanese people that a warm, bleeding body is alive, and that to take organs from a brain-dead person is therefore to assault or even kill the person. Then again, in Greece, the attitude that death is 'ugliness', 'darkness', 'chaos', 'blackness', leads to a denial of death in the doctor–patient relationship, and this tends to make death lonely, frightening, and difficult to face (Dracopoulou & Doxiadis 1988). In certain African contexts and among many indigenous peoples, the importance of a holistic model of health and disease that takes account of spiritual and other factors puts a vast range of issues (such as responsibility for health care, and the concept of well-grounded medical intervention) into a completely different light from that encountered in a developed or contemporary Western context. In view of these diversities, is there any universal grounding of debate in bioethics, or do all conclusions in bioethics have to be linked to a particular context? Should we say, for example, that female circumcision is wrong in the United Kingdom or Australia, but acceptable in some African contexts? Or is a more general viewpoint possible?

In New Zealand, European and Māori approaches to life, death, meaning, and therefore to biomedical issues, have had to achieve some rapprochement. This has happened because the British colonists formulated the founding document of the country as a treaty of mutual respect between two races that promised to safeguard the sovereignty and treasures of the Māori people. In Australia there is increasing awareness that traditional Aboriginal concepts of health have to be taken into account in both clinical and research ethics. In both these settings the European is seen as the latecomer with an intrusive culture that needs to accommodate a different worldview. In contrast, the case of female circumcision of Third World immigrants to European societies is generally regarded as going beyond culture, and has become an issue of human rights.

The writings of Alice Walker projected female circumcision into the Western consciousness as no scholarly discussion ever could.

circumcision is a taboo that is never discussed. How then do the chiefs know how to keep it going? How is it talked about?

My mind is a blank. Surely no one ever told me anything except that . . . this thing M'Lissa did to me expressed my pride in my people . . .

But what did you think, I asked M'Lissa. When I came into the Mbele camp asking to be 'bathed.'

I thought you were a fool, she says without hesitation. The very biggest . . .

Of course she took the outer lips, because four strong eagle-eyed women held me down; and of course the inner lips too . . .

What my mother started, the witchdoctor finished . . . he showed no mercy. In fright and unbearable pain my body bucked under the razor-sharp stone he was cutting me with . . . [Walker 1992, pp. 217, 227, 206].

When we read of the practice, its inhumanity seems obvious. The more it is examined, the more it appears as systematic brutality towards, and abuse of, women. Alice Walker's character seems to undergo a profound disillusionment based on a deep need for cultural identification. But so enmeshed is it in cultural beliefs about the roles of the sexes, cleanliness, being truly a woman, and cultural identity that it is actively pursued and promoted by women in Northern Africa and Southern Arabia. What is more, the Western and international voices that condemn the practice are often branded as chauvinistic and culturally insensitive. Kopelman (1994) argues that there are common goals relating to human well-being that allow us to enter dialogue and that relativism about practices such as female circumcision is implausible. Given the debate, can we find ground on which to move towards a sustainable view on such an issue?

The experience of the Australasian countries is of wide relevance to cultural diversity and ethical reasoning, because in each case there is a marked contrast between the cultures involved. Each indigenous culture is a pre-metallic, clan-based, hunter–gatherer society living in a close relationship with the land (in the case of the Māori this kind of life is mixed with rudimentary agriculture). European society is post-agricultural, post-industrial, based on the nuclear family, predominantly urban, and committed to enlightenment individualism with its idea of progress. In New Zealand the difference between the two settings led to a formal treaty being concluded between the sovereign Māori people of Aotearoa and the British Crown—the Treaty of Waitangi. The existence of this treaty and its ratification by a quasi-governmental body charged with supervising its implementation makes the New Zealand situation instructive for a meeting of cultures in which some semblance of mutual respect is honoured—in principle at least.

The Māori ethos 'involves the laws of tapu: genealogies, history, traditional knowledge, carving, preparing flax, in fact, nature itself. Tapu is something that teaches you how to respect the whole of nature, because Māori things involve the whole of nature' (Pewhairangi 1992). Post-colonial suppression of Māori language, culture, and political structure, and then increasing urbanisation, have destroyed much of the cohesion of traditional beliefs and values, and the best we can do is formulate certain generalities, relying on more traditional sources, to give a sense of *taha Māori* (the Māori perspective).

New Zealand Biculturalism

Although we will focus for a time on New Zealand society as a mixture of two very different cultures, the issues that arise are not peculiar to New Zealand because many societies must develop medical ethics in a way that reflects the beliefs and concerns of more than one tradition of thought. The challenge of biculturalism in New Zealand is an instance of the difference between post-colonialism and cosmopolitanism or multiculturalism in a post-industrial Western or developed context. Multiculturalism tends to have a haphazard, compromised character, whereby different traditions agree to live and let live, but indigenous peoples throughout the world are not always happy with this state of affairs. The Treaty of Waitangi, for instance, promised that the value and integrity of the Māori people would be considered important in the development of a bicultural society, not just a society that tolerated different cultures on a modified or tolerantly liberal view.

It has been interesting to note the convergence between the concerns of certain strands of philosophical ethics and the concerns of Māori people. Both medical ethics and Māori thought recognise the importance of respect for the individual as a being with a dignity and standing of his or her own. Both recognise the fact that health care is concerned not solely with physiological interventions. However, there are some distinct emphases that a Māori perspective on health introduces, emphases that should be included in our understanding of clinical ethics. All cultures have their strengths and weaknesses and it is very easy to fall into one of two equally problematical stances. The first of these is that Western medicine has an exclusive claim to truth and that it encompasses the knowledge and methodology required to understand the causes of suffering. The second is that there is no right view and that every traditional approach to medicine has equal standing with the Western tradition. The first of these standpoints neglects fundamental insights discernible in the philosophy of science, and the second neglects the pragmatic and interventional nature of medical science (Gillett et al. 1995).

The traditional Māori perspective is similar to other indigenous perspectives. For instance, the African perspective regards physical ills as bound up with mental or spiritual ills (Gbadgesun 1994). Thus, the Māori or African patient may feel himself, not merely to have suffered a physiological or anatomical injury, but to have been wounded and weakened in his soul or essential being as part of his illness. The physical body, for such a patient, is symbolic of the meeting of the physical and spiritual that lies at the heart of a holistic conception of life. Secularised humanism, which frames many discussions in contemporary medical ethics, is, therefore, not open to any health care ethics that aims to respect *taha Māori* and many other kinds of indigenous world views. In fact, a belief in the inherent spirituality of life is probably more prevalent in many

cultures than is its denial, and this may pose significant difficulties for established health care ethics (with its embedded presumption of secular humanism)
as it tries to engage in multicultural discourse.

In sickness and death the inseparability of the physical and the spiritual is
made vivid in traditional Māori thought. Death is, in fact, both the ending of a
life and the reaffirmation of the identity of the person who has died. This identity reaches far back in time and locates the person in a meaningful context so
that death is not seen as being futile or meaningless. Notice the contrast
between this view and what we are told about medicine in Colombia and some
other areas of South America: 'the tendency in medical practice has been
towards what some ethicists have called 'diseuthanasia' which means the unnecessary prolongation of life by all means possible, in some cases against the wishes
of patients and immediate family members' (Llano-Escobar 1988). In a context
where death has an established place in the propriety and rhythm of life
'diseuthanasia' is unlikely to arise.

Sickness, the forerunner of death, has a very special meaning for Māori
patients, in that the sick person is highly dependent on sources of strength aside
from her own *mana* (the divinely given power of the individual), which is
wounded or diminished. For a Māori person, a potent source of *mana* is
belonging—or the connections between the life of the individual and the life of
the *whānau* (extended family). This belonging allows a patient in a weakened
state to draw strength, courage, and the ability to face illness from the fact that
'My relation and I are part of the same tree, we share the same ancestry and
claims of that ancestry are very real' (Dansey 1975). This emphasis on close
support of the dying person contrasts markedly with the situation of dying
Greek patients, who may be 'isolated in small rooms, away from the public,
other patients, friends, and relatives ... All this is a terrible ordeal for the
terminally ill patient' (Dracopoulou & Doxiadis 1988). How reminiscent is this
of the situation where many patients find themselves avoided or cut off because
of their terminal condition? The contrasting attitudes here emphasise the need
to find some basis for rapprochement between cultural practices.

The Māori patient also lives with a sense of wholeness as a human being.
Given the close connection between body and soul, the treatment of one's body
as a mere thing may carry the implication for the patient that his *mana* or individual dignity is similarly reduced, and that the professionals either do not care,
or believe he is nothing, and that there is no hope for him. The Māori patient is
in this respect like many people on unfamiliar 'turf'. A Māori woman, or indeed
any woman, may not feel confident that she fully understands what is happening to her in the course of gynaecological treatment. She will attempt to read,
from the universal body language of her caregivers, the messages that are hard to
evaluate from their words. She, like many patients, will be asking 'What does this
mean for me?' The meaning of her illness, for her, will often not be addressed by

her caregivers, who may be obsessed with diagnosis, evidence-based medicine, and management.

It is unacceptable to treat a Māori person as a set of distinct functioning units, and equally unacceptable to treat this person as detached from his or her 'belonging'. But the same problems are encountered in the Western individual who is reckoned to have his or her own agenda and interests and to be individually competent to make sound decisions. This powerful image (of autonomy and decision-making capacity) tends to dominate medical ethics and results in individuals being treated without reference to the underlying spiritual and inclusive reality that, for many cultures, shows itself in the harm or illness that has occurred. The sources and significance of this harm, which at one level manifests itself in physical disease, range far beyond the sick individual. Consequently, the understanding of illness may be embedded in layers of meaning that can only be unpacked in the context of a *whānau* (or family grouping with its traditional belief system and ways of thinking about human life). In the African context, we find that such convictions may also be critical in terms of the thinking of the patient: 'human beings have to find a way of avoiding the forces of evil. Fortunately they can depend on the support of ancestral spirits to help them in this struggle because the ancestors have acquired greater power in the land of the dead' (Gbadgesun 1994). The Western-trained doctor is not necessarily able to connect with these understandings of disease and yet may have to defer to traditional ways of discussion and interaction in order to be effective. The problems are illustrated in the following case.

> James is a 38-year-old Māori carpenter admitted with severe central chest pain. He is found to have ECG evidence of a myocardial infarction. Over the next few days this is confirmed with enzyme studies and, after considering the history, the doctors decide that he ought to have a coronary angiogram. The junior doctor explains everything to James, who appears to agree with what is proposed and has no questions to ask. Later she finds that James refuses to sign the consent form, and she is puzzled. The cardiologist in charge of the case is asked about it and says something derogatory about the intelligence of Māori patients in general, claiming that they never seem to know what they want. He confronts James in an aggressive manner and later the nursing staff find James making moves to leave the ward because he does not like that 'specialist fella' and would rather go home.

It is instructive to listen to some of the perceptions and concerns of James during these events. (We have expressed these in words that have been used by Māori patients in real discussions.)

> They say it's something wrong with my heart. That is a pretty tapu kind of thing. They tell me that my heart is weak and bits of it might die off. What happens when your heart has already started to die. They want to put some tube in it with this X-ray dye stuff and they

say it might even make it die a little bit more. I don't know about that, maybe taking the pictures of my heart will really screw things up in there. Anyway, I can't say anything to these doctors, but I'm not too sure about it and I'm not going to sign this form. I've got to talk to somebody, maybe the old man or Aunt Rangi, I think I will go home and talk to them so that that big fella doesn't get so mad any more. I will come back and see that young lady doctor when we have all had a talk about it.

James's concerns, which to some extent speak across the barriers of power, education, and culture, reflect the fact that he is worried about the impact of this disease, not only on his physical body, but on his soul or being-as-a-person. The fact that his heart is affected has deep and uncertain significance for the kinds of harms he is suffering, and he is worried about those deeper meanings of his sickness. This intensifies the importance for James of doing things properly, and for that he must have assurance and personal strength. But any illness weakens a person both physically and psychologically (and, for a Māori person, it indicates a state of spiritual weakening). James cannot express these concerns in what is, for him, the alien and lonely context of a Pākehā (European New Zealander)-controlled hospital setting. In that setting he has no status or standing. He does not know how things are done or where he stands because he is not in a place where he belongs. This forces him to search elsewhere for the critical help and guidance he needs, although he knows that his final decision might be to choose the care plan that the Pākehā doctors offer. His situation, made graphic in the context of his own cultural meanings, is common to many whose culture is different from that of the educated elite who staff specialist units, or the educated middle class who staff hospitals in general.

We should also recall the fracturing and dispersion of Māori and many other indigenous peoples in a post-colonial setting. For many people who have suffered the breakdown of their culture, the only sensible way to get health care is the Western way. The difficult cases that most often arise in such contexts are those in which the wishes of individuals differ from those of their most obvious support group. In such cases patients may not wish others from their culture to be involved, and the health care team may be in the unfortunate situation of trying to protect the patient's wishes against those cultural representatives they would normally try to cooperate with and involve. As things stand in most Western countries, it is not permissible for health care workers to go against the principle of individual autonomy (involving privacy and confidentiality) or against the express wishes of their patients, except in rare cases (child abuse, AIDS, dangerous use of a motor vehicle). It would, however, be wise for the health care workers in this situation to involve someone who can attempt a reconciliation—which may, in itself, be a very healing thing to do. These problems of departure from cultural norms are, of course, present in many multicultural settings.

Is There Hope for Transcultural Rapprochement?

Signs of hope for some transcultural rapprochement are not too difficult to find, both in general and in the New Zealand case. The philosophical development of these provides an interesting framework for ethical thinking.

There is common human outrage at certain actions, for instance the wanton destruction of children, whether by soldiers in war or by any other person in civilian life. We acknowledge unusual cases that violate this norm and, when we do, we look for reasons why an otherwise morally incomprehensible type of act is condoned. For instance, the Japanese practice of '*mabiki*, which means to "thin out" . . . was the only way for the poor to keep their families small enough to feed without an effective birth control method' (Kawashima 1988). It was (and is) also applied to the seriously malformed newborn where the motivation was to avoid the shame of having such a child. In these cases, one where the wish is to protect children already born, and the other to avoid dishonour, an over-powering reason is found to set aside the moral implications of the parent–child bond. Often invoked is the idea that the child is a gift of the gods, which we must humbly offer back to them, before we assume that the child is ours to raise and nurture. Despite these exceptions, there seems to be widespread acknowledgment of the special value of the parent–child bond.

The idea of human rights has international appeal, and there is also broad agreement as to the content of the rights. Most societies agree that each human being deserves respect and justice. Different cultures weight this differently according to the needs and involvement of the community to which the individual belongs, but all of them recognise the value of the individual human being. Even if this ideal is often transgressed, and even if the forms according to which it is recognised vary markedly from place to place, serious transgressions are usually recognised as wrong, and excuses are made or justifications offered. The perceived need to excuse anomalies merely reinforces the basic claim. However, we should note the anomaly that women are often regarded as inferior and that women's rights vary greatly between cultures. Thus, in many cultures, women are still oppressed and disenfranchised to the detriment of their health and well-being. But we in the West cannot claim any great distinction in this area. It is not too many years since these same abuses were rife in our own countries, and in some forms are still present. This transcultural constant—the oppression of women—can be hidden by recent changes in its manifestation, but it requires explanation in universal human terms. The constant feature is not one we morally endorse, but it points to a significant commonality between diverse moral contexts.

There are a number of cases where different cultures share the same value under different names. Two such issues have arisen in the New Zealand context and both illustrate deeply held intuitions that cross cultural boundaries.

The first concerns reproductive choices and parent–child relationships. European ethicists have debated many issues concerning assisted reproductive techniques and the rights of adopted children. One of these has concerned the right of a child to know the identity of his or her genetic parents. The ethical debate has weighed the rights of biological parents to privacy and confidentiality against the need for a child to find out about his or her origins. We have eventually settled on a 'right to know' for adopted children, and have justified this by talking about 'genetic bewilderment' (Otago Bioethics Research Center 1991). The matter has been handled differently within Māori culture. There is a strong sense of *whakapapa* or lineage underlying the identity of a traditional Māori person. Belonging to a particular hereditary group has always been important in Māori concepts of self-worth, identity, and duty. Thus the question of belonging and of origins is of central importance for a Māori person in a way often submerged in Western liberal individualism.

This may vary from setting to setting; in some indigenous cultures, for instance that of the Torres Strait Islanders, intrafamilial adoption is widely practised. The significance of this is unclear given that lineage is not necessarily tied to a narrowly defined nuclear family unit. For the Pākehā it has taken the growing awareness of different voices—such as the voices of adopted children—and the development of complex reproductive technology to rekindle our interest and revive our intuitive awareness of roots and their fundamental role in the life of a human being. In fact, although expressed differently from the images found in many traditional cultures, similar beliefs and values about lineage and its importance are rife in Western society, and the debates surrounding reproductive technology merely highlight what was true but unseen in our own attitudes.

The second example is the traditional Māori sense that one's head is *tapu* or sacred in a special way. *Tapu* denotes a place or body part that is imbued with special significance or is set apart for some spiritual purpose. The head is the most sacred part of the body with the brain the conductor of responses and reactions. As such, it is the repository of our experiences and vital to the *mauri* or principle of life of the person. The deeply held value central to this idea is obvious when talking to any patients approaching neurosurgical procedures; the universal intuition is that there is something awesome about the idea of a brain operation. This has to do with the thought that the brain is the essential 'me' or 'you', and that doing things to it is trespassing on the 'holy of holies' of human life, the dwelling place of the personhood of a person (which we also see in the PVS debate in Chapter 12).

The same value is recognised in the many cultures where brain death is recognised as a valid criterion of death. A dramatic New Zealand case that highlights this value occurred when the brain of a Māori person was removed at a postmortem examination, which meant that the brain was not in the head when the *tangi*, or funeral rites, were held. A key part of the *tangi* is the opportunity for those present to talk to and farewell the dead person. One can, therefore, understand the outrage of the extended family when they found that the one to whom they were talking had an empty head. It would be missing the point to observe, as a 'rational and scientific' Western commentator might, that a dead brain is functionally the same as no brain at all in terms of its biological role in personality and relationships. The symbolism here is too powerful. We know what the hurt and anger was all about; we know how stupid and degraded the family felt that this important ceremony had at its heart an emptiness that seemed to destroy its central meaning. This common intuitive recognition of what was wrong with the pathologists' actions crosses the divide between the mind-set of the contemporary Western individualist urbanite, and the pre-metallic, land-based Māori in a way that is completely missed by so-called scientific descriptions of the facts.

However, there are voices objecting to an emphasis on the head or brain that devalues the whole person. Brain death and transplantation from brain-dead donors has been an extremely contentious issue in Japan (Omine 1991). But here, again, there is an intuitive appeal in arguments about the implausibility of calling a person dead when he or she is warm, bleeds, and can be a source of living organs. We do not just have to scratch our heads and wonder what sort of people would think such a thing; we appreciate their moral conflict.

A further experience illustrating the convergence between different religions and cultures was found by the British Medical Association working group on euthanasia. Members of the group took submissions from major religious bodies on the active ending of a human life (British Medical Association 1988), and every one of them (Roman Catholic and Protestant Christian, Jewish, Islamic, Hindu, and Buddhist) took the view that life is a gift that was not ours to give and take. Each group warned of the danger of hubris in the face of something too great for us fully to comprehend. The phenomenon of hubris, of bulldozing through the mysteries of life, birth, and death with progressive and ready remedies, is one that many thinkers regard as suspect in the conduct of clinical practice and particularly in decisions about the end of life (Gormally 1994).

There are many images associated with death that, while particular to a given culture, are instantly recognisable by others. For instance, there are two vivid Jewish images about our role in relation to a dying person. One is that of the faintly burning candle that we must not disturb in case we cause it to go out, even to the point of entering the room quietly and gently rather than banging the door. The second image is of a woodcutter working outside the window of a room where someone is dying; the dying person longs to slip away, but the unmistakable sound of the woodcutter at work keeps pulling the person back to the here and now. These are vivid and readily understandable images; taken together they convey a certain set of attitudes towards death and dying. As images they have a deep-seated or intuitive appeal that arguments about euthanasia often lack, but it is an appeal that does not seem confined within a particular cultural boundary.

At this point we are beginning to see some hope of cultural rapprochement in the many shared intuitions and images (Gillett 2000), even though the complex issues that arise when they conflict are resolved differently in different settings.

A Possible Basis for Ethics

The guiding thought for the pursuit of a wide consensus in ethics is the idea that as human beings we share more than a biological form; we develop through shared human experiences. The experience of nurture is plausibly basic because it is a necessity for all human babies. The child then extends his or her competence in the world by catching on to the conversations of others and entering into life with them. Arguably this is the most fundamental life skill of a human being. We can conclude, therefore, that there is a kind of belonging that is central in childhood, even though the child must also develop as a person in his or her own right. This gives rise to the need for an individual to define himself or herself not just as part of a human group, but also as a distinct individual. Different cultures may emphasise these two components in different ways, but the twofold nature of identity is shown by the naming practices in every culture that signal both kinship and individuality.

In the light of Chapter 1, we are beginning to flesh out a neo-Aristotelian conception of the human form. Aristotle argued that humans were rational and social beings, and that these two qualities distinguished them from other animals. As such, they formed the ground for certain basic human dispositions or 'virtues'—truthfulness, perceptiveness, prudence, kindness, friendliness, and justice (Nussbaum 1993). Some of the boundaries are detectable, but it is our being as biological members of the species *Homo sapiens* that forms the basis for the development of a worthwhile culturally embodied life. This idea takes note of both our embodiment and our acculturation in a way that allows us to go beyond pure animal needs in assessing what is of central and universal value in human life.

This kind of foundation for ethics—in shared human experiences—suggests that to jump straight to moral beliefs or principles as a shared basis for ethics may be to go too far. The experience of becoming an engaged human being creates in us sensitivities, dispositions, and, ideally, skills of thinking that human beings bring to moral judgments. We will, for instance, notice and react negatively to distortions and disruptions of the parent–child bond. Similarly, we will respond to the oppression and abuse of human beings because their feelings are discounted or ignored. These responses are part of our growing among, and needing to be valued by, others.

Human experiences are conveyed in narratives that allow us to enter the perspective of other human beings. For instance, one might be caring for a young Samoan or West Indian man who is losing control of diabetes. At a certain point this young man refuses to continue his insulin treatment, although he realises that he becomes quite ill when he neglects it. What is happening here? If we take the time to talk to this young man and begin to explore his self-image, his heroes, the things he really wants to do, we will almost certainly unravel an experience that we can understand.

Personal narratives or stories take shape within a culture and articulate the experiences of a given life into a more or less meaningful whole. To understand such a narrative is to buy into the experience of the individual involved as a person, who belongs in certain ways. This makes evident cultural beliefs, personal commitments and the position of that person in the situations that make up his or her life. We may find that in certain ways the narrative that we hear is dysfunctional or fragmented, but even so it allows us to appreciate the subject at its centre and what life and the course of medical care mean to that person. It enables us to understand how that person may find a medical encounter either destructive or constructive.

When this kind of understanding becomes part of our equipment, cultural boundaries no longer obstruct the delivery of sensitive and informed health care. Increasingly, as we listen to the stories of those for whom we are paid to care, we will appreciate what it is for this person to live a culturally embodied, worthwhile life, and act accordingly. Where we fail to do this, problems will arise: there will be silence rather than communication, resistance rather than cooperation, anger and resentment rather than appreciation and respect. If one attends to these subtle indicators, corrective listening and heeding can be reinstated in the clinical relationship even across cultural divides. However, the problems that arise in health care settings do not always result from the clinical relationship involved.

We have argued for the possibility of grounding ethics in a way that respects and draws on the insights of different cultures. In doing so, we have discussed common human experiences and the diverse cultural narratives in which we articulate those experiences. Where such narratives are understood, and the underlying intuitions grasped, we have noticed some striking convergences between quite disparate cultures. This goes some way towards defusing the claim that there can be no common ground for health care ethics between people from different cultures, but it is not the end of the story.

A common argument for the cultural relativism of values is the claim that morality merely reflects the dominant or majority social or cultural mores.

If ethics really springs from common and very basic human experiences of living among others, this is not inevitable. Anyone might recognise in the reaction of a person from a different group something that he or she would also feel strongly about. This glimpse of shared humanity carries the spark of genuine reflection and reform. It is evident in the phenomenon of social or moral reform by a minority group in a society, or even by an individual. The great example of this is the anti-slavery campaign that over a period of years managed to reverse, in the United Kingdom then in the USA, a position held by the majority and sustained by powerful financial interests. A reformer or group wanting to achieve such reform has to find something more basic than social convention or agreement to appeal to, and it follows from the present discussion that this something is a moral sense shared by human beings at a deeper and more universal level than the norms of their own society.

History and Transcultural Ethics

The voices of New Zealand Māori, Australian Aborigines, and native North Americans have also made us aware of the importance of the history of dealings between peoples and cultures. For instance, we cannot separate the need for biculturally informed health care ethics in New Zealand from the history of European colonisation. The Māori inhabited a land as part of what they saw as an organic relationship fundamental to their being as a people. The land is in part the source of Māori being and identity (Cooper 1987). The term *whenua* means both land and placenta in Māori. The European viewed the land as a useable and tradeable commodity, and therefore alienated the land from the identity of those who lived in it: a very strange view for Māori to comprehend. This was viewed as a betrayal, and conveyed to Māori an attitude they regarded as degrading and destructive of the fundamentals of human existence. The individualism of the colonists and their economic stance towards others merely confirmed that view. The Pākehā was seen as a user and abuser who had no real commitments except to gain an advantage. Similar stories could be told in other settings where indigenous groups are making their voices heard.

We cannot separate this history from the ethics of post-colonial health care. Almost all indigenous groups have markedly worse health statistics than those of more recent settlers, suggesting that the colonising cultures have not acted with respect and care. In New Zealand the dominant culture is accused of not having fulfilled its promises to protect the integrity of the Māori people (Royal Commission on Social Policy 1988). Similar complaints would carry the same moral force when made by other indigenous peoples.

This means that a prominent question for an individual from any colonised people is that of trust and safety: 'Can I trust what you as a member of the colonising race tell me about my health and well-being? Do I feel safe with you? Do you understand my need?'(Rimene et al., 1998) Once one understands the background of dealings between races, these questions become understandable and not just an expression of sullen hostility and non-cooperation.

The facts of colonisation and historical intercultural abuse imply that ethics needs to go beyond knowing a culture and respecting its meanings, an area of philosophy prominently championed by Peter Winch (1958). To an interpretive or hermeneutic knowledge of the realities of another culture we need to add an understanding of social disempowerment and marginalisation, a strand of thought that is prominent in the work of Foucault (1981) and many feminist thinkers who 'share a recognition that women are oppressed in our society' (Sherwin 1996). They also acknowledge that 'the concept of autonomy, rather than working to empower the oppressed and exploited among us, in practice often serves to protect the privileges of the most powerful'. Foucault helps us identify how a particular cultural view, such as that of Western scientific medicine, or positivist science, becomes dominant because it offers knowledge, and therefore power over phenomena in which those who control a situation have interests. Thus, for instance, the practices associated with institutionalisation and the diagnosis of insanity can mean that people who violate social and behavioural norms are discounted. This approach is highly compatible with the ethic of care, and quite distinct from the perspective where reliance is placed on propositions or rules such as the overriding value of individual autonomy. We saw this in Stalinist Russia, where dissidents would be labelled as being psychiatrically ill and therefore suffering a 'disorder'. This discounted their legitimate criticisms of the political regime and its depersonalising practices. We might be led to see the same situation in relation to an ethnic group whose unease about and criticism of the dominant culture is discounted as being an aberration, due to the backwardness or the lack of enlightenment of their culture.

The move towards a transcultural ethic must, therefore, be based on an appreciation of the history that has produced the present relationships. This can only be understood through a sharing of experiences, an openness to the narratives of others, a willingness to participate in the ordeal of the other, and an attitude that pays attention to our common experiences of humanness. This is highly congenial to the ethic of care, and is quite distinct from a basis in universally agreed propositions or rules, such as individual autonomy. A different basis for ethics arises from basic human fears and beliefs, which while differently expressed in different cultures are common to them. If we can learn the trick of seeing through different eyes then an apparent ethical impasse can often become a common and shared endeavour. For instance, in the case of female circumcision there seems to be a great deal of silence, oppression, and abuse required to maintain the cultural practice. The fact that women's voices from the very context in which it occurs tell a different story from the official line, tends to confirm that there is something deeply wrong (Walker 1992). Therefore, it is not merely the arbitrary imposition of Western norms and prejudices that militates against recognising this practice as an example of ethically acceptable cultural diversity. We also have the narratives of the abused and oppressed, which move us to object.

All too often in modern clinical life, we arrogantly believe that we do all that is required when we treat each individual as an economic and self-governing unit. Patients are often scared and uncertain, needing trustworthy help and guidance, and we must respect those needs and aim to empower patients to cope with them and preserve their individual dignity. Trying to understand the fears and concerns of patients who come from minority or displaced cultures will, we believe, open our eyes to the fact that, at heart, people are not ideal, rational, liberal, economic units, and that both medicine and ethics must apply themselves to beings who are needy and vulnerable. Such beings require care, consideration, and relatedness as much as any other benefits we might confer on them. This insight allows us to come to some conclusions in many of the difficult areas of health care and cultural disagreement, such as female circumcision. It does so, by engaging us with the suffering that we otherwise would not see, and by teaching us to recognise values that contemporary Western culture may have submerged.

4
The Human Body

Introduction

Although health professionals deal daily with human beings, and therefore with their bodies, the significance of the human body itself could readily be overlooked because we emphasise patients rather than their bodies. And yet there are circumstances under which we need to consider the human body in its own right. This is particularly so when dealing with a dead body, and when confronted by decisions regarding what should or should not be done to a dead body. Similar considerations also arise when dealing with living people who wish to donate organs (such as a kidney), since this is an act that may have repercussions for the future functioning of their bodies. We need to consider, therefore, what we think of the human body, what value we place upon it, and in what ways we should respect it.

An instructive place to start is with the relationship between a person and that person's body. This is an issue that permeates all our thinking about the significance of the human body, and the way the question is answered has important repercussions for how we respond in practice to dead bodies, whether they be of someone we have known or not. It is relevant for clinicians and ethicists when deciding, for example, about the use of organs from those killed in road accidents. It is also relevant for those who dissect dead bodies in medical schools.

Dissection is an activity that itself raises a number of issues concerning whether bodies should be dissected and whether prosections (dissections of specific regions of cadavers) should be prepared for display in museums. These are important ethical issues, since the process of dissection involves the dismemberment of a corpse, an activity that society does not allow the general public to indulge in. The act of dissection 'depersonalises' the body and herein lies a danger, since it would be easy to conclude that the depersonalisation or reductionism of dissection gives us a warrant to do what we like with dismembered hands, kidneys or brains, even if we would not contemplate acting in this manner towards intact cadavers. Such a *laissez-faire* attitude towards the dismembered remains of cadavers becomes possible only if we deny the relationship they once had with the bodies of living people. As long as there is awareness of this relationship, limits will be placed on how the remains of people are to be treated, including the introduction of ethical constraints (such as obtaining informed consent for the use of body parts). Even the way in which bodies are obtained for dissection is accompanied by its own set of ethical considerations. This can best be illustrated by an extreme example—the way in which bodies were obtained in the early years of medical education in the United Kingdom.

Obtaining Bodies for Dissection

Historical Developments in the United Kingdom and New Zealand

Early dissections in the United Kingdom (from the sixteenth century onwards) were of criminals executed for murder, with the result that dissection became recognised as a punishment, since it was something over and above execution itself. In 1752 an act of parliament gave judges discretion in death sentences for murder, and this was to substitute dissection for gibbeting in chains. Since gibbeting was regarded as a grim fate, dissection became recognised as being a punishment that was as bad as, if not worse than gibbeting. The intention of both was to deny burial to the wrongdoer. The dissection had a further punitive element because it did something to the body beyond that already inflicted on the scaffold.

This means of acquiring bodies could not match the ever-increasing demand, and as a result another means of obtaining bodies emerged, namely, grave-robbing. The earliest grave-robbers were surgeon-anatomists or their pupils, and by the 1720s the stealing of bodies from London graveyards had become commonplace. Bodies stolen in this way, the so-called *resurrected corpses*, were predominantly those of the poor. There was often a close liaison between the surgeon-anatomists (or medical schools) and the body snatchers (resurrectionists). The latter provided several thousand bodies annually, supplying the overall needs of the medical schools (Richardson 1988).

The *Anatomy Act 1832* was prompted by the need to stop the resurrectionists, and it reflected the prevailing medical opinion that the most uncontroversial source would be the use of 'unclaimed bodies'. This made poverty the sole criterion for dissection, since the Act abolished the use of dissection as a punishment for murder. In the 100 years after the Anatomy Act was passed, 57 000 bodies were dissected in the London anatomy schools, and fewer than 0.5 per cent came from anywhere other than institutions housing the poor (either workhouses or asylums). In the early years of the twentieth century, as workhouses provided fewer bodies, asylums provided comparatively more. It was not until the late 1960s onwards that the number of bequests increased so dramatically, that as a source they alone were all but sufficient to meet the needs of British medical schools.

Developments in New Zealand stem from the beginnings of the University of Otago Medical School in 1875. Over the period from 1876 to 1886 practically all the bodies came from Dunedin Public Hospital, after which the hospital played only a minor role until recent times. By 1900 the Benevolent Institution (the poorhouse) had become the major source of supply, and this continued through to the early 1920s (Jones & Fennell 1991). In the early 1900s a third source of bodies emerged, namely the mental hospitals. One in particular proved a prolific source of bodies, especially from 1916 to 1930. Other mental hospitals augmented the supply from this hospital from around 1920 to the late 1950s. The first record of a bequest was in 1943, but bequests became more frequent only during the 1950s and were not the major source of supply until the early 1960s. The unclaimed poor provided practically the entire supply of bodies between 1889 and 1902, and from then until 1915, made up an average of 50 per cent. When this supply began to dwindle, more bodies became available via mental hospitals, so much so that in the first half of the 1900s it was the outcasts of society languishing in mental hospitals that provided most of the bodies for dissection in New Zealand.

Current Legislation in the United Kingdom and New Zealand

In the United Kingdom today, there are two Acts covering the use of human cadavers: the *Human Tissue Act 1961* and the *Anatomy Act 1984*. The Human Tissue Act makes provision for the use of the bodies of the deceased for post-mortem examination, therapeutic purposes, and for the purposes of medical education and research. The Anatomy Act covers the acquisition of bodies for 'anatomical examination', where anatomical examination is defined as the examination by dissection of a body (or a part of a body) for the purposes of teaching, studying, or researching morphology.

The Anatomy Act of 1984 has little in common with its predecessor of 1832. Current legislation stresses that the donation of one's body for dissection is very much a voluntary act. However, the person lawfully in possession of the body after death may authorise its use, if they have no reason to believe that the deceased expressed an objection to his or her body being used for such purposes, and provided that no surviving relative objects to such use. The same provisions apply for the continued possession of parts of a body after anatomical examination. Legal recognition of the right to choose what happens to one's body after death is likely to reflect societies' changing attitude towards the significance of the dead body.

British legislation pertaining to the use of human cadavers forms the basis for the *New Zealand Human Tissue Act 1964*. This Act contains a number of points of interest. The first is that, while the voluntary element in donation of bodies is paramount, it is still possible for medical superintendents of psychiatric hospitals and superintendents of penal institutions to authorise the use of bodies for anatomical examination unless the deceased person has expressed an objection to this or a surviving spouse or relative does so. A second point is that, even where an individual has agreed before death to donate his or her body, the deceased person's wishes can be overridden by the objections of a surviving spouse or relative. Third, there is no reference to the length of time the remains may be kept before burial or cremation, and it is explicitly stated that 'any part of the body may be retained indefinitely for further study'. Emphasis is placed on avoiding unnecessary mutilation of the body, and also on carrying out the examination in 'an orderly, quiet and decent manner'.

Persons and Bodies

The major stipulations in these acts raise an important ethical query: why do we think in these ways? Why is the treatment of cadavers considered to be of ethical significance? One answer is that the cadaver has *intrinsic* value: it is an end in and of itself. An alternative response is that the cadaver has *instrumental* value: it can be used as a means to an end.

The closest we come to recognising a cadaver's *intrinsic value* is when we argue that a person and his or her body are more or less inseparable, and that the intrinsic value of a living person (shown especially in his or her autonomy) is bestowed upon the cadaver at death. We recognise each other's bodies, and while this applies supremely during life, some very important aspects of identity continue following death. May (1985) has expressed it like this: 'while the body retains a recognizable form, even in death, it commands the respect of identity. No longer a human presence, it still reminds us of the presence that once was utterly inseparable from it.'

Robert Wennberg, a philosopher, refers to this as the 'overflow principle': 'we don't treat human corpses as garbage, because the corpse is closely associated with persons: it is the remains of a physical organism that at one time supported and made possible personal life' (Wennberg 1985).

The *instrumental value* of a cadaver emerges when it is recognised as the source of memories and responses, leading to the conviction that a corpse should be respected and treated in a 'decent' manner. As we remember a person who has died, we respect the person who *was*. All that remains of the person is the corpse, and yet our respect for that person and for the memory of that person leads us to respect the person's remains; this link is not readily broken. Furthermore, relatives and friends of the deceased are now grieving the death, and the cadaver is an integral part of the initial grieving process. The cadaver's instrumental value is also evident when it serves as a source of organs, or provides opportunities for teaching and clinical practice.

It is important to recognise both the cadaver's intrinsic and instrumental value. Separation of these sources of value is artificial, since both contribute to society's recognition of the cadaver's significance. From this it follows that the manner in which cadavers are treated is of moral interest (Jones 1994). In view of this, we respect a person-now-dead when account is taken of that person's wishes while alive. Only in this way do we recognise a continuum between the two, and hence the cadaver's intrinsic value. Similarly, when account is taken of the wishes and feelings of still-living relatives and friends, the cadaver's instrumental value is recognised.

Occasionally, one encounters the situation where a student recognises the body of a close family member in the dissecting room, or has reason to believe that this could occur. In view of the issues just discussed, it is important to ensure that this situation does not arise, or if it does to remove the body until the student is no longer working in the dissecting room.

On the negative side, we show disrespect to a person-now-dead when we allow that person's body to be dissected in the absence of any consent on the person's part prior to death, or where there are no close friends and relatives to argue the case for the deceased. In other words, dissection of an *unclaimed* body is a form of exploitation, since those with greater rights and opportunities before death are protected from this. It may also follow that the manner in which unclaimed bodies are treated actually differs from the manner in which bequeathed bodies are treated.

In order to throw further light on these possibilities, it is helpful to consider the moral values governing organ donation (Vawter et al. 1990). The first value normally used is that of *autonomy*, according to which each individual should have autonomous control over the disposition of his or her body after death, regardless of social need or the public interest. Donation implies that, prior to their deaths, the people concerned made a *free and informed decision* to allow their own bodies to serve as the source of transplanted organs. In acting in this way, they are *giving* the thing that is more closely identified than anything else with what they are and represent.

A second set of moral values focuses on the *interests of family members*, who can in some jurisdictions override the wishes of the deceased, even if the latter has specified that his or her body is to be donated for teaching, research, or therapeutic purposes. Whenever this occurs, it brings with it an apparent clash of moral values—between the prior autonomy and interests of the deceased and the actual autonomy and interests of the living. To emphasise the latter at the expense of the former implies that living family members have greater interests, and are more readily harmed than is a dead person. This emphasises the instrumental value of the cadaver at the expense of its intrinsic value, leading to an imbalance between the two; this in turn may have detrimental ethical consequences in other areas of decision-making.

Underlying the previous values is a premise: the *giving* of one's body is preferable to coercion. This highlights our third value, *altruism*, according to which it is better to give than to receive, and the good of others is better than self-interest (May 1985).

A fourth value stems from the common desire to find solace and meaning by using body parts to help others. This may be especially pronounced with premature or unexpected deaths, and is sometimes referred to as the *redemptive aspect* of organ donation. The death of one person can be interpreted as conferring life on another; out of a tragedy can come new life and hope, when organs are freely given to another in need of them. This value is intimately linked to the autonomy of the donor and to the altruism signified by the donation.

Use of Unclaimed Bodies

The values we have discussed play a significant role in society's regulation of organ donation. To what extent do they apply to the source of cadavers used in the dissecting room? The *bequest* of bodies for dissection parallels the *donation of organs* for transplantation. But what of the use of *unclaimed bodies* for dissection, where the wishes of the deceased are not taken into account, and altruism does not enter the picture? The use of unclaimed bodies in the dissecting room does not directly correspond with any procedure we use today in the realm of organ donation (Jones 1994). What, then, are the problems with the use of unclaimed bodies?

The crucial one revolves around the *absence of altruism*. The 'unclaimedness' of these bodies stems from the weakness, vulnerability, and frequently dereliction of the people when alive, and this unclaimedness mirrors their 'unwantedness'. This may be acceptable if cadavers are regarded as of instrumental value alone, but it fails to account for any intrinsic value they may have. The interests of the person-now-dead have been made subservient to other interests (the educational needs of health science students). But is this taking the argument too far, if for no other reason than that a dead body lacks interests? These people who are now unclaimed bodies were not necessarily mistreated during life, and there is no general ethical objection to dissecting dead human bodies.

All this is true, but the use of unclaimed bodies involves a fundamental lack of consent on the part of anyone with an interest in the person, in addition to which such people generally come from disadvantaged sectors of society. Taken together, these considerations provide forthright hints that the process may be unfair, allowing possibly the exploitation of one individual by another, or one group by another.

Another problem with the use of unclaimed bodies is that it rests on the assumption that the *instrumental value of cadavers outweighs their intrinsic value;* that is, the good emanating from dissection outweighs the autonomy of individuals. With this in mind we have to ask whether the benefits of dissection for health science students are so great, either in terms of anatomical knowledge gained or as a means of self-discovery about death and dying, that society is morally justified in jeopardising the autonomy of a limited number of disadvantaged individuals. To date no one has attempted to argue this case.

Of course it may be argued that what is done to a few disadvantaged individuals has no repercussions for the far greater number of individuals who are not likely to end their lives as unclaimed cadavers. It may be possible to assess these few, generally elderly, individuals in isolation from the very much larger number of young individuals who are killed in road accidents, and who may be candidates for organ transplantation. The manner in which bodies come to be in dissecting rooms cannot be isolated ethically (and should not be isolated procedurally) from how human bodies come to be in operating theatres as organ donors, or how the tissue comes to be in research laboratories. There is a delicate ethical thread linking all three areas.

A further issue revolves around family interests. In an attempt to justify the use of unclaimed bodies, it may be argued that when such bodies are used there are *no family interests*, and hence such interests cannot be infringed by use of the bodies of the deceased without prior consent. But does a willingness to ignore the previous interests of those who have now died lead to a neglect of the autonomy of similar individuals when alive? There may well be a link between treatment of the living and treatment of the dead. At the other extreme, if the value of people after death is perceived as being greater than the value accorded them prior to death, is there not a moral compulsion to improve their conditions while alive?

A final issue concerns the *redemptive element* that was referred to in dealing with organ transplantations. Where does this element feature in our moral evaluation of the use of cadavers in the dissecting room? The force of this value is weakened when bodies are donated at the end of a long life rather than following a premature or unexpected death. Death is less of a tragedy in the former case: it may have been expected; it may be seen as a natural conclusion to a long, fulfilled life, or even as a release from prolonged suffering. Although bodies being dissected do not directly give new life or new hope to individual patients or even to groups of patients, in the long term healing and wholeness do come through the medical expertise of the students-as-future-doctors. This provides an important ethical impetus if it can be demonstrated that there is a close correlation between dissecting cadavers (or studying prosections) and future medical expertise. In the case of unclaimed bodies there is a hint of a redemptive element, although the lack of any altruism diminishes its role.

The use of unclaimed bodies continues to this day in countries where too few bodies are made available by prior donation, or where the legal system directs that unclaimed bodies automatically go to anatomy departments. The willingness of society (and the medical profession) to utilise bodies in the absence of informed consent from the donor prior to death, suggests that greater emphasis is being placed on the educational value of dissection and on possible future medical benefits stemming from dissection, rather than on the autonomy of the disadvantaged within society.

At the other end of the scale is the use of bequeathed bodies with a memorial service preceding their burial or cremation as dissected remains (Bertman & Marks 1989). While these services take a variety of forms, their aim is to honour those who have donated their bodies to an anatomy department for the purposes of teaching and research; they also constitute a formal and public demonstration of the department's appreciation of such bequests. Whether secular or ecumenical, such services bring together the altruism of the donors, the gratitude of the students and faculty, and the memories of close relatives and friends, and are fitting symbols of the positive use to which bodies can be put after death. In the words of one student: 'If studying human anatomy is our initiation into the science of medicine, the Convocation of Thanks (memorial service) is our initiation into the art of healing' (Andersen 1994).

Underlying everything that has been written up to this point, there has been one basic assumption, namely that cadavers are gifted to health science students, who then use them for teaching and research purposes. Unfortunately, there are many examples in the United States where body parts obtained in this way (generally by private organisations) are passed on to 'for profit' companies. This has led to charges that some groups act as body brokers, and that the altruistic intentions of the donors are misappropriated. This is a tragic situation that could bring the whole of the cadaveric bequest system into disrepute.

In summary, it is preferable to err on the side of confining the source of cadavers to bequests. An easy acceptance of the use of large numbers of unclaimed bodies may indicate a disregard for the welfare of a small section of the population. Nevertheless, what is done with dead bodies for *good* reasons is not the most important of all ethical matters. A balance is needed at this point, a balance that emerges in other areas, where ethical strictures against the use of organs from both adult and foetal cadavers for transplantation purposes have to be weighed against the potential benefits accruing to debilitated patients.

It may appear that the issue discussed in this section is of relevance only to a small segment of the population—those involved in the teaching of gross anatomy to medical, health science, and science students, and to the students themselves. Such a conclusion would be misleading, since the ethical considerations that apply here are relevant in many other contexts where human material is used.

Cadavers in the Dissecting Room

Perceptions of the Cadaver

How do those who utilise cadavers, such as medical students, actually perceive them? More specifically, how do they view cadavers in the dissecting room, since this is one of the traditional arenas in which human anatomists function? Sadly, the literature on this subject is relatively limited. Hafferty (1991) has conducted the most extensive study in this area, on what he terms 'death and the socialization of medical students'. As a sociologist, he had to acquaint himself with the dissecting room environment before embarking on his study. He writes:

> Of all the sights I encountered that first day in lab, one of the most vivid and memorable was that of forty-four cadavers, all similar in their characteristic lifelessness, but all identifiably different in physical appearance. Some appeared more humanly evocative than others, but none was so distinctively unfamiliar or alien-appearing that the term 'human' seemed totally inappropriate. On the other hand, none closely resembled anything I had previously considered human. My definitional boundaries were stretched and shattered by these new objects. It was these reflections that first led me to think of the cadaver as an ambiguous entity: human but not human [Hafferty 1991, p. 81].

Leon Kass, following the sudden death of a wonderful old man, wrote:

> There he lay, peacefully, a frail figure . . . as if in a pleasant dream . . . I asked myself, 'Where *is* he? Where did he go? Where is that mind, that learning and understanding, those unwritten books that no one will now write?' . . . The body, the still warm and undisfigured body, identical in looks to what I had seen the day before, mocked me with its unintentional dissembling and camouflage of extinction. Here, there was vastly *less* than meets the eye. The dead body may be more than what our science teaches, but it is also less than what it appears to us to be. The body may be more than stuff, but the man seems to be more than his body [Kass 1985a, p. 21].

For Kass there are two possibilities. The first is that we are only physical beings; we are our bodies and nothing more. Alternatively, we are more than our physical beings; we are more than embodied matter, having some intangible and unseen dimension. Limited as these options are, they suggest that dead bodies are very much like us and very different from us, simultaneously. They are sufficiently like us to be recognisable as human beings and also as individuals. Yet, they are sufficiently unlike us to leave the distinct impression that they now exist at a level of being far removed from the one to which we, as living entities, identify with. For example, these dead bodies are no longer able to move, speak, or communicate with us, and in this sense we feel cheated. What, then, is the relationship between the dead body and the person who was once associated with that body? Consider the following, from Nicholas Wolterstorff's book *Lament for a Son*.

Born on a snowy night in New Haven, he died twenty-five years later on a snowy slope in Kaisergebirger. Tenderly we laid him in warm June earth. Willows were releasing their seeds of puffy white, blanketing the ground. I catch myself: Was it *him* we laid in the earth? I had touched his cheek. Its cold still hardness pushed me back. Death, I knew was cold. And death was still. But nobody had mentioned that all the softness went out. His spirit had departed and taken along the warmth and activity and, yes, the softness. He was gone. 'Eric, where are you?' But I am not very good at separating person from body. Maybe that comes with practice. The red hair, the dimples, the chipmunky look—that *was* Eric [Wolterstorff 1978, p. 8].

Hafferty (1991) in his analysis of the way in which medical students relate to dissection, noted that students are upset to varying degrees by the dissection of different parts of the body, with most anxiety being provoked by dissection of the head, face, arm, neck, pelvic, and perineal regions. This is the 'human referent' aspect of dissection reminding us that the cadavers really are (or were) human beings. They were once living people who did things, had goals and purposes in life, meant something to other people, and were just like us. Hafferty concluded that the greater this emphasis on regarding cadavers as formerly living human beings, the greater the emotional upset experienced by the students.

For other students though, the dead body is an aesthetically repulsive object, the death, formalin, and smell all conspiring to repel the sensitive, and forming a substantial barrier to academic learning. What then is the benefit of struggling to come to terms with the distress of the dissecting room complete with threatening cadavers, when anatomy can be learned from clean, aseptic books with glossy colour pictures, or even better from computers? One possible answer is that the study of the dead human body is a far more relevant introduction to the study of living patients than is the study of inanimate, two-dimensional diagrams, or photographs. Ultimately, the study of *somebody's* body is more appropriate than of *the* body for students in the health professions. Moreover, Hafferty contends that dissecting room learning is more than the mere accumulation of anatomical knowledge. It forms the basis upon which medical students develop their view of the privileged position they will one day assume as medical professionals.

Besides the possibilities just mentioned, Hafferty noted that students perceive dead bodies in a variety of ways: as biological specimens, as formerly living human beings, or as an amalgamation of features—formerly living human beings, learning tools, and of value for future clinical situations. For most students, the cadaver is an ambiguous entity: not only is its identity unclear, but it even changes in character in different situations. Of those who perceived the cadaver as a former human being, some considered them surrogate future patients and others as a 'future me'. The human referent of the 'future me' is a haunting and anxiety-promoting presence that has implications for the way in which students react to the issue of donation and dissection of their own bodies.

A complementary perspective on the issues surrounding the perceptions of a cadaver is offered by Howard Carter, a professor of comparative literature and humanities. Carter spent sixteen weeks researching his book *First Cut* in a traditional anatomy dissecting course at an American medical school. Needless to say this is an outsider's account of this unusual process, prompted by a curiosity as to what may have happened to the body of his father a few years previously following its donation to a medical school (Carter 1997).

Like Hafferty (1991), Carter recognises that students approach a cadaver in various ways. The first response he detected was that of disgust and aversion, which, in his experience, was usually fleeting; the second is reduction of the cadavers to biological exhibits; and the third is a reassertion by the students of the humanity of the cadavers. For Carter, dissection does not dehumanise the cadavers, since the students make connections between the implied personhood of the cadavers, their own bodies, and future patients.

Carter is impressed with the nature of the relationships that develop between students and their cadavers, relationships that are often cemented by the naming of the cadavers. These relationships bestow loyalty and honour upon the cadavers, and point to a growing understanding of how the students themselves will relate to other people's bodies, both dead and alive.

Carter detects an 'intimacy' between the students and their cadavers that forms the basis of knowledge about the innermost part of our being and the inner workings of our bodies. Knowledge of this kind is underrated and undervalued in our culture, as is our avoidance of death. For him, this is a great loss, which is compensated to some extent by these students, as they come to know the textures and qualities of the body through direct sensory experience of cadavers.

Carter views the anatomy course as a rite of passage, preparing students for the intimacies of the consulting room. They come to realise that the body is a gift, and as they take this gift apart they learn to do so with reverence and responsibility, an important preparation for future encounters with the living bodies of patients. It is here that he makes peace with his father's bequest. He recognises that his father's body served as a passive teacher following his death, allowing students to make their own discoveries among his tissues and bones.

For Carter, anatomy represents an intellectual approach that leads to comprehension and wisdom. All this occurs in a dissecting room, with its almost unique status, conveying vistas of humanity and deeply perplexing questions that lie well beyond the narrow confines of the learning of anatomical vocabulary.

Students' Experience of Dissection

A number of groups have attempted to gauge the emotional effect that the dissecting room situation has on medical students. These studies have concentrated on their inaugural experiences within a dissecting room and offer considerable insight into a variety of responses to such an environment. One study in this field, conducted by Charlton and co-workers (1994), sought to determine whether undergraduate medical students' attitudes to death and dying were influenced by the experience of dissection. The students were presented with a series of vignettes, both immediately before and several months after exposure to dissection. Following dissection the concern induced by the vignettes was minimal compared to that induced by the identical situation prior to experiencing the act of dissection. In other words, students rapidly develop a coping mechanism enabling them to view dissection as distinct from dealing with living human beings. The authors suggested that this form of coping or detachment mechanism may have detrimental effects on their subsequent ability to empathise with living patients. In their view, this empathy may be enhanced if the students were given greater scope to explore and discuss the complex set of emotions aroused by dissection.

In one such initiative, the experience of human dissection becomes a focal point for an exploration of issues such as detachment, empathy, medical virtue, and group dynamics (Coulehan et al. 1995). Students were requested to write a short narrative on their own reactions to the experience of dissection, or a story about the life of the cadaver they were studying. Seven commonly occurring themes arose out of these essays. These included: initial apprehension, detachment, curiosity about the person, need to relate to the cadaver, self-questioning about the ability and/or motivation to donate one's own body, gratitude, and religious/existential reflection. This exercise may provide students with an understanding of 'clinical distance' and 'detached concern', as well as a means of recognising empathy, gratitude, humility, and cooperation in medical practice (Coulehan et al. 1995).

There is a series of American studies that emphasises the traumatic nature of human dissection. Some of these studies have included reports of academic difficulties attributed to the inability to deal with, or suppress, feelings that surfaced during dissection (Bertman & Marks 1989), and feelings of anxiety and disgust (Gustavson 1988). Further studies have reported both physical and psychological reactions to dissection. Along similar lines, a study conducted on Nigerian medical students has found that 25 per cent of students are initially highly distressed by their dissecting room experience, with 5 per cent remaining 'very upset' after the completion of around 100 hours of dissection (Nnodim 1996). Most seriously, Finkelstein and Mathers (1990) noted that 5 per cent of students suffered from marked disturbances including nightmares, intrusive visual images, insomnia, depression, and learning impairments. These reactions were likened to those of post-traumatic stress disorder. In contrast, a British study by Evans and Fitzgibbon (1992) suggested that most students adapted quickly after the initial few weeks in the dissecting room.

What is worthy of further consideration is the underlying basis of the strong effect on a person that the dismemberment of a cadaver can have. The ability of a student to relate to a cadaver is often hindered by the defacement and reductionism involved with its dissection and dismemberment. This dismemberment is, however, a gradual process. Most people do not respond to a dissected arm, leg, or even a dissected head in the same way they respond to the whole body. What this illustrates is that we appear to associate a person with their body, more or less as a whole, rather than with their dismembered parts. The impact of a horrific scene (such as a major road accident) stems in part from the knowledge that a dismembered arm once belonged to a particular body; we still associate it with a person and that person's body. As dissection proceeds, the task of continuing to think any longer of the cadaver as a whole becomes increasingly difficult. Eventually, a point is reached when it is virtually impossible to regard the fragmented remains as a person. In other words, our analysis and dissection have robbed the cadaver of its personal associations.

And yet, there are limits to reductionism, since cadaveric remains have historic connections, that is, dismembered hands, hearts, and brains once had an intimate relationship with the bodies of the living.

This still leaves unanswered some fundamental questions. Should bodies be dissected at all? Should the *deliberate* defacing of a cadaver by dissection be allowed? Should prosections be prepared for display in museums? Answers to these questions depend on whether dissection can be justified for teaching purposes. If it can, these uses of cadavers can be justified under stringent ethical conditions.

Autopsies

The Relevance of Autopsies

Dissection, as discussed above, has many features in common with the autopsy (also known as a postmortem examination or necropsy), which is the most commonly encountered procedure affecting cadavers. An autopsy can serve numerous purposes including the establishment of truth, detecting change, providing information, instructing learners, and promoting justice (Lundberg 1984). In the majority of cases, the major reason for performing an autopsy is to establish truth; that is, to identify definitively the basis of the disease process(es), and to determine the cause and manner of death (Emson 1992).

They are carried out when someone dies unattended or without having been under medical supervision. Seemingly in contrast to this, they are also performed for deaths in a hospital setting. In this instance they serve as a quality control device for pre-mortem diagnosis and treatment decisions, which some authors consider is the single most important reason for conducting an autopsy. Autopsies are also performed on late foetal, neonatal, and infant deaths, with the intent of assisting in parental counselling should there be implications for future pregnancies. Additionally, they are useful for monitoring the effectiveness of new diagnostic and therapeutic technologies.

The utility of an autopsy is not limited to diagnostic or detective work. Surveys of medical students have shown that they are considered important teaching tools and a valuable means of acquiring new information concerning disease processes, and of improving future patient management (Botega et al. 1997). A list taken from Jones (2000) highlights the research areas that have been illuminated by the study of human tissue obtained from autopsies:

- an understanding of infectious agents such as human immunodeficiency virus, Epstein-Barr virus, and Creutzfeldt-Jakob disease;
- the pathogenesis of Alzheimer's disease;
- the possible causes of sudden infant death syndrome and common errors in determining cause of death in infants;
- an assessment of the body's reaction towards titanium hip implants;
- methods of determining drowning as a cause of death;
- risk factors related to coronary artery disease and myocardial infarction;
- the effect of various agents on the body; for example, aspirin, alcohol, and oral contraceptives.

Despite the substantial gains accrued by autopsy, in recent years there has been a dramatic decline in the number performed. Reasons given for this decline vary (see Brown 1984 p. 447), yet there is evidence to suggest that the decline is not due to a reluctance on the part of the public to consent to the procedure. A survey by Sanner (1994a) found that 84 per cent of people questioned would accept an autopsy being performed on themselves, and 80 per cent would give consent for the procedure to be carried out on a close relative. Along similar lines, there appears to be a huge demand in the United States for autopsies carried out by private companies at the request of bereaved relatives (Marwick 1995).

The above observations suggest that the grounds behind the decline in post-mortem procedures may be attributed to physicians. This could stem from a fear that errors in diagnosis or treatment may be revealed with ensuing legal action, or that physicians may be unwilling to approach grieving family members for consent for an autopsy.

Autopsies and Consent

In a contemporary autopsy, pathologists are required to remove and inspect major organs, and analyse body fluids, tissues, and cellular components. As a matter of course, an autopsy entails the disfigurement of a cadaver, even though this may be limited to internal disfigurement (such as the removal of organs for subsequent study). Such an action warrants a discussion of consent issues, concerning consent prior to death by the person-now-dead, and after death by the next-of-kin. Any such discussion introduces the role of cultural factors in autopsies.

Autopsy is abhorrent to people in some cultures, such as the Chinese and the New Zealand Māori, who place special significance on the integrity of the body (and especially the brain) when buried. Consider the following incidents taken from Jones (2000).

> Mr M, a Māori, who received his dead son's brain in a clear plastic container, is entitled to compensation, according to the ruling of an appeal authority. Mr M's son died as a result of a cot death at the age of two months. Mr M went to the hospital to collect his son's body and carried it out, but with his son's brain in a clear plastic container. The chairman of the appeal authority said Mr M was handed the remains of his son in a disgraceful, tactless, and offensive manner to a person of Māori descent. It was declared that the hospital managed the autopsy in a culturally insensitive way.
>
> Māori elders complained about the treatment of human remains after the body of a man was returned to his family minus his brain. One elder commented: 'In Māoridom it is very hurtful and emotionally stressful for pathologists to hold on to someone else's brain. It is considered 'culturally insensitive' to Māori for organs to be removed without any discussion with the family.' In one case, a funeral was delayed for two weeks until the deceased's brain was returned to the family. The coroner has defended the practice, which he said was often to allow the precise cause of death to be determined. He did not believe there was anything insensitive about it: 'The problem stems from inability on the part of an ethnic group to recognise that their particular burial customs can't always be made to fit into the processes of forensic investigation. There are no racial connotations. The work is done to enable me, and sometimes other agencies, to arrive confidently at the cause of death.'

These incidents bring into conflict several considerations, not simply ethical and scientific considerations, but the expectations and customs of diverse cultural groups. Dissection and autopsy, while not accepted with ease by most, are commonplace in many societies. They have their basis in the underlying presumption that when the need dictates and with adherence to certain strictures, the body can be reduced to its component parts. Along these lines, the body can be buried incomplete, since this poses no threat to the dignity of the deceased.

However, what is legitimate for one culture may be culturally insensitive for another. Where two attitudes co-exist within a society, cultural sensitivity requires that both are treated with deference. Needless to say, this will have repercussions for the way in which a body is treated after death, influencing postmortem procedures, such as the time taken to carry out studies on the brain and other organs. In this way, the competing demands of contrasting groups, one emphasising medical needs and the other cultural, can be met in most cases. However, removal of the brain is fraught with considerable controversy, as evidenced by numerous examples of public outcries at the removal of brains from dead bodies without the relatives' consent. Consider the following passage from Jones (2000).

> The pathologists who took her dead son's brain during a coronial autopsy left Wendy Stride with an awful legacy. Although the brain's removal was beyond her control, it meant she could not honour the last wishes of her 19-year-old son, Timothy. A month before his death in a road accident, Wendy and her son had a discussion about donating one's organs for transplantation. At that time, Timothy clearly expressed his feelings that he wanted to leave this world intact, and by cremation.
>
> At the time of his cremation, the family believed Timothy's body was indeed intact, but two years later they learnt to their horror that his brain had been removed following the accident. Mrs Stride says the family was outraged about not being told of the removal of the brain, since this denied them the chance to honour Timothy's last wishes. For the family, this is a hurt that will remain with them for the rest of their lives. Mrs Stride said: 'It was my son's heart and brain that made him what he was and I am sure most parents would feel the same'.

Mrs Stride's response cannot be readily dismissed, since it tells us that both she and her son felt there was something special about the body—certainly the dead body, and one assumes about the living body as well. Mrs Stride's anger at the disrespect paid to her son's body points to the depth of our moral intuitions, and to the value we generally place on other human beings like ourselves. Strictures of this nature stem from an overriding need to maintain the dignity of the cadaver, and ensure that relatives are included within the sphere of decision-making.

But what about the perspective of the pathologist? In the above illustration, the brain would have been of value in ascertaining the cause of death, in training other pathologists, and possibly in research. Should society be concerned with the removal of organs, when the body is to be cremated anyway a few days later? When ethical issues such as this enter the arena, tension may rapidly appear between ethical and cultural considerations, and the needs of therapy and research.

What, then, of consent? According to some jurisdictions, for example the New Zealand *Human Tissue Act 1964*, permission is given for organs to be 'retained indefinitely for further study'. The United Kingdom's *Human Tissue Act 1961* allows for the removal of parts of the body 'for therapeutic purposes or for the purposes of medical education or research' (Nuffield Council on Bioethics 1995). However, current emphases on consent issues have limited autopsies far more than this. Although the consent required to carry out autopsies for audit or teaching and research purposes should probably be far more stringent than that required for coronial purposes when the cause of death is unknown, this should not preclude legitimate attempts to use postmortem tissue for teaching and research purposes.

There appears to be an all-pervasive unwillingness to obtain consent for autopsies, even when there are compelling reasons to do so. In many cases it seems as if 'ethical' considerations are used as justification for not asking for consent. This stance may itself be unethical, if it results in the burial or cremation of valuable tissue for which consent would have been provided. An intensive effort must be made to seek informed consent for autopsies, and for the removal of organs for teaching and research, either from the next-of-kin or the patient prior to death. The requirements of the procedure must be clearly specified, including details of the organs and tissues to be removed and the future uses to which they will be put.

There are some contexts in which this readily occurs, for example, within support groups for Huntington's disease. In these cases, people are more than willing to provide consent for autopsies and the subsequent use of the brains for research into the disease process. One can only hope that this special situation will set a precedent for the realisation of the value of human tissue for an understanding of human disease.

The autopsy procedure and the procurement of tissue for subsequent teaching and research have been placed in jeopardy, principally due to a lack of effort in obtaining consent for the procedure. The instances above, in which brains have been removed without consent, only to be followed by public outcry and private distress, epitomise the tragedy of unethical attitudes. With a little care and thought, these instances could have been avoided. To do so, a middle ground needs to be reached between the need for consent and the potential significance of the work to be carried out. Failure to undertake research and teaching on the basis of an unwillingness to ask for consent is of grave concern. In the final analysis, the loser will be the medical profession and patients.

Use of Biopsies from Surgical Operations

A surgical operation, whereby tissue is removed from a patient, is carried out for the well-being of the patient. The tissue being removed is unneeded and unwanted by the patient and will normally be incinerated. However, consider a case where the tissue is no longer unwanted and in fact may be of some benefit to research. Is consent required in this case? If so, is this of the same nature as consent to bequeath one's body, or consent to remove material from a body at postmortem?

Let us examine each one of these scenarios in turn. A body is bequested with the sole intention of making that body available for teaching and research purposes. Consent has been given prior to death and the interests of the deceased are served by acceptance of the bequest. A postmortem serves a different purpose, principally to determine the cause of death with consent only being given for those procedures considered necessary to meet this end. At no point is it acceptable to remove organs or tissue for other purposes, either teaching- or research-related.

When patients consent to an operation, they do so in good faith. They consent assuming that an operation will be of direct benefit to them by providing either extended quantity or improved quality of life, or possibly both. Consent covers the surgical procedure itself and the ongoing medical procedures associated with it that will benefit the patient. It does not cover what is to be done with any material removed from the body, unless this is specifically included. This then raises the question of who owns the tissue once it is removed from the patient. Biopsy material is removed by a hospital with the intent of benefiting the patient by providing an accurate diagnosis of a suspected ailment. Does the tissue then become the property of the hospital? The fact that the tissue in question is superfluous to the wants and the needs of the patient seems to relegate it to a category of its own. However, the question of consent still remains. Should consent be required when the tissue has been removed for the sake of the patient's health? One could argue that the hospital has done the patient a favour by removing the diseased tissue, and therefore it should be relinquished to research as a gratuity for services rendered. It would seem that the potential benefits that may emanate from the research should outweigh the need for consent. Regardless of the viewpoint adopted, any form of consent required is likely to be of a very weak variety.

Can the Dead Body be Abused?

Can cadavers or dead people be treated in unethical ways? Who is being treated unethically, now that the person himself or herself is dead? In what sense can a dead person, someone who is no longer with us, be abused? Is it the memory others have of that person that is being abused? Alternatively, it may be the human race that is somehow demeaned when one of its kind (even though now dead) is treated in a less than human way. But what is a less than human way? What does this mean when one is thinking about a dead person? Three illustrations may help.

Teaching on the Clinically Dead

The clinically dead have for many years been used by students and clinicians alike to learn a variety of clinical procedures. Those health professionals involved in emergency care often use fresh cadavers to practise and teach certain non-invasive or minimally invasive techniques. The most common of these techniques are lifesaving procedures, including endotracheal intubation and central line placement. The long history of this practice suggests that its place in clinical medicine is widely supported, or at the very least has not raised undue concern within the medical profession. However, these procedures may in fact be of concern to those outside the realm of the medical profession. This includes the general public of whom some will be future patients or the relatives of future patients. It is these people who have been kept in the dark about such procedures.

Despite the potential for concern, there are a number of compelling arguments for the use of the clinically dead in training procedures. Iserson (1993) contends that the use of the newly deceased as a training tool is morally and ethically justified because there are no effective alternatives available. Iserson continues by stating that the use of the newly dead for education is not disrespectful, but is in fact a way of showing increased respect because 'it promotes the real value that the dead body symbolises rather than the sanctity of the symbol for its own sake'. As mentioned, the practices are only minimally-invasive or non-invasive and therefore do not induce disrespect by disfiguring or marring the body.

It has been suggested that the use of fresh cadavers affords physicians and other health care workers the opportunity to gain competence in techniques that are either difficult or impossible to learn by any other means. In these terms, Burns and co-workers (1994) consider these practices justifiable, given certain provisos: the institution must evaluate carefully who has a legitimate need to master the technique; only non-mutilating procedures should be permitted; the use of the newly dead must be the culmination of a structured training program, and candidates should be required to master the basic techniques on mannequins and other teaching aids, only using the newly dead to refine their skill.

Training procedures carried out on the newly dead normally take place within a short period of time following death. Such immediacy is a necessity as the onset of *rigor mortis* would preclude the completion of these procedures. The need for prompt action dictates that the procedures are carried out without gaining the consent of, or even notifying, the deceased's relatives. To illustrate this point, consent from patient's families is not required by a large proportion of hospitals involved in the use of the newly dead for training purposes, including many hospital departments in both Australia and New Zealand (Ginifer & Kelly 1996).

A major argument used in support of using the newly dead in teaching without prior consent concerns the nature of the request. Many clinicians are reluctant to further burden grieving relatives with what may appear to be an insensitive and inappropriately timed request, leading to an exemption from the requirement of informed consent (Orlowski et al. 1990; Iserson 1993). These people argue that the benefits to be gained from the act outweigh the harm done either to the relatives, by dismissing their wishes, or to the cadaver itself. However, even when the nature of the benefit is not in doubt, the ease with which the interests of the cadaver and relatives are overlooked is of concern (Jones 2000).

Comparisons between these training procedures and complete body dissection have been drawn. The seemingly innocuous nature of non-invasive procedures may be deceptive, since what is done to dead bodies in the teaching of endotracheal intubation and what is done to other bodies in complete body dissection may amount to an indignity in both instances (Jones 2000). Neither procedure is of gain to the newly dead, although society as a whole can be expected to reap the benefits from both procedures. Nevertheless, from an ethical perspective the gulf between the two procedures needs to be recognised, namely, between a body that remains intact, and one that will cease to exist as a recognisable entity.

This perceived gulf has repercussions for the way in which the public responds to the procedures. A destructive procedure like whole body dissection is unlikely to elicit overwhelming consent from the public, whereas a minimally invasive procedure like endotracheal intubation may well be acceptable to many. An example of this is a study by Benfield et al. (1991) which found that a number of parents consented to their newly dead children being used in teaching intubation skills but not to an autopsy.

Despite such perceptions, failure to obtain consent ensures that these procedures remain private, and hence are readily open to exploitation. If the newly dead are being used for training procedures in hospitals without consent, then the public should have a right to know, regardless of the repercussions for the medical profession. In the end, obtaining consent from next-of-kin is the best option, even if it does limit the extent of clinical experience available.

Research on the Clinically Dead

In France in 1988 a young man was left brain-dead after a car accident, and his body was kept alive on a respirator and subsequently used for a medical experiment. The doctor involved had placed the patient on sabotaged medical equipment. He was attempting to determine whether the effects were the same as in similar circumstances on an earlier occasion. The doctor behind these experiments called such patients 'almost perfect human models, who constitute intermediaries between animal and man'.

These experiments led to storms of protest, and the doctor was suspended from his duties. Objections were based principally on the lack of informed consent by the patient. To some, the patient was treated as an object rather than as a human subject, which indicated an attitude that is sometimes claimed to exemplify medical imperialism. To others, of course, the existence of brain death opens the door to experimentation with techniques of reanimation.

But these responses do not bring the matter to a close. Let us assume that informed consent for this type of experimentation had been given prior to death. Would there, then, be any ethical objections to it? What would be the difference between this experimentation and dissecting a cadaver? It is difficult to see that there is any difference, as long as there is no deception of the relatives, and the nature of the experimentation is known and agreed to by an appropriate ethics committee.

In 1978 the Department of Transportation in California had contracted with several university laboratories to test designs for automobile airbags in actual crashes of cars at varying velocities. Since dummies had proved unsatisfactory for measuring the degree of protection for living passengers, some researchers had, with the consent of next-of-kin, substituted human cadavers. One congressman wrote to the Secretary of Transportation charging that 'the use of human cadavers for vehicle safety research violates fundamental notions of morality and human dignity, and must therefore permanently be stopped'. And it *was* stopped despite the department's protest that prohibiting the use of cadavers would set back progress on safety protection for many years. Similar crash test research using cadavers has also been conducted for many years in France and Germany.

The question raised by this instance is: what is the difference between these experiments and dissection? Next-of-kin had given their consent for the experiments, and no attempt was made to carry them out in a secretive way. Why, then, the outcry? Was this on ethical grounds or emotional ones?

Undoubtedly there are major differences between the airbag experiments and dissection, in that the cadavers in the former are violently smashed to bits, whereas dissection is carried out in laboratories by medical technicians or students. Dissection is analytical and scientific, while smashing bodies is violent and destructive, a difference that some regard as having symbolic importance (Feinberg 1985). The result in both situations is destruction: generally far greater destruction in the case of dissection than in that of the airbag experiments. If this is the case, it should be viewed as a relative matter, since what societies are prepared to tolerate varies from one period to another. After all, dissection was not tolerated by most societies just a few hundred years ago, so that what we deem unacceptable today may be considered quite acceptable a few years hence.

We have to decide whether people's intuition in this matter is a reliable guide, since the expected safety benefit of experiments such as these has to be balanced against the offence experienced by some people. Undoubtedly some people are offended by dissection, but they are able to steer clear of it (unless they are students in medical and some other health science fields). It is difficult to see why human dignity should be jeopardised by airbag experiments but not by dissection. The features they have in common far outnumber the features that separate them.

The Age of the Neomort

In a now famous article Willard Gaylin has taken a science fiction look at what society could do with cadavers (Gaylin 1974). Gaylin imagines institutions of the future where brain-dead bodies, now euphemistically called 'neomorts', are maintained and put to various important medical uses. The bioemporiums would resemble a cross between a pharmaceutical laboratory and a hospital ward. He envisages hospital beds lined up in neat rows, each with a freshly scrubbed neomort under the clean white sheets. The neomorts would have the same recognisably human faces they had before they died, the same features, even the same complexions. Each would be a perfect natural symbol, not only of humanity in general, but also of the particular person who once animated that body and had his or her life in it.

Using such 'preparations', medical students could be taught the techniques of rectal or vaginal examination without fear of disturbing or embarrassing real patients. Experiments could be performed to test the toxicity of drugs by judging their effects on real human bodies without endangering anyone's health or life. Other neomorts could be used as experimental subjects, in place of live animals such as dogs and mice, since the use of animals is itself associated with ethical issues and one advantage of using neomorts is that they feel no pain. Other neomorts could serve as living organ banks or living storage receptacles for blood antigens and platelets that cannot survive freezing. From others could be harvested blood, bone marrow, corneas and cartilage, as needed for transfusion or transplants by patients. Still others might be used to manufacture hormones, antitoxins, and antibodies, to be marketed commercially for the prevention or cure of various medical ailments. Again, it has been suggested that neomorts could be used as incubators for human embryos produced by reproductive technology.

Enticing as this vision may appear, these brain-dead individuals were once people and still bear a proximity of relationship to what they were. A science fiction vista of this order demonstrates the extent to which our moral imagination is linked with what we might one day allow. While preparations of this type may bypass problems currently experienced with the use of living patients and animals in research procedures, they fail to provide a simple remedy devoid of adverse moral repercussions, and perpetuate neglect of cadavers.

Unlikely as this scenario is, it refuses to go away. Human reproductive cloning, especially with the prospect of producing 'brain-less' human specimens, reminds us that the public imagination will not easily let go of such an unnerving vision. The temptation to use others for our own benefit is an enduring one, even if a more likely (and ethically acceptable) way forward will use specifically produced tissues and not whole people. Neomorts are deceptive fantasies that may become feasible technologically but will solve none of our ethical dilemmas.

Archeological Human Remains

The return of skeletal remains by anatomy departments, medical schools, and museums to native tribes for subsequent reburial has become commonplace in recent times. This trend has been prompted by the development of ethical guidelines and policies, stressing mutual respect and cooperation between archeologists and indigenous peoples. In a number of jurisdictions, legislation has been passed to regulate the storage, study, and repatriation of human skeletal material. In Australia, federal law states that skeletal remains that pre-date 1770 are to be controlled by Aboriginal authorities.

One example of the repatriation of human remains was the return of nine Tasmanian Aboriginal skulls to Australian government representatives by the University of Edinburgh in early 1991. Remains of Aboriginal skeletal material have also been relinquished by other European universities and museums, and by such institutions in Australia. One particularly contentious case was that of the human remains from Kow Swamp, which were handed over by the Museum of Victoria. These bones were estimated to be between 10 000 and 15 000 years old. Bones of similar age (14 000 years) from Coobool Creek in the Murray Black collection (1800 skeletons) have also been given back to Aboriginal communities (Ewing 1990).

In the United States, the remains of Native American people have been returned by universities for reburial, often following protracted and bitterly divisive negotiations. Such contentious repatriations include: the return by the Smithsonian Institute of a large collection of skeletal remains and funerary objects to Kodiak Island, Alaska (Bray & Killion 1994), the return of skeletal remains to West Virginia, and the return of a 10 000-year-old skeleton to Idaho (Meighan 1993). In other cases, such as that of the 'Kennewick Man' in Washington state, legal wrangling between scientists and indigenous peoples is ongoing.

The tension in cases such as these is between scientific interest and the provision of valuable clues to humanity's past on the one hand, and the sacred feelings and beliefs of indigenous peoples on the other. Some maintain that human skeletal artefacts provide essential information on problems ranging from the organisation of tribal societies, to the origin of certain diseases (such as rheumatoid arthritis). It is also argued that these remains are part of the world's heritage and are not simply of significance to the direct ancestors of the people who happen to live in an area today. The indigenous position stresses the religious and cultural importance of respect for the remains of tribal ancestors; it may include a desire for restitution in the face of past mistreatment, or may be part of a struggle for rights and recognition. It is sometimes asserted that much of the material is not used, and that any information derived from these studies is not passed on to, or shared with, the indigenous communities themselves. Although this controversy is far removed from clinical medicine, it does raise important ethical considerations, some of which are of relevance in a broader context.

The first point it raises is that respect for the beliefs and feelings of indigenous peoples is crucial, since this means respecting them as human beings. Inherent within this is respect for their ancestors now dead, provided that a traceable line exists. This last point is important. If the remains are ancient and thus so far removed from modern-day people that no traceable link exists between the two, then they should 'belong' to humanity in general, rather than to any local interest (Jones & Harris 1998). This factor of age is one of three variables to be taken into account when assessing a claim. The remaining two variables are: the time the material was unearthed, and the manner of the individual's death. Each specific example of skeletal material will fit anywhere along the continuum of each variable, resulting in a variety of permutations or outcomes.

A fundamental premise is that there is an ethical interest in human material because of the close association that is generally recognised between such material and an identifiable person. This probably does not apply with anything like the same force when no link with any known person or group of people can be established. Nevertheless, it is still material of human origin, which tells us something about its associations, even when these have been forgotten. Some indigenous groups also recognise it as an essential part of their history and ancestry. In other words, even ancient human material does not become nothing simply because links with the present have been lost.

An additional point is that there is a place for the scientific study of archeological human remains because this is a particular application of the more general principle, that the study of human material is important and ethically acceptable. However, in this instance, no one has consented to the study of these remains since none of the direct descendants could do so. This either renders any study of archeological human remains unethical, or makes consent irrelevant. Jones (2000) contends that consent should be sought whenever possible, since the remains in question are still human ones. A compromise is to seek proxy consent from present-day descendants, if any can be identified. The issue of consent becomes far less demanding when one is dealing with remains of a pre-historic nature, which lack clear associations with the living. What is of pre-eminent significance in cases such as these, is the contribution the material can make to the understanding of human development and culture.

A final consideration is the question of whether material resulting (in part, at least) from past mistreatment of some indigenous peoples should be studied at all. Take as an example the situation in Australia, where some collections of Aboriginal skeletal remains were obtained through the horrific acts of grave robbing, contract killings, and massacres (Monaghan 1991). This touches on the moral complicity argument, according to which, those who use material or data obtained unethically are themselves implicated in the unethical practice. According to Jones (2000), a case can be made for the study of archeological remains in spite of past atrocities, as long as the myriad factors relevant to this material are taken into account. However, scientific work, either ongoing or sporadic, is necessary to justify the maintenance of these remains within universities or museums. Where descendants of the material can be identified, one way forward is to allow a defined time for scientific study of the remains prior to reburial, but only if this has been agreed to by the indigenous communities.

New Zealand and Australia are examples of countries where an attempt is being made to address these important issues. In New Zealand, the Ngai Tahu tribe has produced a policy on the treatment of human remains, which gives them the right to manage the remains from their tribal area. The document also permits scientific investigation of ancestral bones when justified and if conducted with sensitivity. In Australia, the National Health and Medical Research Council (1991) has published *Guidelines on Ethical Matters in Aboriginal and Torres Strait Islander Health Research*. Although the guidelines do not deal directly with Aboriginal remains, they do underline the need for sensitivity to Aboriginal views and customs.

PART II

Clinical Ethics

5
Genetic Dilemmas

Introduction

In this chapter we move into an area frequently referred to as 'genetic engineering', which for many years has been the inspiration for exciting science fiction and alarmist futuristic scenarios. Since genetic engineering is often regarded as having the potential to manipulate human nature itself, it encapsulates people's fears regarding future abuses of science. For many, it is going where humans have never been before, and where humans should not go.

It may come as a surprise to many that gene therapy is not a new concept; speculations regarding its feasibility have been around since the 1960s, although the techniques and ideas necessary for development were inappropriate at that time. Unsound practices also served to sidetrack it until more recent times (Culver 1993).

Present-day human genetics is far less monolithic than is frequently imagined. Genetic technology ranges from genetic screening and the use of DNA probes, on the one hand, to pre-emptive intervention and selective abortion on the other; from genetic counselling to somatic cell gene therapy and, in the future, possibly to germ line gene therapy. It also encompasses the Human Genome Project (HGP, with its production of the complete nucleotide sequence of the human genome). Cloning, once considered a nightmarish fantasy of irresponsible scientists, now occupies a central place in serious ethical debate. By contrast, eugenics (enhancing desirable human dispositions and characteristics by genetic means) continues to play little part in serious discussion of genetic developments.

Molecular medicine encompasses three broad areas: the study of genes and gene products, the detection of abnormal gene expression in diseased states, and the therapeutic modification of abnormal gene expression. DNA technology has already succeeded in elucidating the genetic basis of a number of single-gene (monogenic) disorders, including cystic fibrosis (CFTR gene), Huntington's disease (IT15 gene), fragile X syndrome (FMR1 gene), familial hypercholesterolaemia (gene for the low-density lipoprotein receptor), familial hypertrophic cardiomyopathy (gene for heavy chain myosin), and Duchenne muscular dystrophy (gene for dystrophin). While work on the genetic basis of multigene (polygenic) diseases is inevitably more complex, rapid progress is being made in the search for the genes involved in conditions such as heart disease, hypertension, diabetes, osteoporosis, and, particularly, Alzheimer's disease and some forms of cancer. Two susceptibility genes for breast and ovarian cancer have been identified (BRCA1 and BRCA2), one for Alzheimer's disease (APOE), and one for heart disease (AGT). In fact, molecular diagnostic tests for susceptibilty genes for breast and ovarian cancers are now commercially available in the United States.

Although the initial goal of gene therapy was the replacement of mutated genes in germ line cells and the cure of inherited genetic diseases, a far greater impact may be achieved by replacing deficient proteins in differentiated somatic cells. Trials of somatic gene therapy commenced in 1990, with the bulk of these having malignant cells as their targets, especially melanoma, ovarian and breast cancers, glioblastoma, and various forms of leukemia. Other conditions for which studies are ongoing include cystic fibrosis, certain brain tumours, coronary disease, AIDS, and Duchenne muscular dystrophy.

Clinical Illustrations

In order to place this technology in a human setting, let us consider a set of illustrations concerning a couple, Rebecca and Rex, whom we shall follow over a period of a few years.

> In their first pregnancy some years ago there were reasons to suspect that the foetus might have cystic fibrosis. At sixteen weeks an amniocentesis was carried out, and a small amount of amniotic fluid was removed so that some foetal cells could be tested using a recombinant DNA-based gene probe for cystic fibrosis. They knew beforehand that, if the test produced a positive result, they had a choice to make; either continue with the pregnancy knowing that the child would be afflicted with this debilitating and distressing condition, or have an abortion. If the pregnancy had occurred more recently, this testing could have been carried out at eight weeks, with a chorionic villus biopsy. The choice, however, would have been exactly the same. In the event, the test for cystic fibrosis turned out to be positive, and Rebecca and Rex decided not to abort. As a result, Catherine was born.

The dilemma here is whether a foetus with the gene for cystic fibrosis is to be valued less highly than a foetus without this gene. But this is only the beginning, since an affected foetus will become an affected child and adult, and this affected person will, on present knowledge, have a limited life-span. Is non-existence preferable to the continued existence of a foetus in this situation?

A little into the future, we revisit Rebecca and Rex, who are now hoping to have another child.

Understandably they are worried about the prospect of another child with cystic fibrosis. On this occasion they are informed that the embryo itself can be genetically tested before it has a chance to implant in the uterus. This is the technique of embryo biopsy. They are told that *in vitro* fertilisation (IVF) will have to be the method used, and that one cell will be removed from an early embryo and tested with the same genetic kit as used previously. If this shows that the embryo does not have any indication of cystic fibrosis it will be implanted in Rebecca's uterus in the normal way. On the other hand, if it tests positive for cystic fibrosis, it will be discarded and the same procedure will be carried out on a second embryo. This will be repeated until a negative result is obtained.

What might Rebecca and Rex be doing if they move in the direction of discarding genetically impaired embryos? The choice is no longer between the value placed on a foetus and the value placed on a person; it is now the value placed on a four-cell or eight-cell embryo as opposed to the value placed on a person. Some would argue that a willingness to discard a human embryo is equivalent to the taking of human life. On the other hand, it may be closer to the sort of decision about non-existence raised by contraception. Clearly, if Rebecca and Rex used contraceptives, so that they did not have children, they could not be said to be taking human life.

There is a final scenario for Rebecca and Rex, one that pushes them yet further into the future. This time they are again advised to use IVF, but the emphasis on this occasion will be on testing the embryos with the intention of correcting any genetic defect that may be found. Hence, there will be no question of an *in vitro* abortion; instead, if the first embryo tested is positive for the cystic fibrosis gene, that gene will be replaced or will be overridden in some way by insertion of some other gene. This is the realm of germ line gene therapy.

In practical terms germ line gene therapy would be far more difficult and costly than refraining from implanting defective embryos. Nevertheless, if germ line gene therapy were feasible, we would have to consider what potential objections may be raised against it.

And so this couple have made their choices. They have two children—Catherine, who has cystic fibrosis, and Rachel, who does not. Rachel was the result of implanting a healthy embryo following gene-testing. Two embryos were discarded prior to this. Rebecca and Rex could have avoided the birth of Catherine, who is now thirteen, is far from well, and has a poor life expectancy. That would have meant a late abortion. Two individuals with cystic fibrosis could have existed, but do not. Rachel is healthy. Underlying the possibilities inherent in these scenarios is the multifaceted realm of genetic technology, to which we now turn.

Somatic Cell Gene Therapy

Somatic cell gene therapy, which was first approved in humans in 1989 and first used in 1990, involves the correction of gene defects in patients' own cells, the cells in question being somatic cells (that is, ordinary body cells). The strategy involves gene replacement, gene correction, or gene augmentation, the genes being introduced via retroviral vectors. Foreign genes are introduced into cells so that their DNA can be transcribed into messenger ribonucleic acid (mRNA), which converts the information encoded in DNA into proteins capable of being synthesised. The most efficient methods to date have utilised viruses, which are altered to contain the gene of interest, with their normal infective machinery being used to carry the gene into cells. Viruses acting in this manner are referred to as vectors, and include retroviruses, adenoviruses, and adeno associated herpes simplex viruses.

Besides these vectors, it may be possible to inject DNA directly into human cells, encased in structures such as liposomes that can act as a vehicle for certain genes. At present none of the vectors is trouble-free; all have disadvantages as well as advantages in experimental and clinical practice.

The aim of somatic cell gene therapy is to modify a particular cell population and so rectify a specific disease in a given patient. As such, it is similar to procedures like organ transplantation, but is far more powerful than any indirect genetic therapies. However, there are technical difficulties associated with the expression and appropriate regulation of new genes in somatic cells. Enormous care has been exercised, both procedurally and ethically, in conducting studies on human patients, and very specific guidelines have been elaborated. There are approximately 300 clinical trials under way worldwide on a diverse range of disorders including cystic fibrosis, inherited genetic diseases, coronary artery disease, and AIDS. Despite the effort being poured into this emerging field of medicine, no form of gene therapy can yet be considered an outright success. Problems with delivery mechanisms, lack of sustained gene expression and toxicity have dampened initial enthusiasm for this form of therapy. A number of trials have reported encouraging results, and expectations for the future remain high. However, they were dashed somewhat in late 1999, when eighteen-year-old Jesse Gelsinger died four days after receiving gene therapy treatment for a rare metabolic disorder.

Cancer Gene Therapy

Cancer has been described as a disease of the genes, since genes are responsible for regulating the growth and division of cells. Loss of this control results from genes switching off prematurely or ceasing to function after a period of time.

However, five or six genetic changes are generally required to induce malignancy, indicating that cancer is a multigene disorder.

The goal of cancer gene therapy is to enhance the patient's anti-tumour response. Of various major approaches the first example is the use of suicide genes, or 'Trojan horse' vectors. These kill the cells in which they are located by producing what is, in effect, a cytotoxic agent. Second, is the use of lymphocytes, such as tumour-infiltrating lymphocytes (TIL) harvested from tumour biopsy specimens and infected with retroviruses containing human cytokine genes. A third approach has concentrated on increasing the immunogenicity of tumour cells by inserting appropriate genes, such as interleukin-2 and interleukin-4. Fourth, direct manipulation of oncogenes or restoring tumour suppressor genes may prove useful, since some genes may be critical at particular stages in the development of a cancer and the reversal of a single event may prove beneficial for therapy.

An increasing range of cancers are now the subject of experimental gene therapy, including advanced melanoma, cancer of the breast, colon, bladder, prostate, ovary, and pancreas, as well as leukemia and non-Hodgkin's lymphoma. DNA testing for the detection of predisposition to cancer is also available and widely used. This would allow individuals at high risk to take preventive measures. Debate currently revolves around colon and breast cancer, since small percentages of patients with these conditions carry altered copies of particular genes. In the case of colon cancer about 10 per cent of patients have an altered MSH2 gene, and 80 per cent of people with this modified gene have a predisposition to develop colon cancer. This constitutes a well-defined high-risk group that could be assisted considerably by diagnostic tests and colonoscopy as required. In the case of breast cancer, 5 per cent of women with this condition have inherited an altered copy of the BRCA1 gene on chromosome 17. Women with this mutation have an 85 per cent risk of breast cancer and an increased risk of ovarian cancer. Genetic counselling and surgery may be of value here, although the benefits have not as yet been fully established.

Responses to Somatic Cell Gene Therapy

What, then, are we to make of somatic cell gene therapy? Its aim (the treatment of those with serious genetic conditions, and hence the enhancement of the welfare of individuals) fits within the traditional medical ethos of curing where possible and always caring. However, the boundary between alterable and unalterable conditions has been shifted by somatic cell gene therapy. Many conditions that were, until recently, in the unalterable category have now entered, or will shortly enter, the alterable category. Clearly there is no virtue in living with a deformity or debility that could be rectified. On the other hand, the existence of a deformity or debility does not reduce an individual's life to meaninglessness, and it is imperative that the pursuit of physical perfection is not placed above the enhancement of specifically human characteristics. Genetics epitomises an inequality in biology, and it is crucial that we come to terms with the total genetic burden of humankind. In our attempt to reduce this burden, somatic cell gene therapy will undoubtedly play an important role, but it is a partial role. Other contributions include moves to establish just social systems that protect and support the genetically disadvantaged, and community efforts that endow the genetically disadvantaged with meaning as human beings of worth and dignity.

Ethical issues of significance to somatic cell gene therapy include the need to balance any potential benefits and harms, and to assess the safety and effectiveness of new techniques. There must be unequivocal evidence from animal studies that the inserted gene will function adequately and have no deleterious effects; there needs to be assurance that the new gene can be accurately placed in the target cells and that it will remain there long enough to be effective; that it will be expressed in the cell at the appropriate level and only in that tissue; and that neither it nor the retroviruses will harm the cell or the patient. It is important to assess the benefits of gene therapy against current alternative therapies (such as bone marrow transplantation and chemotherapy for cancer), and to ensure that the interests of patients are paramount.

Some of the ethical issues can be summarised using a set of questions proposed by the National Institute of Health (1985), which are still relevant today. What is the disease to be treated? What alternative therapies are available for treatment of the disease? How safe is treatment with gene therapy likely to be for the patient, for the patient's offspring, and for other people who come into contact with the patient? How effective is treatment with gene therapy likely to be for the patient? What procedures will be followed to ensure fairness in the selection of subjects? How will patients (or their parents in the case of children) be properly informed about the proposed study, and how will their consent be elicited? What steps will be taken to protect the privacy of gene-therapy patients and the confidentiality of medical information about the course of their treatment?

These questions, together with the stipulations they carry, are in line with important ethical principles developed to protect patients and their welfare in other clinical areas. They also constitute the basis of the protocols within which current gene-therapy trials in the United States and Europe are being conducted. These include the 1993 report from the Nufffield Council on Bioethics, a 1995 Council of Europe policy, and 1997 recommendations from the United States Task Force on the Ethical, Legal, and Social Implications of Genetic Testing (ELSI Task Force on Genetic Testing 1997).

Germ Line Gene Therapy

Germ line gene therapy involves inserting a gene into the germ line (sperm, eggs, and embryos) so that, when the modified individual reproduces, all off-spring will have the inserted gene instead of the original defective one. It is attempting to manipulate an early embryo so that the individual into which it will develop is not affected by a fatal disease. Animal experiments have shown that this form of gene therapy is associated with high risks, because gene expression may occur in inappropriate tissues. Since the foreign gene is inserted randomly into the host DNA, some facets of normal embryological development may be disrupted, with serious adverse consequences. Furthermore, any damage to the DNA caused by this procedure will stay in the germ line and be passed on to subsequent generations.

Germ line gene therapy is not permitted by existing official guidelines. Were it to become a safe procedure, there would be various arguments in favour of its use. For some genetic disorders it may be the only possible form of treatment (for example, brain cells in hereditary central nervous system disorders, which are not open to genetic repair after birth). Germ line gene therapy would also dispense with the need to repeat somatic cell gene therapy in different gener-ations of a family with a genetic disorder, by eliminating the defective gene from the population and so improving the efficiency of the therapy.

In assessing these arguments, it is pertinent to point out that germ line gene therapy involves obtaining embryos via IVF, determining which ones require treatment, and then carrying out the therapy. However, as we have already seen in the case of Rebecca and Rex, an alternative and simpler procedure would be to refrain from implanting defective embryos. This achieves the same therapeu-tic aims without running the risks of inserting a new gene into a defective embryo, making it far less problematic ethically. However, this simpler course of action may be rejected by some on the ground that it is unethical to select healthy embryos and reject defective ones.

Negative and Positive Eugenics

Negative eugenics involves the elimination of defective genes, and hence elimin-ation of the prospective possessors of these genes from the population. While negative eugenics does not actually change individuals, its potential for changing the genetic make-up of a community is considerable. Strictly speaking, negative eugenics is not an illustration of manipulation, since it does not modify individ-uals who will be born. However, it is a means of selecting healthy as opposed to unhealthy individuals, via the abortion of foetuses thought to be carrying defec-tive genes. In this sense it is implicated in manipulation of the population, although viewpoints vary considerably regarding the ethical status of abortion in this context. Ethical considerations to be taken into account in the decision-making process include: the severity of the genetic disorder and its effect on the possibility of meaningful life for affected foetuses; the physical, emotional, and economic impact of the birth of a child with the genetic condition on family and society; the availability of adequate medical management and special educational facilities; the reliability of the diagnosis; and the increase in the load of detrimental genes in the population as a result of the carriers of genetic diseases reproducing.

Positive eugenics has invited a great deal of idealistic support, with visions of improving attributes such as intelligence and personality. This emphasis on improving human design stands in stark contrast to conventional medical approaches with their emphasis on rectifying abnormalities and combating disease. This form of eugenics has a long history, going back to the ancient Greeks like Plato, who believed we could breed for desirable human qualities in much the same way as we breed for desirable qualities in plants and animals. In the nineteenth century neo-Darwinian ideas were introduced, envisaging social policies that favour reproduction of the select.

Although current emphases are on genetic approaches, the concept has changed little. The difficulty has always been to identify, and then to promote, only those genes considered to be desirable. It is not surprising that eugenic approaches have proved disappointing, since traits such as intelligence are controlled by an estimated ten to one hundred genes, as well as by environmental factors. Quite apart from deciding which traits to promulgate, control of this order lies outside the realm of feasible science, even though it is being increasingly involved. Consequently, positive eugenics is both unscientific and unethical; any attempts to impose it on society (no matter how crude) would be at the expense of individual freedom of choice. One illustration of this was the Nazi eugenic program in Germany in the 1930s; the terrible consequences of this program serve as a painful reminder of what can happen if such technology falls into the wrong hands.

Cloning

Cloning has been defined as the production of a cell or organism with the same nuclear genome as another cell or organism (Australian Academy of Science 1999). In other words, cloning is the production of one or more carbon copies of any given cell, or animal, including a human. It was in fact the successful cloning of a sheep, the now famous 'Dolly', in 1997 that represented a major breakthrough in the cloning arena. Dolly's special status stems from the fact that she was the first vertebrate animal to be cloned from a cell of an adult animal as opposed to a cell from an embryo. Dolly was the brainchild of Ian Wilmut and colleagues at the Roslin Institute, in a collaborative effort with PPL Therapeutics. The birth of Dolly provided the impetus for further cloning and since then, cattle, mice, and most recently pigs, have joined the ranks of 'clonable animals' (Wilmut et al. 2000).

How is it then that scientists have been able to mastermind such remarkable acts? Cloning may be carried out by two distinct methods, embryo splitting and nuclear replacement. Embryo splitting is the artificial division of embryonic cells at a very early stage of development, and replicates the natural process that can give rise to identical twins. Nuclear replacement involves the introduction of genetic material (a nucleus) into the cytoplasm of an unfertilised egg or embryo, whose own genetic material has been removed. Unlike the embryo splitting technique, nuclear replacement has the potential to create a clone of an adult organism, as was the case with Dolly.

The production of cloned animals has stimulated much interest and consternation worldwide, due to the implications this may have for human cloning. There are various potential uses of cloning techniques and a discussion of these will help to identify both the scientific and ethical issues involved. From a scientific viewpoint, cloning opens up numerous potential research and therapeutic opportunities. For example, it may increase our understanding of the fundamental processes of cellular differentiation, thereby making possible its reversal, and hence providing a means of controlling pathological and aging processes. Cloning technology also has the potential to improve the efficiency of production of transgenic livestock, which could be used both for the production of organs or tissues for transplantation into humans (see Chapter 8), and for the production of human proteins in cow's or goat's milk. At the Roslin Institute and PPL Therapeutics, a transgenic sheep (Polly), carrying a human gene for Factor IX (used in the treatment of haemophilia), has been developed. The pharmaceutical possibilities are enticing.

By far the most controversial use for cloning technologies is human reproductive cloning, which tends to dominate the popular discussion of cloning. The thought of the production of genetically identical human beings induces fear and outrage. Unfortunately, much of this discussion is misleading and unhelpful, since it ignores a fundamental distinction between the different types of cloning. The focus of popular attention is on *human reproductive cloning*, that is, the creation of genetically identical human beings. It tends to ignore *human therapeutic cloning*, which is the production of stem cells, tissues, or organs for the benefit of medicine and humankind and which does not involve the creation of genetically identical individuals. Besides this, there are also the routine procedures for cloning human cells and genes, as well as cloning human skin to treat burns patients (Human Fertilisation and Embryology Authority & The Human Genetics Advisory Committee 1998).

Therapeutic cloning techniques have the potential to revolutionise the treatment of damaged tissues and organs. It may soon be possible to use adult human cells as the starting material for the growth of self-compatible tissues or organs, which could subsequently be incorporated into an individual's body without the risk of rejection. An alluring example is the use of neural tissue to treat patients with Parkinson's disease, and muscle tissue to treat those with heart disease.

Since human therapeutic cloning does not involve the creation of genetically identical individuals, it appears to largely circumvent the ethical minefield surrounding human reproductive cloning. However, therapeutic cloning may make use of early human embryos (although this can be avoided by using adult somatic cells), precluding its acceptance by those who do not approve of manipulation of human embryos under any circumstances. In the United Kingdom, the *Human Fertility and Embryology Act 1990* allows research on embryos of up to fourteen days development under strict licence from the Human Fertilisation and Embryology Authority. Under these circumstances, many have argued that embryo research involving nuclear replacement technology, but not resulting in cloned individuals, does not raise any new ethical concerns in relation to the special status of the human embryo (Human Fertilisation and Embryology Authority 1999; Department of Health Report 2000).

Currently, human reproductive cloning is banned in many countries, including the United Kingdom, Australia, and throughout most of Europe. In the United States, current law prohibits the use of federal funds for the purpose of human cloning, yet there are no federal regulations on the use of private funds for this purpose. The general consensus worldwide from organisations such as UNESCO, WHO, the Council of Europe, and the Australian Academy of Science is that human reproductive cloning is unsafe and unethical and should be strictly prohibited (Council of Europe 1996; UNESCO 1997; Australian Academy of Science 1999).

It has been suggested that there may be compelling reasons to make 'a copy' of another human being. For example, the cloning of a dying child for the sake of the parents, the cloning of an individual to act as a compatible organ donor, or the cloning of one member of an infertile couple to create offspring (Human Fertilisation and Embryology Authority & The Human Genetics Advisory Committee 1998). In such circumstances, if human cloning were safe and/or possible (and all immediate scientific problems regarding life span and susceptibility to cancer had been overcome) would there be any inherent ethical objections to it?

Let us take the example of the cloning of a dying child. Such an act encourages parents to produce one child in the image of another, and yet the parents would not be 'getting back' the same child that was lost. Cloning under these circumstances may encourage society to view children as interchangeable commodities (Annas 1998).

Regardless of the motives for human reproductive cloning, the most widely expressed fear is that the resulting individuals (clones) would be psychologically harmed, with a diminished sense of individuality and personal autonomy. This is a pragmatic argument, which may or may not turn out to be valid. Such an argument requires critical assessment, since even human clones will be exposed to different environments, different cultural pressures in different generations, and therefore vastly different experiences; they would also have different mitochondrial DNA. In practice, they will be far less like one another than natural identical twins, who generally demonstrate as much individuality as anyone else. In other words, a dissimilar genetic identity is not essential for human beings to feel, and indeed be, individuals in their own right.

Central to the way we regard human clones are our motives for bringing them into existence. If they are produced 'to order', their value in the eyes of their progenitors would appear to lie in the extent to which they replicated a previous person or were able to carry out certain predetermined tasks. The danger here is that they would not be valued as unique individuals, but simply in terms of their ability to perform specified functions or demonstrate specified traits. If cloning is used to treat human beings solely according to their functional value to society, the intrinsic worth and dignity of human beings is undermined. But is this inevitable?

Genetic Screening

Genetic screening was revolutionised in the late 1970s by the advent of the recombinant DNA technologies, which in turn have led to the development of DNA probes for detecting large numbers of human genetic variants and genes with known functions. The amount of information stemming from these procedures is enormous, and its use demands serious ethical assessment.

Knowledge of this order paves the way for various forms of testing. The first and most general form is predictive testing, that is, tests to predict whether a genetic disease will appear at some time in the future. This general testing can be subdivided into more precise forms. The first of these is *presymptomatic testing*, that is, testing individuals before any symptoms have appeared in order to determine whether they are carriers of a particular genetic condition. Since these people have no symptoms of the condition, they are not ill and may know nothing about their susceptibility to a genetic disease prior to the testing. Whether or not they eventually become ill depends on their genetic constitution. The second form of predictive testing is *prenatal screening*, that is, tests to establish a foetus's genetic predisposition to a particular disease, for instance Huntington's disease. This form of predictive testing is far more powerful than presymptomatic testing since it is carried out much earlier, with the result that an affected foetus may be aborted (or perhaps treated or even cured).

Both forms of testing look ahead to what may happen to an individual's health at some time in the future, possibly in the remote future. This is a type of medical and even social foreknowledge, which carries with it the possibility of control at a number of levels. Such knowledge may be highly desirable, since it may help individuals to avoid disaster and suffering. It may also direct preventive health services towards groups at risk of certain diseases. On the other hand, it forces those afflicted with discernible genetic disease to confront their predicament and to make choices they would not otherwise have to make, and may prefer not to make. Ignorance may be a valid stance.

Principles of Genetic Screening Programs

Genetic screening can be regarded as having three goals: to contribute to improving the health of people who suffer from genetic disorders; to allow carriers for a given abnormal gene to make informed choices regarding reproduction; and/or to move towards alleviating the anxieties of families and communities faced with the prospect of serious genetic disease (see Nuffield Council on Bioethics 1993). Presymptomatic genetic testing in children and adolescents raises additional considerations. Wertz et al. (1994) have proposed the following guidelines:

1 the test is capable of detecting conditions for which treatment or preventive measures are available;
2 the test has no health benefits for the minor, but may be useful to the minor in making reproductive decisions now or in the near future;
3 there are no medical benefits and no current reproductive benefits from the testing, but parents or the minor request it;
4 testing is carried out solely for the benefit of another family member.

Multiplex testing, where numerous genetic diseases could be detected, is also a possibility. It may be argued that this form of testing is inappropriate, since it could be carried out in the absence of any effective cure for most of the diseases, and/or in the absence of efficient screening and counselling expertise. Information overload for the affected individual is itself a difficulty, since this may result in the counselling process becoming misleading or meaningless. Important principles include the following:

1 *Prior consent*
   Consent is necessary because of the emphasis we place on the autonomy of individual people. Genetic screening involves obtaining information about a person that is as significant as information about that person's liver or

lifestyle. As a general principle it would be unethical to undertake genetic screening on an individual in the absence of prior informed consent.

2   *Confidentiality*

Once informed consent has been given for genetic screening, the results of that screening must be confidential between the subject, the investigator, and whoever commissions and interprets the results.

3   *Handling of genetic information*

There is a distinction between the storage of personal genetic information about specific people, and the storage of anonymous genomic information in public data banks. Information about identifiable people relates to those people, and may well be relevant to their welfare and well-being. As such, it should be shared only with those to whom it refers, after having been obtained after informed consent and kept confidential by those who gathered it. In terms of the human genome in general, personal information is irrelevant, and these constraints do not apply. This is impersonal data, just as information on the structure and function of the liver is impersonal information.

4   *Stigmatisation of the genetically disadvantaged*

In principle, there should be no stigmatisation of those with genetic disadvantages, as long as confidentiality is ensured in practice. However, if society is to place greater weight on genetic aberration than on other forms of aberration, problems could ensue. But this issue is not confined to genetic questions, and does not even arise from genetic advances. It stems from society's view of the dignity of humans and the value placed on individuals regardless of their health, or their value to society, or their cost to it.

In more general terms, we can say that unsolicited and sensitive information about an individual should not be forced onto that individual. A right to be informed does not entail a duty for the doctor to inform the patient against the patient's wishes. A person has the right to refuse testing and thus to prevent knowledge about himself or herself from being generated. Second, information should be given to a patient in a way in which the patient can make sense of it and appreciate its relevance for his or her own life and condition.

In the third place, information given a patient is 'owned' by that patient, and he or she can grant or refuse third person access to this information. The issue of who should have access to the information is further complicated by the implications that genetic information may have for the siblings, spouse, parents, or children of an affected individual. The sharing of such information should probably be done only with the consent of the patient, and only if the third parties want the information, and it is relevant to them in some important respect.

A fourth point concerns information in the workplace. The concern here is that employers may use genetic screening as a basis for discrimination against employees with health problems, a fear that has already been borne out. This is a more sophisticated means of discrimination than is currently available. It is also conceivable that employers may wish to use genetic screening to detect whether workers are genetically susceptible to unavoidable hazards in particular occupations. A program of voluntary testing of this nature to inform workers of their risks is ethically defensible. Against this, compulsory genetic testing would violate deeply held notions of individual autonomy, and could be used in socially undesirable ways. Such consequences have to be guarded against, even though compulsory testing could benefit individuals, by protecting them from exposure to diseases to which they are genetically susceptible.

The use of genetic information by insurance companies raises difficult issues. On the one hand, patients wish to safeguard their right to privacy concerning their genetic status; on the other, the insurance company has a right to genetic information relevant to determining insurability. In its excellent report *Genetic Screening: Ethical issues*, the Nuffield Council on Bioethics (1993) recommends that insurance companies adhere to their current policy of not requiring genetic tests as a prerequisite to obtaining insurance; it also recommends that a temporary moratorium on requiring the disclosure of genetic data be instituted. When use of genetic information is under consideration by insurance companies, issues of equality and fairness immediately come to the fore, but we must ask whether the traditional policies of insurance companies are based on these same principles. In other words, would the use of genetic information by these companies signify as radical a departure from current practices as is sometimes suggested? If it is ethical for companies to weight insurance premiums against those who smoke cigarettes or who have a known history of heart disease, is it any less ethical to do the same to those with known genetic disease? Any differences revolve around the precision, or lack of precision, of risk prediction in the different conditions.

Genetic Screening for Susceptibility to Disease

Genetic screening for susceptibility to common diseases such as some cancers, cardiovascular disease, diabetes, and mental health disorders such as Alzheimer's disease, bipolar disorder, and schizophrenia may soon be a reality. This approach differs from the highly selective predictive testing for a small number of uncommon genetic disorders within known families, as described above, by screening the general population for susceptibility to common, multifactorial disorders. It has been suggested that the elucidation of genetic factors predisposing some people to common, multifactorial disorders will lead to a paradigm shift in health care, allowing identification of people at increased risk of certain diseases. This could result in health benefits if those at high risk were to modify their lifestyles in appropriate ways. Alternatively, it may precipitate stigmatisation of those who are shown to be susceptible to the diseases in question.

These general screening tests are likely to be costly, the tested individuals may not alter their behaviour sufficiently to achieve noticeable benefit, and a more equitable improvement in a population's health could probably be achieved by firm government action to promote healthy lifestyles and discourage unhealthy or hazardous activities. Furthermore, those not at risk may actually be adversely affected by complacency arising from their non-risk status, a status that in turn may lead them to ignore obvious indicators of a healthy lifestyle.

Ambivalence dominates every facet of this discussion. If screening for susceptibility has clearly demonstrable benefits, it is to be encouraged. On the other hand, if it leads to fatalism, this itself may exacerbate the risk factors. Yet again, the close relationship between susceptibility tests and commercial interests may lead to the testing being driven by market forces, and to a culture of geneticisation.

Emphasis on individuals with genetic diseases or predispositions may in itself pose ethical dilemmas. If this is done at the expense of social action and expenditure, the brunt of the problems created by genetic disease is borne by individuals rather than by society. For instance, in a workplace characterised by toxic chemicals in the environment, emphasis on individuals may lead to them relinquishing their jobs, while failing to direct attention towards the organisation's responsibility to remove the health hazard (Levitt 1995).

Patenting of Human Genes

Is it morally acceptable to patent human genes? Patents may be issued on individual human genes as well as on micro-organisms into which human genes have been inserted. They may also be issued to anyone who invents or discovers a new and useful process, manufacture, or composition of matter. Within these terms, the discovery of a human gene or gene fragment, and the products (proteins) and mutations of these genes, would come under the category of 'manufacture', or 'composition of matter'.

The significance of this debate can be illustrated by reference to the patenting of the genes BRCA1 and BRCA2, linked with inherited breast cancer. Regardless of the case for or against patenting, the respective arguments in this instance are instructive. Considerable scientific and financial resources have been ventured by biotechnology companies in the search for a diagnostic test that in turn could prove of considerable value in genetic counselling. A diagnostic test can be devised once identification and characterisation of the gene have been achieved, and it is the test that can be patented. However, more than one research group (including university-based groups) has devoted time and effort, and also made significant contributions, to the search for these genes. If the competition and sharing of information involved in such efforts were to be threatened by patenting, the whole nature of the scientific endeavour could be altered in molecular genetics research.

This area is characterised by frequent disagreement between industrialists and environmentalists. Large pharmaceutical companies, in particular, contend that they must be free to patent genes and human cells where these have been isolated and characterised outside the human body. They argue that they need to be able to profit from the resulting new diagnostic techniques or therapeutic treatments to cover the very high development costs. Allied with this pragmatic approach is the argument that neither isolated genes nor large quantities of purified proteins occur naturally, and they should as a result be patentable. The contrary position is summed up by arguments opposing ownership of human life and commercialisation of the human body, leading to the position that parts of the human body, including genes, cannot be patented when they remain in the human body (Butler & Gershon 1994).

At a more global level, there is concern that patents on living organisms remove distinctions between living and non-living matter and so undermine the unique status traditionally accorded to life—including human life. In more specific scientific terms, the case is frequently put that genetics research should be a cooperative search for new knowledge, rather than a self-interested pursuit of profits. Once patenting comes to the fore, researchers may become increasingly reluctant to share information, thereby diminishing its transfer between laboratories. It is also feared that patenting will slow the development of gene therapy by forcing royalty agreements from researchers developing screening kits. A clear illustration of these tensions has been evident for the last few years in the different approaches adopted by the private and public consortia working on sequencing the human genome.

Although these arguments have not delved overtly into ethical considerations, they have helped to clarify important issues. An ethical assessment raises matters such as the integrity of nature, the dignity of human beings, and autonomy and fairness (Holtug 1995). Few objections can be mustered on the basis of the first three issues, unless some form of genetic reductionism is also espoused, and patenting is to apply to naturally occurring genes within the human body. In terms of fairness, the interests of the worse-off patients (that is, those with severe health problems) are the ones to be protected. What then remains unresolved is which course of action will best accomplish this—patenting genes and gene products, or not?

Vigilance in this area is essential. Commercial interests could readily dominate the genetic scene and restrict freedom of investigation, pricing genetic therapeutic products out of the reach of ordinary people or even whole societies.

On the other hand, if these investigations do not take place, the potentially beneficial products will not be available to anyone.

Human Genome Project

The HGP was initiated in 1990 as an ongoing fifteen-year program (although it will have been completed by 2003). The aim has been to analyse and sequence all the DNA on all the human chromosomes. Simple as this appears, it brings biology into the realm of 'big science', both in terms of the worldwide effort required and of the costs involved. The former is characterised by collaboration between bodies such as the National Institute of Health (NIH) and the European Union, loosely held together by an international group of scientists called the Human Genome Organisation. The eventual cost of all these efforts may well reach US$3 billion. Where have such large sums of money come from? The HGP has been publicly funded with the intention of making the data freely available to researchers around the world. Running neck and neck with the HGP in the sequencing race has been a privately funded company, Celera Genomics. Concerns had been expressed in some quarters over the involvement of this company, which has not accepted any public money and is therefore under no obligation to make its data public. Celera's president, Craig Venter, has agreed that the data should be made public, but many still fear that this eventuality will be commercially driven and constrained by strict conditions and burdensome licensing.

Despite the often acrimonious competition between the two rivals throughout the project, they reconciled their differences for the joint announcement of the draft map of the human genome in June 2000. Prior to this, the inaugural results of the HGP appeared in the form of the first complete sequence of a human chromosome, number 22. Chromosome 22 is one of the smallest chromosomes but it is nonetheless thought to be gene-rich. At least twenty-seven human disorders are believed to be associated with this chromosome, including cancers, trisomy 22 (the second most common cause of miscarriage) and schizophrenia. Following on from this milestone, the complete sequence of chromosome 21 was released in May 2000.

The primary goal of the HGP was, and still is, to improve human health. The mapping of the human genome is likely to revolutionise the practice of medicine. It offers the promise of improving our lives and health through uncovering the genetic triggers for many diseases—from Alzheimer's to diabetes and heart disease. Once this is done, exquisitely sensitive diagnostic tests can be devised that make diagnosis sure and treatment swift. Analysis of the human genome may yield genes that are promising drug targets, allowing the development of more effective drugs. Pharmaceutical companies will also be able to tailor drugs to a person's genetic make-up, boosting effectiveness while dramatically reducing side effects. The advent of 'personalised medicine' is also envisaged, where treatment and preventative programs are tailored to an individual's genetic profile. Doctors will then prescribe a personal regimen of immunisation and screening, in addition to lifestyle measures, to prevent the most likely diseases throughout life.

However, such optimism must be tempered slightly. We now know our complete genetic code, but we may not understand the meaning—or the 'translation'—of that code for many years to come. Knowing the code for a gene is not the same as knowing what protein it produces in the body, or what that protein does, or what happens when something goes wrong with that particular protein. This sort of information transports us into the realm of proteomics, the latest trend in the post-genomic era. The ultimate goal of proteomics is to catalogue and analyse every protein in the human body, a project as enormous in magnitude as the mapping of the human genome. A host of biotechnology firms including Celera Genomics have launched proteomic programs. Such a flurry of private activity raises the issue of intellectual property disputes similar to those that have plagued the HGP.

The HGP raises a great number of ethical questions. These have been classified into three categories: individual issues, societal issues and species issues (Annas 1993). The principal individual issues are those of autonomy and confidentiality. Autonomy requires that all genetic screening be voluntary, with all participants providing their fully informed consent. Confidentiality requires that no information be disclosed to anyone else without the individual's consent. On an individual level, the questions raised by the HGP are a matter of degree rather than kind, since autonomy and confidentiality are also issues of fundamental importance in individual genetic screening programs.

Society-based ethical issues revolve around questions of resource allocation, commercialisation, and eugenics. What percentage of research budgets should be devoted to this project and its future offshoots? How much should be spent on identifying and treating genetic diseases, as opposed to other conditions that cause disease, such as poverty, drug and alcohol addiction, poor housing and education, and inadequate access to reasonable primary health care?

'Who "owns" the information that results from the project?' is one of the questions provoked by commercial considerations, and 'can such products be patented?' is another. The other societal issue is that of eugenics. Society will be forced to decide whether or not the genetic knowledge resulting from the HGP should be used to *improve* the species, and to examine thoroughly the moral and philosophical concerns that this change in direction would provoke.

The HGP also poses ethical questions for the human species as a whole, as it could undoubtedly alter the way we think about ourselves. The reductionism that is entailed by the HGP could conceivably have a number of consequences.

First, it could lead to people being viewed as products capable of being manufactured, with the result that people could be 'made to measure'. Second, our actions might come to be viewed as genetically determined rather than as a matter of free will. Some individuals accused of crime have already used the defence that their genetic composition predisposed them to commit the crime and thus they should not be held accountable for their actions (Annas 1993). Third, knowledge gained from the HGP may lead to the construction of a 'standard' human genome. If this occurs, one must then ask what variation society would view as permissible before an individual's genome was labelled as substandard or abnormal.

Another gene-mapping project that warrants discussion in this context is the Human Genome Diversity Project (HGDP). The aim of this project is the reconstructing of the recent history of *Homo sapiens*, from a comparison of the genomes of different human populations. This project would map DNA from approximately twenty-five individuals representing 500 of the world's 5000 or so different ethnic groups. The project was proposed in 1991, with support from the Human Genome Organisation, but it has as yet obtained little funding due partly to controversy surrounding its procedures and implications. Criticisms of the HGDP stem from concerns that the project mainly targets indigenous peoples, who will then be alienated from the control and use of their own genetic material and information. The procedures concerning how—if at all—intellectual property rights would be claimed on biological material derived by the project remain to be clarified. The Department of Commerce in the United States has already filed patent claims on cell lines taken from people from the Solomon Islands.

Furthermore, indigenous groups believe that the HGDP is aimed primarily at benefiting scientific knowledge rather than assisting the indigenous people themselves. Many think the HGDP will not be of any benefit to them. The fear is that the genetic reductionism inherent in this project threatens to destroy any mythologies of human origins different from those of the dominant world cultures, and may also increase discrimination against indigenous populations. Since 1992 there have been a number of statements by indigenous groups outlining their opposition to the HGDP. In New Zealand, Māori have endorsed one such statement known as the Mataatua Declaration. Originally developed and tabled in the United Nations (June 1993), the Mataatua Declaration calls for 'an immediate halt to the Human Genome Diversity Project until its moral, ethical, economic, physical, and political implications have been thoroughly discussed, understood, and approved by indigenous peoples'.

The leader of the HGDP, Professor Luigi Cavalli-Sforza, has assured indigenous groups that protocols addressing these concerns are being drafted. It remains to be seen, however, whether these protocols, when finalised, will be sufficient to calm the very real fears of many people.

The shaky financial position of the HGDP, coupled with poor political support, has seen a reduction in the size and scope of the project. It now appears that the ambitious goal of a DNA repository and database is unlikely to be realised and as a result, there are considerable doubts over the long-term viability of the HGDP.

Similar ethical concerns have been raised over the use of genetic data in Iceland. Iceland's genetically isolated population has attracted geneticists and medical researchers alike, on the grounds that it is a fitting place to investigate the genetic factors involved in many medical conditions. This has led to the passing of a controversial law that gives a private company the exclusive rights to an electronic database of the nation's health records. This database consists of genetic, health care, and genealogical information on every person in the country. The law has outraged many with regard to issues of consent (which is presumed), and patient privacy. The main criticism, however, is the granting of *exclusive* control of a database of all Icelanders to a single company. There are fears that the licence-holder will veto the use of the database by Icelandic scientists if their proposed research is judged to threaten its commercial interests. Many are also uncomfortable about handing over data with no real idea of how it is to be used in the future.

General Ethical Questions

The notion of 'playing God' raises its head in most scientific domains, the intended message being that this is dangerous territory (Boone 1988). But is genetic technology tinkering with nature or even with people in a uniquely dangerous way? Is it *interfering* with nature? In one sense, it is; but is this of any ethical interest? Frequently it is taken to imply that the interference is going beyond acceptable limits. That may or may not be the case; but it is difficult to see how genetic technology *per se* does this. Nature has given us genetic combinations that lead to Huntington's disease, diabetes, and heart disease, but few would argue that these constitute a good. Medicine has traditionally done its best to cope with genetic conditions, and these have not, in themselves, been regarded as transgressing the boundary of acceptable human endeavour. Humans have intruded into nature throughout recorded history, whether it has been by draining swamps infested with malaria-bearing mosquitoes or by using antibiotics. What is of far more importance is whether such intrusions enhance or diminish the *human condition*. What is required is that we determine the sort of interference with nature and the genome that will advance *human welfare* and the *integrity of the planet*, while respecting the dimensions of what it means to be human. This calls for a great deal of enlightened ethical discernment, and an awareness of the tentative path along which we are travelling.

In spite of these points, somatic cell gene therapy may be considered unethical on the grounds that it represents the beginning of a slippery slope, its inevitable concomitant being germ line gene therapy and eugenics. This is an understandable viewpoint, since so often one innocuous process leads to another far less innocuous and originally quite unintended process. Implicit within the slippery slope argument is the assumption that permission to allow one kind of intervention extends to allow all kinds of intervention. However, this is not the case in moral reasoning, where there is an immense gulf between two sorts of measures. For instance, there is a considerable moral chasm between gene therapy to treat disease (such as cancer or heart disease) and gene manipulation to alter human behaviour or morality. This is the boundary between the two worlds of therapy and of eugenics or genetic enhancement, where there is a logical stop sign. The major challenge of an ethical approach to gene therapy is to recognise this moral gulf.

What this means is that gene therapy represents a path governed by a therapeutic rationale. There is the possibility of stopping between somatic cell gene therapy and germ line gene therapy, since there are major ethical and biological issues of concern at this point, even though both are governed by a therapeutic rationale. However, the move to genetic enhancement and eugenics is a move away from the world of finding cures to diseases that kill, disfigure, and limit basic human capacities, to a world of idealistic attempts to perfect the human species and improve fundamental human attributes. Any move into this latter world would be placing ourselves on a slippery slope towards perfectibility and manipulation. That is not where we are at the moment, although some in the bioethics community are arguing for a closer look at genetic enhancement.

Genetic knowledge confronts us in a poignant way with ambiguity. On the one hand, we want to know all; our curiosity drives us to search and to keep on searching. Genetics shows us a great deal about why we are as we are, but it also enables us to know something about what we will be like in the future. And it is this ability to foresee and potentially control the future that is so alluring. But are we afraid of too much self-knowledge? Will this challenge our view of who we are?

Alongside this ambiguity rests another: the prospect of greatly increased control and all-pervasive intervention in people's lives. Such intervention and control may be used exclusively for good, but there is always the prospect that this may not be the case, and we recoil from it (Van Tongeren 1991). Here then is ambiguity once more: we may be able to control others, but they equally will be able to control us, and they may not do it with the best of intentions. Alongside this perspective stands another: the tension between perfection and imperfection. Grand genetic vistas allude to perfectibility, improving humans in unspecified ways. While such vistas are not on any current genetic agendas, they still feed the imagination. But even in the imaginary realm there is ambiguity:

do we want perfection, with its elimination of challenges; do we want total genetic control? Too much genetic control challenges our conception of what it means to be human, and possibly our sense of self-identity. Such idle speculation does little more than stultify discussion of genetic developments.

Such general considerations do not tell us whether or not we should enter into any particular genetic ventures. If it is true that an ability to do something, makes that something inevitable (it *must* be done), then we have limited the ethical possibilities open to us, because we have lost a fundamental element of what we are, and of what we ought to be.

6
Issues Before Birth

Introduction

The ethical issues raised in the previous chapters revolve around society's view of the human body after birth. Complex as some of those issues are, they are grounded in a strong consensus that the human body is to be treated with respect and that under all normal circumstances human life is to be protected. However, when we turn to life before birth and to embryos and foetuses, a similar consensus does not necessarily hold. To many people it is not self-evident that embryonic and foetal life is to be given the same degree of protection as human life after birth. Additionally, considerations such as the autonomy of the mother emerge as being of major ethical significance.

The moral and legal status ascribed to human embryos and foetuses is far from easy to determine, and different people reach different conclusions. What is more, this status is arrived at on both biological and moral grounds, and neither provides definitive guidance. We shall look first at the biological component.

Biological Definitions

Embryo and Foetus

The term 'embryo' is traditionally used to refer to the human conceptus from fertilisation to eight weeks gestation, although in recent ethical writings it is sometimes confined to the period up to implantation (that is, two weeks gestation). This pre-implantation phase is also known as the pre-embryo stage of development. While the precise terms used are somewhat arbitrary, any deviation from the traditional embryo–foetus distinction at eight weeks gestation should be undertaken only with care.

The foetal period is further subdivided into previable and viable periods. The term 'previable' refers to a foetus showing signs of life but not having the capacity to survive after separation from the mother. A foetus is generally considered to be previable when under twenty weeks' gestation and weighing less than 400 grams (although these figures are relative and vary from one country to another). The term 'viable' refers to a foetus having the capacity to survive and sustain independent existence.

Fertilisation and Pre-embryonic Stage

Fertilisation is the fusion of a sperm and an ovum. This is achieved by penetration by the sperm of the outer layers of the ovum *(corona radiata* and *zona pellucida)*, which becomes engulfed within the cytoplasm of the ovum. These processes induce the ovum to complete its maturation. One aspect of this is the joining of the male and female pronuclei (syngamy), which marks the completion of fertilisation twenty-six to thirty hours after its commencement. The process of fertilisation usually takes place in the uterine tube and the fertilised ovum is known as a *zygote*.

The moment of zygote formation is taken as the beginning of embryonic development. Once it has occurred, the ovum becomes active and the genetic individuality of the embryo is established by the combination of genes from each of the parents. The zygote is still capable of splitting to form two individuals, a potential that remains for up to two weeks after fertilisation.

The first cell divisions of the fertilised ovum produce a cluster of equivalent cells *(blastomeres)*, which in the early stages are not integrated into a multicellular organism. This non-integrated state persists for a few days after fertilisation, during which period one or more cells can be removed without affecting the outcome of development—a complete individual is still capable of being born. After this the outer cells begin to differentiate to form a surface layer, the trophectoderm, which becomes the trophoblast once implantation occurs. It is the trophoblast that establishes the uteroplacental circulation. Of the inner cells, some are destined to form the foetus (embryo-foetus), while the remainder (embryo-placenta) represent forerunners of extra-embryonic tissues (Jones & Telfer 1995).

The first blastomeres appear within thirty hours of fertilisation, while by three days a ball *(morula)* of sixteen or so cells has formed. The morula enters the uterus shortly after this. It lies free in the uterine lumen for one or two days, by which time it consists of fifty to sixty cells. During this time a fluid-filled cavity gradually develops within the morula; when this is established the whole structure is known as a *blastocyst*. Some of the cells form a structure that, later on, will form part of the placenta.

At about six days the blastocyst adheres to the wall of the uterus, following which some of its outer cells begin to invade the uterine wall. This is the beginning of *implantation*. Two or three days later the amniotic cavity makes its first appearance. By twelve to fourteen days implantation is complete, and a primitive placental circulation has developed. At this stage the embryo is still a flat two-layered disc, although the first indication of the future head end of the embryo appears at about this time. The *primitive streak* develops as a midline thickening at fifteen to sixteen days, after which early features of the nervous system make their appearance.

The concept of a 'pre-embryo' has acquired considerable significance of late in the scientific and ethical communities, and requires some comment. Its use reflects the view that the early embryo for the first fourteen or so days of gestation is conceptually different from the two- to eight-week embryo. This view stems from a number of its characteristics: much of it gives rise to the placenta and supporting tissue; it is neither a coherent nor a spatially defined individual entity; and its early developmental potential is unrestricted (McLaren 1986). The appearance of the primitive streak is seen by some as marking the onset of individuality (McLaren 1984).

However, even though much of the early embryo is committed to the formation of extra-embryonic tissues, the whole of it is essential for the well-being, growth, and further development of that particular prenatal individual. There can be no future embryo and foetus without the extra-embryonic tissues. To compartmentalise the two as though this were not the case is to fail to do justice to the maternal-foetal environment. As far as the primitive streak is concerned, it is a transitory phenomenon, on its way to being transformed into more definitive features of the early embryo. Its biological significance, therefore, needs to be seen within a developmental context rather than as the sole organiser for an individual being's existence.

Embryonic development occurs gradually rather than in quantum leaps, with later stages being totally dependent on the successful completion of earlier ones. What is significant is the whole, regardless of whether some parts of the whole will or will not continue into postnatal existence. The pluripotential nature or otherwise of cells tells us nothing about how we should correctly treat the early embryo. Neither does the first appearance of the primitive streak convey anything of moral significance. What is more interesting is what lies beyond the primitive streak stage. Consequently, use of the term 'pre-embryo' helps clarify neither the scientific nor the ethical issues at the beginning of human life. An alternative may be to describe the parts of the early embryo that will give rise to the placenta and foetus as the embryo–placenta and embryo–foetus, respectively (Holland 1990; Jones & Telfer 1995).

In spite of this, the fourteen-day boundary with its approximate equivalence to the appearance of the primitive streak, has become enshrined in legislation in a number of countries as the last day when research may be conducted on human embryos. This denotes what are regarded as important ethical distinctions between the pre– and post–fourteen-day periods.

Personhood of the Embryo and Foetus

The difficulties associated with deciding when 'life' begins biologically are more than matched by the difficulties of determining when *persons* come into existence. Of course, in real life the two issues are not quite as separate as this, since there are large areas of overlap between the biological and the philosophical. Imagine the following scene.

> Edith has just become aware that she is pregnant, since she has missed two periods and has had the pregnancy confirmed. An embryo has been in existence for about six weeks. There is no doubt there is new biological life within Edith; either this will keep on developing or something will go wrong and she will miscarry. Either way, she will be aware of it. Edith is delighted at being pregnant, and she refers to this embryo as 'her child'. What does she mean by this term? She knows what children are like, of course; her sister has a three-year-old. But is her six-week-old embryo a child in the same way as the three-year-old is a child? It will probably become a child, but is it one now?
>
> Let us now consider an alternative possibility. Edith never intended to become pregnant, and now wants to have an abortion. For her, the embryo is nothing like a child; it is a nuisance since she has other plans for the next two years and these do not include having a child. An abortion presents her with no moral difficulties, since for her a six-week-old embryo is nothing special in human terms.
>
> A third possibility sees Edith wanting her pregnancy to continue. However, she has no desire to refer to the embryo within her as a child. She hopes everything will continue satisfactorily, but she is unable at this early stage to feel she is carrying a complete new human being. If anything goes wrong, she will probably be upset, but she will not actually consider she has lost a child.

These three scenarios are representative of the three major viewpoints on the moral status of prenatal human life: embryos/foetuses are persons, non-persons or potential persons.

Embryos/Foetuses are Persons

In this position, the embryo is to be regarded (and therefore treated) as a human person from the time of fertilisation. Some argue that, since it is impossible to prove that personhood begins later than fertilisation, moral prudence should err on the conservative side and conclude that personhood probably begins *at* fertilisation. While not all contributions under this heading are theological, such perspectives have proved important for this position. Whatever the precise formulation, the outcome is the same: from fertilisation the embryo is to be treated in the same way we would treat a mature human.

According to this viewpoint, the process of embryonic development is nothing less than the development of a person. There is no stage in human existence when we are not people (Iglesias 1984). Iglesias distinguishes between the process of development *into* a person, and the process of development *of* a person; she favours the latter, with its corollary that embryos and foetuses are to be accorded absolute respect and treated as inviolable. Underlying these conclusions is the idea of *potentiality*: whatever we now are was present in potential form in the embryos from which we developed. Since we *now* have self-consciousness, the potential for self-consciousness must be present in all embryos. The embryo is a minute form of a mature person: all that is required is the opportunity to unfold. It is the adult in miniature; it is an actual person with great potential. With respect to this view, no living body can *become* a person unless it already is a person.

The question, however, is whether the capacity of *a* to develop into A makes *a* exactly the same as A. Quite obviously, the ability of an acorn to develop into an oak tree does not convert the acorn into an oak tree. Conversely, to destroy an acorn is not the same as destroying an oak tree. A three-day-old embryo is not the same as a thirty-year-old human adult. Although the potential is undoubtedly there, the actual adult is far from realisation in a three-day-old embryo.

Alongside this can be placed the limited prospect of an early embryo developing into a child, let alone an adult. The probability of survival from fertilisation to clinical pregnancy has been estimated at 42 per cent (Boklage 1990), a figure that accords with many studies that set pregnancy wastage from fertilisation onwards in the vicinity of 70 per cent. The main factors contributing to this wastage are chromosomal abnormalities. Figures such as these in no way undermine the moral significance of early embryos, but they are a reminder that the chances of a three-day-old embryo becoming a newborn infant are relatively small; its potential for further development is far removed from the realisation of that potential.

In no other area of life do we equate the potential with the actual. For instance, a student commencing a course of study has the potential to pass the final examinations, and this potential may ultimately be realised. In order to accomplish this, however, a great deal of teaching and learning is required, and it is these acts alone that convert potential into actual success. Along the way, however, the student is changed by the learning, so that the student who passes the examination is different from the student who turned up at the first class with a potential for passing the examination (Jones 1987).

Reliance on an embryo's potential does not convert it into a 'nothing', any more than the student in the above analogy is regarded as a 'failed' student, or is excluded from further study on the grounds that he or she has not yet passed the final examinations. Respect is owed to the embryo because of what it is and, more strongly, because of what it may become. This follows, however, from its potential, and not because its potential has been converted into an actuality (Poplawski & Gillett 1991).

When this distinction is ignored, problems may arise if the welfare of mother and foetus come into conflict, as epitomised by legislation that treats mother and foetus as equal (Holden 1994). If the good of two 'individuals' with equal moral status clashes head-on, there is no clear indication which is to give way.

Embryos/Foetuses are Non-persons

One argument in favour of the non-personhood of embryos and foetuses stems from the generally held viewpoint that we do not consider it wrong to destroy either the ovum or sperm before they have united. From this, Singer and Wells (1984) argue that there is no moral obligation to preserve the life of the embryo. Even more provocatively, they suggest that the embryo should be regarded as a thing, rather than a person, until the point at which there is some brain function.

According to this viewpoint, the first few weeks of gestation have no moral significance. In practice, for Singer and Wells this means that the embryo is regarded as a 'thing' for at least the first six weeks of development. The complete lack of any personhood (either actual or potential) places no moral obligations on the human community. The embryo, as a non-sentient being, has no moral rights. The point at which this situation changes is open to debate. Considerable emphasis is placed by some writers on the acquisition by the embryo or foetus of consciousness, or at least a potential for consciousness. This, in turn, depends on some minimum degree of nervous system development. The emphasis here is on the acquisition of *sentience*, that is, the ability to feel pleasure or pain. This, it is argued, signifies that an embryo or foetus has sufficient moral status to make it wrong to do certain things to it, for example, to inflict unnecessary pain upon it.

If this argument is accepted, it has to be asked at what stage of brain development consciousness is manifested. From a neurobiological angle this is a difficult, if not impossible, task; and yet it is an essential one if the embryo or foetus from this point onwards is to be the bearer of moral rights. Stages from six weeks of gestation all the way through to twenty-eight weeks have been quoted as the beginning of a 'brain', or, using different terminology, as the earliest indication of consciousness. Whatever one makes of these widely divergent appraisals, they cast doubt on the advisability of using any of these possibilities as the definitive beginning point of personhood (Jones 1989; Moussa & Shannon 1992). As a last resort the most we can do is draw a quasi-arbitrary line in the development of the embryo.

An alternative case for the non-personhood of the embryo and foetus is based on drawing a distinction between *being a human being* in the biological sense and *being a person* in the moral sense (Tooley 1983). When this is done, it can readily be concluded that not all human beings are persons. This, in turn, raises the inevitable question of whether or not the foetus is a person. If we expect of a person properties such as being able to recall past states or envisage a future for itself, or having personality traits that do not alter too drastically over short periods of time, foetuses are not persons. Nor are young infants, adults in a vegetative state, or adults with severe dementia. On the other hand it has been claimed that the adult members of some animal species, such as some primates and dolphins, may be persons (Singer & Wells 1984).

Tooley (1983) concedes that human foetuses and neonates are potential persons. However, he also argues that potential personhood only allows us to confer a right to life (for foetuses and infants) if we also accept the principle that it is wrong to refrain from producing additional persons. If one assumes that we are under no obligation to produce children (that is, contraception is acceptable), Tooley concludes that the killing of a foetus (a potential person) is no worse than using contraceptives.

In arriving at these conclusions, Tooley has overlooked what one commentator has described as the 'moral obligation to nurture' (Sommers 1985). He fails to take account of the commitments humans have to the welfare and survival of infants and also, to varying extents, of foetuses. The human family has obligations, since the newborn is totally dependent on the voluntary acts of responsible moral agents committed to its care. Without such interactions, neither foetuses nor the newborn would survive. In other words, neurological and behavioural factors alone are not sufficient to tell us how we should act towards foetuses and infants (and also seriously impaired adults), since they fail to take account of the commitments that are so essential to life together in the human community. Even when the neurological and behavioural features of the foetus or newborn are inadequate on a biological scale of values, our commitment to care for one of our own is basic to what we are as humans living together. In other words, the notion of personhood incorporates social and intellectual factors, as well as biological ones.

Embryos/Foetuses are Potential Persons

A third perspective occupies a place somewhere between the above two positions. It views the foetus as a being with the potential for full personhood. According to this perspective, a foetus (as a potential person) has some claim to life early on in development and will acquire a person's claim to life as development proceeds (Langarek 1979). In these terms, a human foetus is a potential person, as opposed to an actual person (a normal adult human being), a being with a capacity for personhood (a temporarily unconscious person), a possible person (a human sperm or ovum), or a future person (a person in a future generation). In practical terms, potential persons such as foetuses have some claim to life, whereas possible persons have no such claim.

Emphasis on this sort of potential takes seriously the continuum of biological development, and does not draw an arbitrary line to denote the acquisition of personhood. At all stages of development the foetus is on its way to full personhood and, if everything proceeds normally, it will one day attain full personhood in its own right.

According to this viewpoint, there is no point in development, regardless of how early, when the embryo or foetus fails to display the potential for personhood—no matter how rudimentary. This bestows upon the embryo and foetus some claim to life and respect. This claim, however, becomes stronger as foetal development proceeds, so that by some time in the third trimester the claim is so strong that the consequences of killing a foetus are the same as those of killing an actual person—whether child or adult. Consequently, the foetus in the last trimester will, when necessary, be treated as a 'patient'. This mirrors most people's responses in ordinary life, where we recognise a difference between the accidental loss of an embryo or early foetus and the birth of a stillborn child. Both entail the death of human life, and yet under most circumstances the loss of a life that 'almost made it' is felt much more acutely than a life that had hardly begun to develop.

Like all intermediate positions, the potential person position satisfies neither extreme. It is seen as being too liberal by those advocating a 'foetus is a person' viewpoint, and too conservative by the 'foetus is not a person' school. Not only this, but the 'potential person' stance is itself open to varying interpretations. Nevertheless, its gradualist emphasis strikes a chord with many people, on biological, philosophical, intuitive, and pragmatic grounds. It assists many through the maze of problems associated with the prenatal and neonatal areas, and provides a useful basis for tackling the specific ethical issues raised here.

Research on Embryos and Foetuses

Embryo Research

Embryo research, like foetal research, has become a reality because of prior human intervention in the reproductive process. The intervention in the case of foetal research is abortion; in the case of embryo research it is *in vitro fertilisation* (IVF) and the production of 'spare' embryos. In neither case, however, does the research follow inevitably from the first step, although without it there could be no research of the types we are envisaging. The embryo research debate, therefore, revolves not around the embryo *per se* but around the pre-implantation embryo outside the human body, an embryo produced by technical means. In looking at embryo research we are concerned with embryos produced by IVF but not transferred to a woman's uterus for subsequent development.

Embryos such as these can be produced in a number of ways. They may be superfluous to the needs of a couple in a clinical IVF program (spare embryos); produced in the laboratory (using donated ova and sperm) with the sole intention of employing them in a research program; or the by-product of another research program aimed at studying, for example, the fertilising capacity of human ova or sperm.

The research imperative stems from the potential value of these pre-implantation human embryos in the furtherance of a wide range of scientific and clinical objectives (Royal Society 1990). Research attention has focused on a number of areas.

1   *Understanding the normal pattern of development and metabolism in the developing human embryo*
    Studies in this area could lead to the development of diagnostic tests of viability, and the discovery of more appropriate methods of culturing embryos.

2   *Treatment of infertility through IVF*
    Of the two major directions of research in this area, the first involves identification of factors affecting embryonic viability, and the second the development of techniques to assist fertilisation. This work is aimed at increasing the success rate of IVF. There have been significant improvements in IVF procedures and pregnancy rates over the last ten years as a result of such research. For example, the live birth rate for IVF in the United Kingdom in 1986 was 8.6 per cent, compared to 16.4 per cent for 1997/98 (Human Fertilisation and Embryology Authority 1999).

3   *Prevention of genetic disease*
    Research on human embryos has allowed the development of tests that can be performed on developing eggs at an early stage to identify those that will be affected by, or be carriers of, serious genetic diseases such as Duchenne muscular dystrophy or cystic fibrosis, and of replacing in the uterus only those found to be free of such defective genes. Research on diagnosing genetic diseases two to five days after fertilisation has made considerable advances and the technique has already been successfully performed with couples at high risk of transmitting x-linked mental retardation. There are only four centres in the United Kingdom licensed to carry out such tests and they are currently practised on a small scale. However, demand is expected to grow as genes responsible for other disorders are elucidated, and experimental techniques are further developed and refined.

4 *Improvement of contraception*
Research on human embryos can aid the development of simple and reliable methods of contraception by improving our understanding of fundamental aspects of human embryology. Recent efforts have focused on the possibility of using the immune system to provide protection against unwanted pregnancy by means of a vaccine against human chorionic gonadotropin, a hormone produced by the pre-implantation embryo.

A future avenue of embryo research involves the isolation of pluripotent stem cell lines for eventual differentiation and clinical use in transplantation (see Chapter 8). Such tissue could be used in the treatment of disorders such as Parkinson's disease, as well as degenerative diseases of the heart, liver, and kidneys.

Research conducted on human embryos is generally carried out using professional guidelines or national ones. In the United Kingdom, a licence must be granted by the Human Fertilisation and Embryology Authority for each act of reproductive research. The Human Fertilisation and Embryology Authority is the only existing agency of its kind and its role is to approve embryo research for a narrow range of applications, such as improving fertility methods. While guidelines differ from one country to another, they tend to have much in common. For instance, research should be scientifically valid and clinically relevant; the objectives should not be obtainable by research on animals alone; consent of both the donors and a local ethics committee must always be obtained; certain lines of work (for example genetic modification) should be prohibited; no fertilised egg that has been experimented on should be replaced in the uterus; and no fertilised egg should be grown for more than fourteen days *in vitro*.

The possibility of research on embryos has, not surprisingly, proved extremely contentious. For some, the human status of these embryos precludes their use in research under any circumstances. For others, the potential medical and scientific benefits in ameliorating mental and physical suffering are so great that they justify unlimited research using human embryos. These responses mirror two of the positions on foetuses (as persons, and as non-persons) discussed previously.

For those in the first group, research is morally wrong because the embryos, no matter how young and undeveloped, are human, and as such demonstrate (or have the potential for) full human personhood. To some in this group, the human embryo (both pre- and post-implantation) should be accorded the same status as a child or adult. This moral principle is considered to outweigh any of the possible medical benefits of the research. For those in the second group, it is morally wrong not to do everything possible to alleviate human suffering, whether this is the suffering of infertility or of a genetic or chromosomal disorder, such as Down syndrome.

Those in the first group disapprove of any research at all on the human embryo. Those in the second group allow research, although they accept an upper limit on the age at which embryos can be used for research purposes. The basis of this age limit is generally the appearance of neurological structures or characteristics signifying the earliest appearance of sentience. For some in this group, research procedures should be restricted as little as possible since the human embryo is essentially a useful tool in the furtherance of scientific and medical advance. It also follows that human embryos may be produced specifically for experimental studies. Between these two anti-research and pro-research extremes there is a medley of intermediate positions. Most reports issued by governmental and medical bodies have adopted an intermediate position, although they have a clear bias towards the legitimacy of some research on human embryos. When this is the case, a fourteen-day time limit on research is generally invoked (as discussed earlier in this chapter).

Before drawing out some of the principles on the use of embryos in research, there is one consideration that deserves more detailed discussion. This is the notion of therapeutic and non-therapeutic research, which draws a distinction between research that may or may not benefit the individual embryo. A futuristic example of therapeutic research is gene therapy, the goal of which is the development of the embryo into an individual with an improved genetic constitution. This is therapeutic research in its simplest form. The distinction between therapeutic and non-therapeutic research has been borrowed from clinical medicine, where it is helpful in distinguishing between different types of research carried out on patients. But is this notion as helpful when discussing research on embryos?

For instance, the information obtained may be relevant, not to individual embryos, but to embryos in general, for example at decreasing the incidence of infertility. This may involve the selection of one normal embryo from among a few embryos, only allowing that one embryo to develop to term; or it may require the sacrifice of many present embryos so that future embryos will benefit. Is this therapeutic or non-therapeutic research? In traditional adult terms it is non-therapeutic, since it is not aimed at benefiting the individual on which the research is being conducted. However, is it legitimate to move from a principle based on adult patients to one involving four-, eight-, or sixteen-cell embryos? This is an important question since only 1–5 per cent of IVF embryos survive to become living human beings, while 30–40 per cent of naturally fertilised embryos within a woman's uterus achieve this goal.

Another type of research aims to benefit non-embryos, that is, to benefit *medicine in general*. Stem cell research using human embryos falls into this category. This is clearly a non-therapeutic type of research since it makes use of particular embryos in order to provide information with general medical applications.

What does this mean in practice? By August 1999 there were twenty-seven approved research projects under way in the United Kingdom. Of these projects, twenty-one aimed to advance the treatment of infertility (including studies of the maturation of embryos and factors affecting embryo implantation), eleven were concerned with genetic abnormalities, seven focused on miscarriage, five on congenital diseases, and one project aimed to develop more effective contraceptive techniques. A number of projects fell into more than one of the above categories. From this, it can be seen that practically all the projects were of potential benefit to embryos in general. The research cannot, by definition, benefit present embryos because of the inadequacy of the techniques, but their goal is to benefit embryos in the future.

What principles are relevant to decisions regarding embryo research? First, gametes before fertilisation are of lesser ethical concern than are their post-fertilisation products. Consequently, unfertilised eggs are not accorded the same value as human embryos at any post-fertilisation stage.

Second, embryos and foetuses deserve special respect since they are the forebears of individual humans like ourselves. This is not a universally held principle, since the status of IVF embryos outside the uterus may differ from that of embryos fertilised naturally and existing within a woman's uterus. For the former, another act, that of transferring them to a woman's uterus and of a woman consenting to have them transferred, is required if this potential is to begin to be realised. By contrast, embryos within a woman's uterus already possess this potential. This leads some to argue that IVF embryos merit no special protection. However, most consider that they merit a limited form of protection allowing research only under stringent conditions, whereas still others contend that IVF embryos merit absolute protection necessitating their placement in a woman's uterus to provide them with the potential to develop further as human persons.

Third, the embryos used for research purposes should be those that are superfluous to the needs of clinical IVF procedures. This, again, is not a generally accepted principle, but it emphasises that the source of embryos to be used in research programs may be of ethical significance. The deliberate production of human embryos for use in research programs has no parallel in any other medical research, since it involves organisms with the potential for full human life being used only as objects and never as ends in themselves. In contrast, the spare embryos from clinical IVF programs are the unrequired by-products of attempts to create new human life. By themselves, they cannot develop further, and so may be compared with naturally fertilised embryos that cannot develop further because of genetic abnormalities or hormonal deficiencies.

Fourth, requests to do research on human embryos should require especially strong justification because of their high moral value. In particular, research on human embryos should be considered only when no adequate substitute is available, and only to procure data likely to be of clinical importance. This emphasises therapeutic research, at least as far as its value to embryos in general is concerned.

Fifth, the burden of demonstrating the acceptability of any proposed research should lie with those putting forward the proposal. To what extent principles such as these will be modified over the coming years, in response to the prospects offered by stem cell research, remains to be seen.

Foetal Research

There is an extensive literature on foetal research that has been carried out over many years. Of this, three major types of research can be identified: research performed in the uterus prior to abortion or normal delivery; research performed in the uterus during an abortion; and research performed outside the uterus following an abortion, and therefore following separation from the mother.

The first type of research is performed prior to abortion or delivery, and includes many non-invasive therapeutic procedures. Such therapeutic studies have often been the offshoot of diagnostic or therapeutic procedures. Examples include the use of X-rays, amniocentesis, and ultrasound in prenatal diagnosis, and studies of foetal behaviour such as breathing patterns, reflexes, and the response to sound. Other studies in this category are not therapeutic in charac-ter: for example, those carried out to investigate the transfer of substances across the placenta. In these instances the substance is administered to the pregnant woman some hours before abortion, and subsequently the aborted foetus is examined for traces of the substance in question. Among the compounds to have been tested in this manner are cortisol and various antibiotics.

In the second type of study, that which is performed on the foetus in the uterus during an abortion, placental transfer studies have been carried out with the aim of discovering whether compounds such as radioactive isotopes are transported across the placenta from the foetal to the maternal side. Other research in this category has focused on aiding normal delivery: for instance, studies into the effects on the foetus of agents that delay or induce the onset of labour, and drugs used for obstetric anaesthesia. Research aimed at learning more about normal foetal physiology also fits into this category.

In the third type of study, abortuses are examined following separation from the mother. Since aborted foetuses may continue to live following abortion by hysterotomy or hysterectomy, some aspects of foetal physiology can be investi-gated. Examples of such studies include work looking at brain metabolism, endocrine function, and the development and physiology of specific organs such as the heart.

The publication of studies like these raised numerous practical and ethical objections. As a result, committees were set up, and reports produced, in various countries in the 1970s and early 1980s: in the United Kingdom, the Report of the Advisory Group (commonly referred to as the Peel Committee) 1972; in the United States, that of the National Commission for the Protection of Human Subjects of Biomedical and Behavioral Research 1975; and in Australia, that of the National Health and Medical Research Council 1984. These reports concluded that experimentation on live previable foetuses was permissible within certain limits, on the grounds that important biomedical knowledge could not be obtained by alternative means. This included knowledge about the transfer of substances across the placenta, and the reaction of foetuses to drugs.

All published guidelines build various safeguards into their provisions. In regard to experiments carried out on the foetus *in anticipation of an abortion*, minimal risk, or no risk should be imposed on the foetus by the research. This is because the foetus may subsequently be born alive, or the woman may change her mind regarding the abortion. For experiments on the previable foetus *during the abortion procedure* or *following an abortion*, even potentially harmful research is allowed. The conditions are that the method of abortion should destroy the foetus before its complete separation from the mother; the foetus should be less than twenty weeks gestational age; the research should not lead to any alterations in the abortion procedure; and the duration of life of the foetus should not be affected by the experimental manipulations.

Research is also feasible on the dead foetus outside the uterus and on the viable foetus either inside or outside the uterus. Most agree that a dead foetus should be treated in the same manner as any dead human individual. In this instance, consent must have been given by the mother. In the case of a viable foetus after delivery, even after an abortion, most argue that the ethical obligation is to sustain its life, and that it is unethical to experiment on it in any way that would jeopardise its life.

The stance of these guidelines appears to be that, once the death of the foetus is inevitable, at the time of the abortion or subsequent to it, the foetus can be exposed to risk. The rationale is that, since the previable foetus is doomed, any harm resulting from the experimentation is of little consequence compared with the much greater harm caused by the abortion. Hence, if abortion is allowable, so is research on the foetus.

In general, the various guidelines adopt an intermediate position on the status of the foetus. They are not based on the view that the human foetus should be accorded the status of a person from the earliest stages of development, thereby debarring any experimentation on it. But neither do they view the foetus as a non-personal organism, since they proscribe causing harm to the living previable foetus. This intermediate position raises a number of general questions that are of help in focusing attention on dilemmas inherent in foetal research. The fact that the foetuses are doomed (they are about to be aborted) plays a crucial role in all aspects of experimentation on live previable foetuses. The argument appears to be that, since these foetuses will never be able to realise their potential as fully developed persons, it is legitimate to use them for the good of medical science, and therefore for the good of other foetuses that will realise that potential. But if this position is accepted, we need to ask whether children and adults who are also doomed (for whatever reason) can be used for the good of medical science. Should experimentation on them be justified for equivalent reasons? If we answer these questions in the negative, because of major differences in the status of prenatal and postnatal human life, we have to determine the ethical nature of these differences.

Another issue concerns the nature of the parental consent required in order to allow experimentation on live previable foetuses. This is generally based on the consent required to experiment on children, that is, the consent of the mother or parents. However, there is a difference between the nature of the consent in the two instances. With children, the consent is for research on a being for whom one expects to shoulder responsibility in the future. With previable foetuses, however, the consent refers to a being for whom the parents will have no future responsibility. In addition, since the parents have consented to abortion, they hardly have the best interests of the *foetus* at heart (except perhaps where the abortion is on the grounds of severe foetal abnormality). It is unlikely, therefore, that any consent they give for non-therapeutic research on the foetus will have the same meaning as consent for similar research on a child they want to live and for whom they hope to care.

Abortion

Of all the ethical issues affecting life before birth, none can be more daunting than abortion. In some countries (such as the United States), the issues involved have become so polarised that the prospects of reaching a satisfactory consensus appear forlorn. In some quarters, labels dominate every aspect of the debate, with 'pro-life' and 'pro-choice' positions encapsulating all possible options within the two opposing perspectives. In other words, the vast complexity of moral discourse is whittled down to a simple decision—either an absolute stance in favour of the unborn or an absolute stance in favour of the mother's right to self-determination. Any mediating position is automatically placed in one or other of these categories.

In attempting to come to a workable ethical stance over abortion we shall suggest that account has to be taken of, first, the wishes of the pregnant woman, second, the ethical demands made on us by the foetus, third, the relevance of the stage of foetal development, and fourth, the conflicting ethical assessments of abortion within society.

The first proposition we shall put forward is that abortion demands serious ethical assessment of the situation of *both* woman and foetus. To make decisions based on the interests of *only* mother or *only* foetus is to deny the serious ethical weight that has to be placed on the personhood of the mother *and* on the potential for personhood of the foetus. This is necessary for two reasons. Firstly, the mother is a person, whose bodily integrity should be respected and valued, and secondly, since the (previable) foetus's continued existence is dependent upon the mother's body, her wishes regarding the use to which her body is put cannot be overlooked or suppressed.

No matter how much protection we may wish to give the foetus, this cannot be absolute because foetuses cannot be isolated from whatever conflicts are inherent in the human condition. Consequently, to expect complete protection for foetuses but less than complete protection for adults is to impose on foetuses an aura of idealism we do not impose on other members of the community. There *are* occasions when the welfare of the foetus will come into conflict with that of the mother, and criteria have to be formulated for taking seriously the welfare of both. We propose that one of these criteria is the extent of foetal development. We would argue that the degree of protection afforded the foetus should vary with the degree of foetal development, increasing as development proceeds. From this it follows that a seven-month-old foetus should be given greater protection than a three-day-old embryo. In terms of a gradualist position, the former is closer to realising full personhood than is the latter (Poplawski & Gillett 1991).

We suggest that foetal protection is to be abrogated where there is, or appears to be, unresolvable conflict. This will usually be between pregnant woman and foetus, although it may also involve the family unit, and could be exacerbated by serious medical circumstances afflicting the foetus or woman. The conflict will be of sufficient severity to jeopardise the integrity of the woman and/or the family. This will undoubtedly vary from one situation to another, depending on the social and religious culture in which the woman or couple is living, the degree of social and medical support available in the community, and the extent of assistance from family and friends.

We do not consider that the dilemma of abortion will be solved by restrictive legislation. This is due to the profound moral differences present in society. Many people will not be persuaded that abortion is murder, because they consider that, at certain stages during its development, the foetus is a non-person. These are legitimate ethical perspectives that are incompatible with the belief that the embryo and foetus should be given absolute protection. Any attempt to enforce legislative restrictions on people who remain unconvinced by ethical arguments is a dangerous way to proceed in a pluralist society where we tolerate a wide range of competing ethical positions and attitudes.

Those with opposing ethical positions on the status of the foetus and the legitimacy of abortion have to appreciate the force of the ethical arguments put forth by the other side. This is particularly important for health workers, who have to deal professionally with people upholding differing value systems. Conflicts of values can be expected to arise between health professionals and patients in this area, highlighting the obvious fact that doctors and nurses are also humans with their own value systems. While they should not attempt to foist their own values on their patients, every effort should also be made to safeguard personal autonomy, so that where there are procedures of which health professionals disapprove, they are not compelled to provide them, or participate in providing them, to patients.

7
Birth and Beyond

Birth Rights

The potential conflict of rights that becomes evident as a pregnancy progresses to full term becomes still more acute as the time of birth approaches. The phrase 'birthright' is usually applied to rights the child acquires at birth, yet at the same time the rights of the woman giving birth also require respect for her own sake, and not only with reference to the child's welfare. The dilemma reaches its most acute form when the birth itself threatens the life of both mother and child, with the possibility that only one can be saved. In the past some religious teaching encouraged women to 'sacrifice' themselves for the sake of the baby, arguing that the stronger moral claim was from the life yet to be lived. Such a view receives little support today. The woman giving birth is seen as the prime decider, and her own wishes, as well as her possible obligations to existing children in her family, are seen as the determining factors. Thus a decision, however painful, to ensure her own survival at the cost of the life of her unborn child would no longer be condemned as 'selfishness'. Rather, it would leave her options open for continued parenting, in a way that the 'sacrifice' of herself could not.

But what of other choices by pregnant women that do not inevitably cause the death of the baby, but may place it at risk in some way? Such questions arise with the increasing opposition to an over-medicalisation of birth and a renewed emphasis on a woman's right to choose its place and manner. There are really two separate issues here. One concerns the question of whether the use of hospital facilities and their associated high technology improves the prospects for the baby's survival and welfare, or worsens them. This question has been extensively explored by Tew (1990), who concludes that the technology has done more harm than good. The factual issue can only be resolved by continued research into the outcomes of different approaches to birth, and an attempt to define more precise criteria for technological interventions. However, a second issue concerns the priority of the woman's choice, whatever the predicted outcomes. Is the woman's right to choose how and when she gives birth an absolute one, whatever this may mean for the safety of the child?

A question of this kind inevitably involves an ethical decision about whose rights should prevail. There have been examples of court-ordered interventions that are tantamount to assault, but have been justified on the grounds that the child's welfare must outweigh the woman's rights over her own body. Is that how the dilemma described above (where birth itself threatens the welfare of both the mother and child) should be decided? Some philosophers would regard the newborn child as not yet possessing full personal status (for example Singer & Kuhse 1985) and so would presumably favour the woman's right to choose. Such a view, however, has serious hazards for the rights of children long after birth, since personhood, if defined in terms of capacity for rational thought, is not gained for some years. We would argue that (unless the mother's life is in danger) the primary medical responsibility is to ensure the safety of the child. The child is the most vulnerable party and has no capacity to ensure its own well-being. However, using court action to force a woman to undergo some medical procedure cannot be seen as an acceptable moral solution, since the assault is so great that it is likely to cause a breakdown in the mother's relationship with the child and so perhaps be equally damaging in the long run. Rather, the doctor or midwife needs to act as the child's advocate, seeking an outcome through persuasion that will respect the woman's bodily integrity, but also involve her in caring about her baby's welfare. The welfare of a child is (in our view) paramount, but at the time of birth and afterwards this welfare is intimately bound up with the mother–child relationship in all its physical and emotional dimensions. This moral assessment of the situation has been backed up recently by the British courts. The Appeal Court has ruled that a woman who was forced to undergo a caesarean section by being sectioned under the Mental Health Act was treated wrongly, since there was no evidence that she lacked competence under the terms of the relevant section of the Act. The legal situation has been summed up by Lady Justice Butler-Sloss: 'If the competent mother refuses to have the medical intervention, the doctors may not lawfully do more than attempt to persuade her' (*Guardian* 27 March 1997).

Dilemmas After Birth

> A child is born with a severe form of cri-du-chat ('cat's cry') syndrome and inherited conditions with severe mental retardation. Against medical advice, the parents request that the heart defect be corrected. This is done and some months later the child is admitted to a paediatric chronic care institution where she is unresponsive apart from occasional mewing cries.

Our impulse in medicine is to furnish help and comfort to the human beings who come to us, and to do so by using whatever technology is appropriate. The ill child, in effect, makes an appeal for love and care, and cannot repay that except by responding to the attitudes that we show. Our care for the human infant is an expression of our membership of a human community in which the dependent members call for our protection. If we were to suppress this deep commitment to members of our own species, we would undermine one of the natural wellsprings of moral understanding; therefore, we acknowledge a creative responsibility for the development of the 'little person' concerned.

However, there are some groups of children about whose potential we must think more carefully before we allow our moral concern to result in 'heroic' medicine. First, there are children who do not have any conscious appreciation of life and will never develop it. They have the physical appearance of human beings, but lack the essential functional qualities of being human, including the capacity for conscious life. If an individual can show neither any awareness of, nor response to, the care and love of other human beings, then we would seem to be on fairly safe ground in concluding that the individual is not equipped to appreciate things as mattering to it. Thus, where there is neither the capacity nor the potential for personal life, our normal medical concern to treat for recovery can be appropriately suppressed. Such children will include those with microcephaly, anencephaly, hydranencephaly, and certain other major deformities of the central nervous system. Whenever we can say that the children concerned have been born without the potential to enter into human relations, we can say that we are released from any obligation to keep them alive.

What of children who do have some capacity for participation in human relationships, but have such severe handicaps that intervention seems to gain little more than prolonged suffering? Often the decision is made to offer no treatment, apart from basic comfort and custodial care, because anything more would be cruel and fruitless if inflicted on the being concerned. This is the issue confronting those involved in a decision about the child with cri-du-chat syndrome. What was gained for anyone in the intervention to correct a heart defect, except (perhaps) some reassurance to the parents that they had done all they could for their child? When intervention also becomes the prolongation of suffering, such a reason should not be the determinative one. Instead, concern for the child must prevail.

> Alice was born with oxalosis. By the age of two she had developed stones in the kidneys and increasingly severe renal failure. For some weeks she drifted in and out of uraemic coma with her parameters being carefully monitored and adjusted by zealous junior paediatric staff. Each day she needed blood tests to check for electrolytes and acid base regulation. Every few days she needed her IV lines renewed and these were increasingly difficult to site. She was usually in pain and her small body was pale and weak. It was eventually decided, in consultation with her parents, to let her drift into uraemic coma and die.

If such decisions are morally justified, should there be a more forthright determination on the part of paediatricians and parents to eliminate handicap by much more rigorously selective treatment policies, or indeed by painlessly killing those who are defective in any serious sense?

> A couple slightly older than average look forward to their first child, only to be devastated when the child has Down syndrome. They refuse to authorise surgery for duodenal atresia, but are overridden by the courts and surgery is performed. Years later they are still having difficulties accepting that their child will not achieve the educational and other goals they had hoped for, but they love him very much.

A number of philosophers have suggested that it is only a sentimental 'speciesism' that brings about such restrictive judgments on parental wishes. For example Peter Singer, in an essay on sanctity versus quality of life (Singer 1983), argues that it is merely the fact that such defective infants are members of the species *Homo sapiens* that makes the imposition of treatment different from what defective dogs or pigs would receive. If we were concerned more rationally with the balance of happiness over suffering, we would not prolong defective human lives needlessly. Singer's challenge forces us to examine more carefully the principled basis for special concern over the lives of young and helpless human beings who suffer from handicaps.

How can we defend the idea that the ethical importance of a human being is greater than that of other animals? Is this judgment just an irrational prejudice in favour of our own species? To meet the challenge, we usually invoke facts about the wishes and desires of the individuals concerned, their conscious appreciation of life, and/or their preferences regarding what should happen to them. But, on any set of criteria of this type, it is plain to see that neonates, possibly infants, and arguably certain mentally defective children, turn out to be less well qualified candidates for ethical consideration than animals such as chimpanzees, gorillas, perhaps dolphins, and even pigs!

It is, however, unacceptable to be told not to grieve over the death of an infant or neonate because it does not really matter any more than the death of a valued family pet. Our concern for other humans goes deeper than mere regard for species membership—it is a fundamental part of our nature as ethical beings. Certain reactions, sensitivities and responses are the basis of moral judgments. Moral reasoning concerns evaluative concepts that are learned through human relationships and involve the understanding of suffering. Thus a person has a tendency to empathy towards others just because they are human; this natural empathy underlies many of our moral sensitivities. Without empathy of this very natural type, and the feelings of compassion to which it leads, a person would not 'catch on' to the reasons why moral considerations are important. Therefore, although we can argue about what is the right thing to do, we also depend on a conviction that certain things are right and that a tendency to do right rather than wrong should constrain our choices.

Another natural response is to take care of the young of one's species. This, too, is part of that foundation in human nature on which moral understanding is built. To harm a child or to exercise wanton cruelty towards another human being betrays a basic flaw in our ability to make any moral judgments at all. If one does not feel the force of the moral imperatives about caring for and protecting children, then one is impaired in one's moral thinking. That is why the death of a child, no matter how young, is a shocking tragedy. We find our noblest and most creatively altruistic tendencies enlisted in our response to children. In a way, all that is best in oneself finds a focus in the appeal of a child. To the shock of death is added the loss of that possibility of sharing and of being a better person, of watching a life unfold and respond to what one has to give.

Yet are there not circumstances in which we should carry the responsibility of a child's death as a necessary and humane action? Ironically, the sanctity with which we endow all human life often works to the detriment of those unfortunate humans whose lives hold no prospect except suffering. Singer is right to the extent that, while a dog or pig, dying slowly and painfully, will be mercifully released from its misery, a human being in similar circumstances may well have to endure its hopeless condition until the end.

These issues were raised in a very dramatic way by a celebrated Australian case in 1989 concerned with withdrawal of active treatment from a gravely disabled infant. Baby M was born with severe spina bifida and her parents (both devout Roman Catholics) argued with the doctors that further active treatment was pointless and should be withdrawn, and also that sedatives should be given to the child. Members of the Right to Life Association intervened on the ground that, if Baby M were sedated, she would in effect die from starvation. The baby did die, but at a subsequent coroner's inquiry the parents and doctors were exonerated from any wrongdoing and the members of the Right to Life Association were severely criticised (see Skene 1991).

Given that treatment decisions for the disabled newborn pose formidable legal difficulties for both parents and doctors, guidelines (which the courts could accept) are clearly necessary if we are to prevent future Baby M cases. The following represents an example of what may be a less contentious decision on non-treatment:

> A nine-month-old child develops vomiting and rapidly becomes unconscious after a minor flu-like illness. The diagnosis is Reye syndrome. She continues to worsen to the point where cerebral circulation is compromised. She has clinical brain death except for occasional extensor spasms and swallowing movements. Respirator and nasogastric feeding support continue for months until the decision is made to turn off the ventilator.

What is the right action to take in this and similar situations? A full consideration of the issue is undertaken in our discussion of euthanasia (see Chapter 12).

A preliminary answer may be attempted in terms of the fundamental orientation of medicine towards saving or salvaging human lives, an orientation that can lead to over-meddlesome medicine but whose elimination could well be a greater threat to human well-being. Doctors and nurses persevere in what can be a very demanding professional task because of a powerful presumption in favour of preserving or restoring life. Faced with a human being whose form has been distorted or defaced, the medical reaction is to expend extraordinary effort on behalf of that individual. The successes of medicine throughout history have been inspired by this impulse. Conversely, to kill or deliberately neglect an individual who is afflicted is to obey a fundamentally different impulse. A medical profession that over-treats out of misplaced therapeutic zeal is certainly to be deplored, but a less ethically admirable approach to paediatric medicine would be one that coldly sought to eliminate human handicap. Between these two extremes, responsible choices must be made, choices focused on the best interests of the individual child as far as we can predict and assess them.

A recent document by the Royal College of Paediatrics and Child Health has offered some parameters to be used for making such agonising choices. They suggest that there are five situations in which withdrawing or withholding treatment may be considered: the brain-dead child; the permanent vegetative state; the 'no chance' situation; the 'no purpose' situation; the 'unbearable' situation (Royal College of Paediatrics and Child Health 1997). Such guidelines may help clinicians and families to order their thinking in the middle of what is inevitably an emotionally fraught situation, but it would be naive to suppose that this alone can 'solve' the dilemmas. For example, the categories of 'no chance', 'no purpose', and 'unbearable' are by no means self-evident and must depend on subjective assessment of what constitutes suffering and of what could be seen as a reasonable chance. Every situation will have unique features and most will entail considerable uncertainty about the likely clinical and social outcomes. In the final analysis there can be no short-cut in the decision-making process. It will require care and support from staff who respect differing viewpoints but hold each other in mutual respect and who are prepared to spend the necessary time with parents to ensure that whatever decision is reached, it is one they feel is the best for their child.

At times, however, there can be irreconcilable differences between the parents' view of what is best for their child and the clinical staff's obligation to act in the best interests of the child. We consider this next.

Parental Decisions Regarding Treatment Options

The parental right to choose treatment for children is based on the intuition that parents are protectors of the child and responsible for its care. This is regarded as the 'natural role' of parents and is recognised universally in legal codes. It is assumed that the parents are training and nurturing the child to bring that child to the point where it can make its own decisions. We act on the presumption that the parents will make decisions in the best interests of the child and, on this basis, empower them to do so. However, in certain situations this presumption cannot be sustained.

> Anna is a five-year-old girl with a heart defect. She requires surgery in which blood will be recirculated and a transfusion given to her. Her parents object on religious grounds to her receiving any blood. The surgeon and physicians involved believe that she will die without surgery and that surgery cannot be performed without blood being given. A petition is made to the court and the child is made a ward of the court for the duration of her treatment because the court believes that the parents are not acting in her best interests.

This decision shows what we believe to be paramount in dilemmas involving children. We believe that the child's interests should come first. In Anna's case that meant overturning her parents' authority because their judgment was thought to be distorted by their religious belief so that they could not rightly discern the best interests of the child.

Other cases are much less clear-cut. In the United Kingdom, a high profile case in 2000 concerned the decision of a court, sustained on appeal, to authorise the separation of conjoined ('Siamese') twins against their parents' wishes. The hospital argued that unless the twins were separated, both would eventually die. However, one twin was totally dependent on the other for breathing and circulation and the separation would inevitably kill her. The parents believed, on religious grounds, that this act of killing was morally wrong and that they should allow nature to take its course. The court found that the killing of the weaker twin was lawful on the grounds that this was the only way to defend the life of the other. This case illustrates the hazards of assuming parental responsibility for such difficult choices. It is hard to see how the parents in this case were acting on mistaken beliefs or out of a lack of concern for their children's welfare. They simply believed that taking one life to save another was morally wrong and in this they were expressing a view shared by a very large number of people. Had, then, the courts, the right to interfere with their parental responsibility, when the issue was so morally ambiguous?

Decisions become still more difficult when a child is old enough to have a view of his or her own, but is under the legal age of consent. In most jurisdictions there is a fuzzy boundary between the age at which a child can give consent to its own treatment and the age at which parental consent must be sought. Most ethicists advise that the child be included as far as possible in the decision-making process, but for children up to at least sixteen years old the parents must give consent to medical treatment. Moreover, the legal situation in England and Wales (but not in Scotland) is that the parents and the courts can overrule a young person's refusal of treatment up to the age of eighteen years.

Once again, the moral issues here are very complex, as two recent legal cases will illustrate. The first was heard in England in 1999 and involved a young woman of fifteen, who had a fatal heart condition requiring an immediate transplant if her life was to be saved. The patient refused to have the operation, giving as her reasons her unhappiness at having another person's heart in her body and an unwillingness to undergo the continuing regimen of immuno-supressive drugs. The parents and clinicians were of the view that this refusal was not in her best interests and took the matter to court. The court overruled the patient's refusal and the transplant operation was performed, at that stage with the compliance of the patient. The second case occurred in 1999 in New Zealand, where a thirteen-year-old boy with a cancerous tumour on his knee refused to have the chemotherapy recommended by his doctors, and he subsequently died. He and his parents had strong religious convictions, believing that God would look after him. His parents were willing to consent to treatment, but would not go against their son's refusal, since they had promised him that they would not force him to have treatment. The parents are now facing manslaughter charges for failing to consent to treatment on his behalf.

Why did the doctors not take this second case to court? An explanation may be found in another high profile New Zealand case, in which parents wanted natural therapies for their child's cancer and eventually went into hiding to avoid a court ruling requiring chemotherapy. Their case elicited huge public sympathy for the parents and eventually their refusal to cooperate led to a discharge of the order. These circumstances illustrate the severe difficulties entailed in losing the cooperation of parents in the relatively ambiguous circumstances of cancer therapy. It is very hard to ensure the welfare of the child if parents are unwilling to cooperate in the treatment. Different understandings of what constitutes the welfare of the child are not easily resolved by courts and—in an ideal situation—the aim should be to find a way of working with the parents that does not unduly affect their child's welfare. In cases where competent young people—who are legally under the age of consent—refuse treatment, the respect for autonomy, which underlies all medical care, must surely be a powerful factor in any decision about recourse to the courts. We need to be very sure that our assessment of the person's best interests is genuinely more accurate than their own assessment (see Huxtable 2000).

Child Abuse and Child Protection

There are, however, other circumstances in which the duty to act in the best interests of the patient is much clearer.

Dion is eighteen months old. He is admitted with fits, vomiting, and irritability. Upon examination, the doctors find that he has haemorrhages in his retina and bruises on his limbs, with a superficially infected burn on his foot. A CT scan reveals a chronic left-sided subdural haematoma and a skeletal survey shows a healing fracture of the left humerus and broken ribs on the right side. The doctors interview the mother and her live-in partner. Social Welfare is informed and the child protection team comes to see the child, who is made a ward of court. Burrholes are performed to remove the subdural haematoma.

The likely course of events in this case is that the child will be removed from the custody of the mother until the child protection team can take steps to remove the danger to Dion, and assure themselves that he will not suffer by being returned to his mother's care. She may have a part in this decision, but she will not be authorised to make decisions for the child as she has failed in the role of guardian. There may, of course, be reasons for her actions or for her allowing someone to injure the child, but these are not material to decisions about the welfare of the child in the short term. The short-term priority is to protect the child from harm and to act in his best interests. Long-term interests can be considered as soon as it is clear that the child is safe and unlikely to be more damaged than he already has been by the physical abuse he has received.

All these decisions are difficult and require careful judgment. The doctor must take special precautions in dealing with child abuse cases. A colleague ought always to be called on (where this is possible) to validate findings and confirm the decision. Those with the responsibility for overall care must in particular give very careful consideration to the diagnosis and its evidential base. Social Welfare ought to be involved as soon as the diagnosis is clear. In this situation information gained by the doctor is not under the normal confidentiality constraints. It can and should be shared with those who are entrusted with the child's protection. Prior to their involvement, it should be used to firmly establish the need for that involvement.

The health care professional should be aware of the tangled loyalties and dynamics of these situations. A doctor, nurse, or social worker may well feel committed to and sorry for a young, perhaps disadvantaged, mother of a child like Dion. This mother may be as needy as her child, and the health care professional may look upon her as a client requiring special support. This should not be allowed to cloud the issue of the best interests of the child. Once the child is safe from harm, the situation can be addressed more calmly and deliberately than is possible in the 'messy' period when suspicions abound and nothing has been done to bring the problem to the attention of those whose expertise is needed. Often, by taking things out of the hands of the non-coping parent or parents, the doctor can relieve the guilt and tension in the fraught and complex situation. In any event we must recognise, in cases of child abuse, that our loyalties clearly lie with more than one person, and that the person most at risk is also the person least likely to be able to safeguard his or her own interests.

The 'Best Interests of the Child' Criterion

The problems surrounding child abuse highlight the fact that children are not possessions of their parents but human individuals in the process of becoming persons in their own right. Thus we have to weigh the wishes of parents against what is best for the child wherever there is reason to believe they are not in full agreement. There are not many situations where this is the case. Often parents will see more clearly than doctors that a child has had enough and that some 'heroic' treatment should be discontinued. (In this they are often supported by nurses, who are closest to the child in day-by-day clinical care.) However, there are situations where the parents will be so upset by what has happened or is happening to their child that they will not make a good decision.

> Barbara is a twelve-year-old girl who is brought into hospital after collapsing at home. She is found to have had a haemorrhage in the right occipital lobe of her brain. By the time she is stabilised it is clear that she is beginning to develop a right temporal pressure cone with dilatation of the right pupil and a steady deterioration in her conscious level as measured by the Glasgow Coma Score. An angiogram shows an AV malformation based in the right lateral ventricle of the brain. The need for an operation to save her life, the fact that she has partially lost her sight, and the risk of some residual damage to the brain are all explained rather hurriedly to the parents in seeking their consent for urgent surgery.
> Barbara is a very attractive girl and, when they are faced by these rather dire prospects (although it is mentioned that her long-term prospects are good) and the need for her to have her head shaved for a brain operation, both parents, the mother most vehemently, say that they cannot consent to surgery and that she should be allowed to die in peace. Words like 'brain damage', 'vegetable', 'like a horror camp victim' and so on punctuate their discussion. The doctors and nurses try to reason with them but to no avail. Eventually, having informed their chief medical officer, they prepare to go ahead with the operation. The medical officer informs the local child protection team. The child is in the process of being made a ward of court when the brother of Barbara's mother contacts the medical team to say that the parents will sign consent for surgery.

In this situation the health care team was forced to take extreme measures to save the life of a girl who would almost certainly fare very well despite her urgent neurosurgical problem. It was likely that she would have a partial visual defect, but otherwise her vision would be intact and she would function normally. It would certainly have been wrong to concur with a decision in which emotional disturbance would cost this girl her life.

> Libby is thirteen. Her parents are separated because of problems between them and related problems involving sexual abuse of Libby and her nine-year-old sister. Libby has a relapsing leukemia that has resisted three cycles of chemotherapy and produced a malignant meningitis also unresponsive to intrathecal care. Libby and her mother have decided that comfort measures are all she can cope with, and the paediatric oncologist agrees. The father contacts the superintendent and says that if anything less than full, active treatment measures are used he will see to it that the Health Board and the doctors involved are sued for manslaughter. He demands to see his daughter and, after an emotional scene, Libby tearfully decides she has to keep fighting.

Here we need to be especially aware of the strain put on Libby by the wider dynamics of her situation. It would seem that the health care professionals involved, particularly female professionals, need to get very close to Libby to enable her to make authentic and undistorted decisions about her own future. It would be unlikely, in this situation, that the father's legal threats would get very far but, on all sides, the decisions would be more secure if discussions could be clearly documented, at least in outline, and clear medical and ethical reasons given for the choices made.

Resource Allocation and At-risk Children

The special regard in which we hold children can lead to unwise resource allocation decisions. It is often possible to obtain large amounts of money by using graphic portrayals of the plight of sick children. This can mean that health care resources are not, in the larger picture, used wisely. To avoid this we need to bear in mind a couple of crucial points affecting resource allocation to paediatrics.

First, money spent is not always to meet a one-off cost as often the intervention prevents or mitigates complications that would later be very costly in health care terms.

> The neonatal unit was threatened with a cut to funding that would mean it could not treat as many children as before. Members of the unit had two choices: they could either accept an overall budgetary constraint or adopt a policy of non-treatment for all children under 750 grams. They pointed out that the latter policy would mean that over three years, approximately one child who might survive with some disability, would instead die. This saving was thought to be minuscule

compared with the overall throughput. It was also pointed out that most of the under 750 gram children who actually survived did so with good quality of life and the policy would condemn these children to die. It was finally pointed out that there were children of birth weight greater than 750 grams who ought not to be treated, and yet the policy would require such children to receive treatment regardless. The alternative was to enable joint decisions to be made by parents and the neonatal team, and to encourage cessation of treatment where the prognosis was hopeless in children of any birth weights.

This example suggests that informed conjoint decisions should remain the cornerstone of health care policy for neonates: parents must be given realistic prognoses; and the option of care, but not heroic intervention, should be endorsed for those children who will either never achieve conscious life or will experience little except suffering. This is a far more sensitive response to shortages of funds than heavy-handed lines drawn across the continuum of birth weights or other parameters.

Unfortunately, spectacular reports from centres in other parts of the world can often prompt a dramatic appeal for some new and unproven therapy to be made available to a child with a tragic condition. This kind of drama often works to the detriment of other sick children because of overall funding restrictions.

The correct ethical response to such an appeal is a careful and measured consideration of the costs and benefits of the proposed high-profile therapy, and a diligent examination of local and often cheaper, but equally effective, alternatives. If this were underpinned by honest, unbiased medical opinion that was open-minded enough to give alternatives a fair hearing, much misleading optimism and disappointment would be avoided. The almost hysterical playing on our natural sympathy for children can only be destructive in the long term and costly for the community concerned. What is more, it threatens the credibility of real medical advances for suffering children. Health care professionals, in particular, ought to be aware of this danger and associated abuses.

Children as Research Participants

Finally we come to a topic that is more fully dealt with in Chapter 13: the use of human beings in research projects. The general issues associated with research are discussed later but, in the case of children, a fundamental dilemma arises: unless the research project can be shown to be of direct benefit to the child (and this would be a rare circumstance), has anyone the right to enlist a child in the project? In all other situations of consent on behalf of children, the guiding principle is the best interests of the child. How can a parent—or any other person—volunteer a child for procedures that are not for the child's benefit and may carry an element of risk?

One way of dealing with this difficulty is to insist that, whatever the legal age for consent, a child should always be consulted about research participation, and no action should be taken to which the child does not give clear assent. This is only a partial solution, however. In the first place, a significant proportion of paediatric research is carried out on neonates, or on children well below the age of understanding. Moreover, even when a child is old enough to be given an explanation, the scope of comprehension may be quite limited, and the influence of parents or other significant adults on the decision-making process will be considerable. One cannot make young children into the equivalent of adult volunteers.

This leaves two options: to ban all non-therapeutic research on infants and young children; or to find some other form of moral justification. If a ban is to be avoided we must develop a broader view of 'benefit' than that which applies only to an individual child. We all, adults and children, have an interest in the progress of medicine through the application of well-designed and effective research. Children, in particular, have an interest in the progress of paediatric medicine, and would be harmed by a ban that prevented whole areas of that field from being adequately researched. Thus, although a specific project might be of no conceivable benefit to the individual child participating as a research subject, the prevention of all such forms of research could well present a hazard. For example, the child acting as a control subject in a study of asthmatic children might never need therapy for this form of respiratory disorder, but could well benefit from an improved understanding of therapeutic measures in paediatric respiratory medicine generally. Children might also, as many adults do, wish to help others like themselves. Arguably, they should not be denied the chance to act altruistically.

Taking this broader view, we may countenance the involvement of children in research provided that some stringent conditions are observed. First, it can never be justifiable to volunteer another to undergo any significant risk for what can be only a very indirect benefit. Thus all paediatric research that is of no direct benefit to the research subjects must carry minimal or negligible risk. In assessing such risks, the dangers of creating anxiety or embarrassment in young children must also be avoided.

Second, parental consent to participation of a child does not of itself legitimise a research project. There is a special responsibility on the researcher, and on those committees vetting the research, to ensure that the project is well designed, safe, and worth doing. Parents may not be in a position to assess this fully and objectively, and may be predisposed to cooperate out of a sense of indebtedness to the medical institutions caring for their child.

Third, every effort should be made to turn the child into a research participant rather than merely a passive recipient of procedures he or she cannot understand. Even if valid consent cannot be obtained, the active involvement of the child should be sought where possible, and research should never be allowed to proceed when the child is clearly distressed by the procedures. Some have proposed that children's representatives be appointed to research ethics committees.

Finally, no research that could equally well be done on adults should ever be done on children. Children should never be used merely because they are accessible (as patients in an institution, for example) and reasonably compliant. Research with children as participants should be necessary for the welfare of children in particular. In this way we begin to teach children the mutual obligations within which we live, and help them to recognise that special form of identification with the needs of others that leads to altruism. The child who learns to care for the sufferings of other children is much more than a mere research subject. The experience becomes a source of learning about the purpose of research and the meaning of the medical enterprise as a whole.

Thus, as we have been stressing throughout this chapter, there is much to be learned from paediatric medicine about the basic moral values that underlie medicine as a whole. When we learn to respect the vulnerability of children, and to enhance the development of their capacities as autonomous moral agents, we see the humanistic roots of medicine from which the whole endeavour of health care gains its stability and strength.

8
Organ and Tissue Transplantation

Introduction

The need for organ donors is vast. In the United States alone, there were 55 789 people on the organ waiting list at the end of 1997, with kidneys and livers being the most sought after organs. An analysis of trends in organ transplantation has shown that for the period 1989–96 the total number of transplants increased in both Western Europe and North America. Alarmingly, some countries such as France and Germany have witnessed reductions in organ donations over a similar period of time.

Surveys of public attitudes to organ donation have consistently shown that although people are aware of the need for donor organs, they are reluctant to donate their own organs or to consent to the donation of organs from relatives (Evans & Manninen 1988). One such study explored the reasons behind the refusal to consent to organ transplantation (Sanner 1994b). These included:

- *the illusion of lingering life*—a feeling that the integrity of the dead body should be maintained, as if the deceased continues to be regarded as a living person;
- *the need to respect the dead* as a way of showing respect for the individual who once was;
- *distrust* of the medical establishment and biomedical developments and of the criteria for brain death, and a feeling of anxiety concerning one's power-lessness;
- *the feeling that transplantation is contrary to nature*, including discomfort at the thought of one's organs surviving in another person's body, or a fear of offending God or Nature.

In the United States, it has been estimated that it may be possible to increase the number of donors available, by identifying and then applying the measures used in states with the highest organ procurement rates (such as Arizona, Florida and Maine). These strategies include the instigation of high profile public and professional education campaigns, more liberal donor selection criteria, and state legislation to stimulate procurement activity.

A crucial ethical requirement when using cadaveric organs for transplantation is the informed and free consent of the donor prior to death.

Consent in Cadaveric Organ Donation

Consent in cadaveric organ donation is paramount, underlying as it does the fundamental ethical requirement to respect individual freedom of choice and self-determination. Consent for donation is normally discussed with reference to two diametrically opposing systems: *opt-in* and *opt-out*. Of these two, the opt-in (*informed consent*) system has predominated in most Western societies until recent years. An opt-in system stipulates that consent is explicitly required for organs to be removed for transplantation purposes. The opt-in position contends that consent is best provided by the donor when still alive—in the form of an organ donor card or data on a driver's licence, or by the person's family after death. In contrast, under the opt-out (*presumed consent*) system, consent is assumed, unless people have expressly stated otherwise during their lifetime. Various intermediate positions between these two extremes also exist.

The strength of the opt-in policy lies with its recognition of the importance of the integrity of the dead body and the respect it accords the autonomy of the deceased. Giving organs for transplantation reflects altruism on the part of the deceased, or their next-of-kin, and directs attention towards the importance of giving rather than receiving.

A drawback of the opt-in position is its focus on the wishes of the deceased to the exclusion of all others, including the next-of-kin, as well as the potential recipients and their families and even society in general. The exclusion of the interests of society is more subtle, but it is important to recognise it, since society is obliged to shoulder the economic burden of those who could benefit from transplants. The inadequate supply of organs for transplantation under the opt-in system has led to considerable pressure to move away from this approach in favour of an opt-out policy.

The presumed consent (opt-out) policy operates in a number of countries including Israel, Singapore, 60 per cent of Europe, and some US states. In order to opt-out under this system, one must carry a 'non-organ donor' card. In France, parental consent for removal of organs from children is presumed, and in Austria, any deceased foreigners' organs may be taken.

An opt-out policy for kidney donation by non-Muslims was introduced in Singapore in 1987, with passage of the *Human Organ Transplant Act*. The donation of kidneys by Muslims is voluntary, as is the donation of other organs for all citizens. Various incentives and disincentives have been incorporated in this policy in order to encourage compliance. For example, non-dissenters of the policy will be given priority access to kidneys; dissenters who withdraw their objections will have the same access as others, but only after two years from the date of their withdrawal; immediate family members of kidney donors enjoy a 50 per cent waiver of all government hospital charges for five years following the donation.

This system can be criticised on the grounds that it is discriminatory (against the Muslim population in this instance), and coercive (Gillon 1995). However, the element of coercion may not overshadow the motives of those who donate their organs for humanitarian and altruistic reasons (Teo 1991), and an opt-out clause exists to protect against coercion. In practice, however, an opt-out clause cannot protect the uninformed, and if individuals and families are not aware of their rights, then presumed consent could become a means of avoiding consent altogether.

The rationale of the presumed consent system is that far more organs become available for transplantation (as demonstrated in Singapore and Belgium). This pragmatic argument is often rejected on the grounds that presumed consent undermines an individual's self-determination. Proponents of presumed consent argue that the value of self-determination is eclipsed by the benefit of the additional lives saved by this policy.

There are those, such as Kennedy (1988), who contend that the debate must be broadened to encompass a whole set of competing interests: the deceased; the spouse and relatives; the potential donor; and society at large. Kennedy's sympathies lie with the potential organ recipient and society at large, since he sees this as the only means by which the needs of those with organ failure can be satisfied. In his view it is inappropriate to place the interests of the deceased above those of the spouse, and in turn to place the spouse's interests above those of the dying and society. But if this type of position is accepted, any preferences expressed by the deceased prior to death are likely to be overridden. If this were to eventuate, it is preferable to increase the supply of organs by other means, thereby retaining ethical interest in the dead body.

Apart from these opt-in and opt-out schemes, there are intermediate positions such as the policy of *required request*, which operates in many states in the United States. According to this policy, hospital administrators or physicians are legally responsible for ensuring that the next-of-kin or legal guardians are asked about their willingness to donate the deceased's organs and tissues after death (Caplan 1984). However, the policy of required request appears to have had little effect on the availability of donated organs.

A related proposal is *mandated choice* under which individuals would be required to declare their preference either for or against becoming an organ donor at a nominated time, such as at the renewal of a driver's licence, or when income tax forms are filed. According to its proponents, this approach promotes individual autonomy in organ donation decisions, and reduces stress on surviving family members and physicians, by eliminating doubt as to the deceased's wishes (Council for Ethical and Judicial Affairs 1994).

Additional possibilities are based on a form of *payment* for cadaveric organ donation. Peters (1991) has proposed that a death benefit be paid to motivate families of potential organ donors. In reply, Pellegrino (1991) has argued that this undermines the consent process, since a family does not have proprietary rights over a relative's dead body and 'as a once-living person it is entitled to a certain dignity'.

A more extreme strategy of payment involves a 'rewarded gifting' system, where people are provided with an incentive to seriously consider selling their organs (for example, Brams 1977). Such incentives could include: payment to the deceased's relatives to cover funeral costs or outstanding medical expenses, health insurance rebates, or tax breaks for those who agree in advance to donate their organs at death. Proponents of this system justify it on the grounds that it may increase the transplantation success rate by matching buyers and sellers to organs in advance, while at the same time respecting individual autonomy and allowing altruism free rein.

Proposals for payment for cadaveric organ donation beg the question as to whether it is acceptable for human organs to be viewed as commodities to be bought and sold (Teo 1992). Discussions of the special moral significance attributed to the human body (see Chapter 4) suggest that to do so would strip the body of human dignity (Kass 1985a). Moreover, under such a scheme, values like altruism and goodwill may fall by the wayside, and one has to question whether this can be justified even for the lofty purpose of saving lives.

Other suggestions to remedy the poor responses to organ procurement have included: educating the public by allaying fears that potential donors may not receive sufficiently aggressive medical treatment in the event of an accident, making a public commitment that cadavers will be respectfully treated, and ensuring that there are fair policies for distributing donated organs (Teo 1992). Other strategies include improving the diagnosis of brain-dead patients to increase the cadaver donor pool, and exploring further the use of animal sources (see Xenotransplantation, later in this chapter).

The success of organ procurement in any given country is likely to reflect the priority given to transplantation in terms of funding and health care resources. For example, Spain has dramatically increased its rate of organ donation through centralisation of transplantation services, information on donors and patients, the appointment of specially trained transplant coordinators, and media management allowing open and positive communication with the general public (Boddington 1996). By improving the efficiency of central distribution systems, many of the perceived failings of an opt-in scheme may be eliminated, while altruism may be maintained as the ethical bedrock of donation.

Organs from Living Donors

The purchase of kidneys from living donors for transplantation appears to be almost commonplace in some countries. Mostly the sellers are poor and healthy, while the purchasers are rich and unhealthy. The reaction of many public figures to this trade in human kidneys has been one of moral outrage, stemming principally from the notion that it is unethical to sell parts of the human body for money.

There has been widespread acceptance that a patient's relatives may donate a kidney for altruistic reasons. They are volunteers, and may well consider it a privilege to do this for a loved one. Donations to patients other than relatives are also approved, provided that donors are made aware of the short- and long-term hazards of the procedure and understand that they are freely and voluntarily giving their fully informed consent to the donation. There appear to be no ethical reasons against this, and perhaps the altruism and risk-taking involved are to be encouraged.

But what about selling organs? It is difficult to see why organ donation for money is inherently wrong, especially if the money is to be used to buy education or health care for a close relative. In this case it could, once again, be an example of altruism, the motives being ones of concern and care for others. In terms of a marketplace philosophy, the selling of organs may serve to recirculate cash from the haves to the have-nots. However, some are far from convinced by arguments of this kind and have compared the selling of kidneys with prostitution. But, as with prostitution, it is difficult to identify the guilty party. Is it the donor who sells part of his or her body in a once-only deal, or is it the purchaser who pays for what he or she cannot live without? Is it the broker who makes possible the exchange, or the transplant surgeon desperate to help the patient? These are not easy ethical questions, especially when framed in a world characterised by frightening inequality in wealth and access to health care at the same time that there is major failure to harvest all potential cadaveric organs.

The one factor in this debate that is ethically unacceptable is exploitation. This is implicit in a marketplace situation, and yet once again the question is: who is exploiting whom? There may be emotional exploitation of a reluctant donor by family members, financial exploitation of a reluctant donor by relatives or a broker, or various forms of exploitation by the medical profession and intermediaries. These dangers are present in any form of brokerage for profit, especially where the financial stakes are high. Not surprisingly, therefore, financial deals for organs almost inevitably mean that money—rather than medical need—determines which patients receive kidneys. While it may be possible to avoid this, it would be horrendously difficult to administer. Consequently, whatever procedures are permitted in this area need to be carried out under stringent guidelines designed to protect living donors from all forms of exploitation.

This debate highlights the tension surrounding any use of human organs for transplantation—balancing the 'good' of the transplantation and the 'evil' of the source of the organs. This applies whether the organs come from dead or living donors, although the ethical issues vary between the two groups. The emphasis in the former is on the tragedy resulting in the death, and in the latter on the risks attached to the donation procedure. The nature of the necessary informed consent also differs in the two cases, although an element of moral complicity is present in both situations.

Use of Anencephalics in Transplantation

Each year in the United States, between 40 and 70 per cent of the children on transplant waiting lists die before appropriately sized organs become available. While the majority of adult organs are donated following motor vehicle crashes, few children become donors in this manner. Such an extreme shortage in 'child-sized' organs for donation has prompted proposals that organs be taken from infants suffering from *anencephaly*, a condition in which major portions of the brain, skull, and scalp are congenitally absent.

Organ transplantation from anencephalic infants is only feasible for live births, which occur in approximately 25 to 45 per cent of cases. In most instances, these infants will die within a few hours or days of birth from cardio-respiratory arrest, but during this brief period residual brainstem function allows circulatory and respiratory systems to function naturally. Consequently, these infants are not dead using a whole brain definition of death (see Chapter 11).

Some physicians have kept anencephalic infants 'alive' on ventilation until brain death is diagnosed and organs are harvested, in order to prevent oxygen deprivation making the organs unsuitable for transplantation. Because there is no possibility of recovery in anencephalic infants, their placement on life-support is solely for the benefit of someone else. In view of the dilemmas inherent in such life-prolonging procedures it has been suggested that whole brain death criteria should be amended to include higher brain death, or that a new 'brain-absent' category be created to cover anencephalics (Harrison 1986b). Anencephalic infants are dying but they are not dead, and it is questionable whether they should be classed as such for the sake of organ procurement.

A number of reasons have been put forward to justify the use of anencephalic infants as organ donors. The first is the overwhelming demand for suitable transplants (Caplan 1987), yet despite the obvious need, this is not sufficient justification for the use of anencephalic infants.

Second, the donation of organs from anencephalic infants may be beneficial for the parents as they are able to feel that their child's life has had meaning

(Harrison 1986a). Studies have revealed that parents are in general willing to donate, however, the procedures involved in organ harvesting may impact negatively on their ability to accept the death of their infant and to grieve appropriately (Stierman 1987). In light of this, claims of a reduction in parental distress through organ donation need to be substantiated.

A third reason used as justification for procurement of anencephalic organs is that these infants are beyond suffering; they cannot be harmed, and, hence, have no interests in the way they are treated (Caplan 1987). Yet, prolonging the biological life of anencephalic infants in order to procure their organs has to be questioned, amounting as it does to the use of the body of *one* to serve the purposes of *another*. In cases such as these, recognising the viewpoint of the parents is important, given the significance of the close relationship between the mother and anencephalic foetus/infant. The parents' wish to maintain a pregnancy to term, with the prospect of donating the infant's organs, constitutes substantial justification for transplantation. However, the strictures already discussed are considerable and will mean that only a limited number of anencephalics will become available for donation purposes.

Foetal Neural Transplantation

Foetal neural transplantation burst upon the public scene in the late 1980s as a promising avenue of research for neurodegenerative disorders such as Parkinson's disease and Huntington's disease. At the same time, it raised a great deal of contention in both scientific and ethical circles. Over the last twenty years, clinical transplantation studies have been carried out worldwide on several hundred patients with Parkinson's disease. These studies suggest that grafts of human foetal midbrain tissue can survive for a long period in the human brain, restore innervation to the basal ganglia, and provide symptomatic relief in patients with Parkinson's disease (Bluml et al. 1999). It remains to be seen whether these and other findings are sufficient to demonstrate that grafting is an effective treatment for the disease.

The controversy surrounding foetal neural transplantation stems from the fact that the tissue used is derived from foetuses made available by induced abortion. In light of this, Gillam (1989) recognises four major positions in relation to the significance of abortion for the foetal transplantation debate:

1   Foetal tissue transplants are wrong because experimental results to date are not good enough to warrant clinical application.
2   Foetal tissue transplants are wrong because abortion is morally wrong and the wrongness of abortion cannot be isolated from any subsequent ethical decision concerning use of the foetal tissue.

3   Foetal tissue transplants are acceptable because there is nothing morally wrong with abortion. Any safeguards that are required are to protect the woman having the abortion.

4   Foetal tissue transplants are acceptable even if abortion is considered morally wrong. Such a separation is feasible because the two procedures are morally separate, as long as safeguards are in place to ensure that the abortion decision is kept separate from the transplant decision.

Position 1, that of *scientific pragmatism*, is familiar to everyone in clinical research. Premature use of new techniques or procedures is unethical as is the initiation of *ad hoc* clinical studies in the absence of a clear protocol, which includes standardised patient selection and surgical technique, and rigorous follow-up by the centres performing the procedure. This position leaves the door open for future clinical developments and by the same token may call a complete halt to them.

Position 2 may be characterised as an *abortion-dependent* viewpoint because the opinion held by some of the abhorrence of the act of abortion taints any possible beneficial uses of the resulting foetal material. The two acts are inextricably linked and this renders someone who uses the material from an aborted foetus an accessory to premeditated killing. Exponents of this position are concerned that clinical use of aborted material will lead to an increase in the rate of induced abortion in the community, and will cause women to become pregnant in order to serve as a source of foetal material.

Position 3, the *clinical benefit (abortion-irrelevant)* stance, regards induced abortion as of limited moral concern when placed alongside the potential benefits of transplantation. Implicit in this stance is a difference in the moral status of foetus and adult; the foetus having a lower status than that of both the mother and the patient. Restrictions are called for, but these reflect the mother's interests rather than those of the foetus.

Position 4 may be regarded as an *abortion-independent* stance. This position acknowledges the profound respect accorded to a foetus on the basis of its potential to become a fully formed human person, yet it allows the use of foetal material in the same way that adult human organs are used for transplantation purposes following morally questionable or tragic circumstances. The thrust of this position depends on one's ability to view as morally acceptable a procedure (transplantation) that would not be possible if it were not for the possibly morally unacceptable procedure (induced abortion).

Of the four positions illustrated, the final one appears to reflect the stance of most members of society. This position, however, has been criticised on grounds of *moral complicity*; that is, the transplantation fails to disentangle itself from the moral evil of the underlying abortion, thereby implicating the scientist in this act. However, the moral complicity argument is being used too selectively, since if it is to be employed in this case, it should also apply to discussions of other areas dependent upon the use of human material. For example, is there complicity in the road toll when organs are used from the victims of road crashes? in homicide when organs are transplanted from murder victims? or in poverty when cadavers of the destitute are used for dissection? In these cases there appears to be moral distance between the evil and the moral good. As a general principle we act on the assumption that good can come (albeit indirectly) from evil and we are prepared to benefit from tragedies. This is an ethically valid stance provided that we are in no way responsible for the tragedies and would have prevented them had we been in a position to do so.

The use of human material in medicine is a reality; while it is not always justified, it sometimes is. The ethical question, therefore, is not *whether* this should be done, but *how* it should be done. The benefits expected to accrue from the use of human tissue and the needs and interests of all groups involved must be assessed and a balance met. Guidelines for the use of foetal tissue include:

1 the foetus must be dead, with the tissue being taken from a foetal cadaver;
2 the abortion is not to be influenced in any way by the prospect of foetal grafting, its manner and timing being unaffected by such procedures;
3 the abortion and the grafting are to be kept completely separate;
4 there is a genuine possibility of significant benefit to a specific patient or patients suffering from a specific (neurological) disease;
5 the benefit expected from the therapy or research is greater than any harm that might be attached to the use of aborted foetuses;
6 this form of therapy is used as a last resort, all conventional forms of therapy having been found inadequate;
7 there is fully informed consent by the pregnant woman to any procedures that might affect her, and appropriate consent (proxy consent according to some writers) for the use of foetal material;
8 the recipient is in a position to provide fully informed consent;
9 there is anonymity between donor and recipient, excluding the possibility of any relationship between them;
10 the research design should be sound so that the study contributes in a substantial way to ongoing understanding of the grafting procedure.

While the existence of guidelines such as these is commendable, they do not guarantee that research of an ethically questionable nature will never be undertaken.

Xenotransplantation

The term 'xenotransplantation' covers all procedures involving the transfer of tissues between different species. It includes therapies, such as the transplantation of pig heart valves into humans, and more recent controversial experiments, such as implanting human foetal neural cells into rats to investigate neuronal growth patterns, and the insertion of human genes into animals to reduce xenograft rejection rates.

The ever-increasing gap between the supply and demand of cadaveric organs for conventional same-species transplantation (allotransplantation) has been the driving force behind the search for alternative organ sources. Xenotransplantation also circumvents the ethical dilemmas associated with the use of human foetal tissue derived from induced abortion.

Research indicates that xenotransplantation is worth pursuing as a therapeutic option. Animal organs, such as kidneys, could be used as replacement or 'bridging' organs for patients who are waiting for human organs to become available. There have been encouraging results with the experimental technique of transplanting foetal neural tissue into patients suffering from neurodegenerative diseases and tranplanting porcine pancreatic cells into diabetics.

Even at the scientific level, there are conflicting viewpoints. Some would like to halt further development on account of costs and unresolved issues. The US Food and Drug Administration has announced a *de facto* ban on clinical trials of xenotransplants from non-human primates to humans, whereas the medical journal the *Lancet* feels the time is nigh to leave the laboratory (Editorial 1999).

Rejection Problems

From a scientific perspective, the biggest obstacle in xenotransplantation is host immune rejection of the transplanted tissue, a problem also encountered in allotransplantation. However, in xenotransplantation there are more 'discordant signals' (resulting from the donor and host cell-surface markers differing from one another), leading to an increase in the activation and intensity of the host's immune response. There are three main types of rejection: hyperacute, delayed graft, and T-cell mediated rejection (Weiss 1998).

The rejection problems encountered in the first transplantations of kidneys from both chimpanzees and baboons into human patients in the 1960s may have installed mistrust into what was a new field of research. The introduction of immunosuppressive drugs in the early 1980s prompted further attempts at transplantation from baboons to humans, all of which culminated in failure (Nelson 1992). The most widely publicised of these was the case of Baby Fae, an infant born with a fatal form of congenital heart disease who, at the age of fifteen days, became the recipient of a baboon's heart. The infant survived for only twenty days, but the surgical team responsible for the operation believed the outcome was sufficiently favourable to warrant further investigation of the procedure (Bailey et al. 1985). They reported that the regime of immunosuppressive drugs they had used had almost totally prevented cell-mediated rejection, and that graft failure had instead resulted from a progressive, potentially avoidable response to the incompatible blood group.

Advances in genetic modification techniques (Weiss 1998) give reason to believe that some types of rejection may be substantially overcome in the future. For example, hyperacute reaction may be overcome by the incorporation of human genes into donor pigs.

For various reasons, many now favour the use of organs from the pig as opposed to non-human primates for transplantation (Nuffield Council on Bioethics 1996). The reasons for this include: those primate species most closely related to humans are endangered, and thus officially protected; pigs are domesticated, have large litters, and can be bred in a pathogen-free environment; the pig has a similar physiology to human beings in terms of the heart, liver and pancreatic islets; and pig organs grow rapidly to the size of human ones.

Passage of Pathogens

Xenotransplantation creates a ready passage for viruses, since both physical barriers and natural host immunity are compromised in transplant recipients. The usual immunological physical barriers, like skin and mucosal surfaces, offer no protection against viruses transplanted into cells placed within the body (Weiss 1998). Since transplant recipients are routinely given immunosuppressive drugs to prevent rejection of the transplant, these patients make ideal hosts for viruses and other micro-organisms. Unfortunately, immunosuppressive therapy has its drawbacks, since it may allow for the activation of latent pathogens, such as endogenous retroviruses, as well as increasing the host's susceptibility to pathogens.

Unknowns in Xenozoonotic Infections

Xenotransplantation is considered by some to be too risky, due to the potential for xenozoonosis or xenosis (the transfer of infection via xenotransplantation). This risk is difficult to assess because of numerous unknown factors. Since viruses such as ebola, and morbilliviruses such as distemper, can cross species barriers to infect humans (Formenty et al. 1999), retroviruses or other pathogens from animals have the potential to infect human cells. It is not known whether these agents will replicate, or even more seriously, cause a communicable disease in graft recipients (Tackaberry & Ganz 1998).

Another problem is that pathogens that may be latent or inconsequentially pathogenic in the donor animal may cause significant disease in a human recipient. Additionally, novel organisms may have unrecognised clinical symptoms, making infectious agents difficult to identify and treat (Weiss 1998).

In the pig genome, there are at least three known porcine endogenous retroviruses (PERVs); two of these have been shown to infect human cells in culture. This may or may not occur *in vivo*. To date, none of the recipients of porcine islet cell xenotransplants nor those who have been extracorporeally attached to pig kidneys, have shown evidence of PERV infection (Paradis et al. 1999). Appropriate biosecurity of source animals may well eliminate most of the risks from infectious agents.

Public Health and Informed Consent

Xenotransplantation could have a serious impact on the general population, since those who have not received organs could be affected by xenozoonotic infections. If this occurs, the people potentially at risk will include those close to the recipients, as well as others further afield. In light of this, it has been suggested that recipients and those close to them will have to be monitored for the rest of their lives (Clark 1999). Widespread public discussion on developments in xenotransplantation should also be encouraged. If the spread of infections turns out to be as wide as postulated by some, then the extent and even nature of informed consent will need to be revisited with the potential for consent being sought from both the recipients and their intimates, and even from the general public.

It is at this juncture that clinical and ethical considerations meet head on, since a balance will have to be found between patients' autonomy and the right of the wider public to be protected from risks of cross-species infections. In other words, the interests of the individual are inseparable from more general interests.

Further Considerations

The 'unnaturalness' of xenotransplantation is espoused as an argument against its further development and use. Yet, anything humans do to alter the natural order is, by definition, unnatural, and so xenotransplantation may be no more unnatural than the use of antibiotics in the treatment of infection, or than many surgical procedures. The ethical issue is not with the unnaturalness *per se*, but with its consequences for the well-being of patients. Each procedure stands or falls on its merits and each can be justified as long as the intended good outweighs the possible disadvantages. Consequently, arguments based on unnaturalness alone are not sufficient to condemn xenotransplantation.

A possibility that appears to elicit the most alarm is the potential for the blurring of species boundaries by xenotransplantation. Consider first the use of organs that serve primarily mechanical functions, like kidneys, hearts or, lungs. In clinical terms, the transplantation of a kidney can be compared ethically to the use of dialysis equipment, since the therapeutic goals are comparable, regardless of whether the organ comes from a human or a pig. If the transplanted kidney functions to keep the person alive and to increase their quality of life, the ethical issues accompanying xenotransplantation and allotransplantation are comparable. This suggests that species boundaries are of limited importance compared to the potential benefits of xenotransplantation. Had the pig been genetically altered to express human proteins in order to prevent graft rejection, species boundaries would still not have become blurred. Only a few out of several million human genes would be inserted into the pig, which would continue to look, behave, and be regarded as a pig.

On the other hand, the transplantation of neural cells from one species to another has the potential to affect personality and personhood, and could possibly have implications for an individual's humanity. Does this form of treatment differ substantially from standard neurosurgery and psychosurgery, which may cause considerable damage, in an attempt to help a patient? Procedures such as these are generally regarded as ethical, as long as they are carried out with a therapeutic rationale and in the best interests of the patient. The therapeutic intent behind xenotransplantation is similar, since it is organs that are transferred not 'pigness'.

It is difficult to see how the ethical issues associated with xenotransplantation are different from those of any neural allotransplantation. A neuron's significance stems from its functional capabilities and from the connections and circuits of which it is a part. Thus, neurobiologically, it may be more important to focus on the brain region being studied, and on the character and extent of the neurons, growth factors, and transmitters being transplanted, than on the origin of the neurons, whether it be human, rodent, or porcine. In light of this, there may be no outright difference between neurons from different species, as it is the environment and context within which they develop and function that are determinative of an individual's ultimate personality (Jones & Sagee 2001).

There is no evidence from allotransplants to date (to alleviate conditions such as Parkinson's disease and Huntington's disease) that the presence of another human's neural cells inside our brains makes us different people, at least not in the sense that worries people philosophically. The pivotal question should be whether the individual will be enhanced or diminished as a person by xenotransplantation.

Xenotransplantation represents for some, another attempt by human beings to deny their own mortality and to make our bodies seem invincible. However, this is not a reality in clinical terms and, like allotransplantation, the goal of xenotransplantation is an ordinary one: organ or tissue replacement.

For others, xenotransplantation threatens to alter a person's identity and perception of their body (Nairne 1996). While the responses of recipients of human organs have been documented, such experiences of recipients of xenotransplantation have not been reported. Concerns centre on a fear of rejection and infection, the intrusive nature of immunosuppression, and a change in bodily image. The psychological implications of breaching what are usually inviolate boundaries between humans and animals will remain unknown until hard data are obtained from xenotransplantion patients.

Animal Welfare

An ethical concern central to xenotransplantation is the use we make of animals for our own benefit. Caplan (1992) concluded that this use of animals can be morally justified on the grounds that, in general, humans possess capacities and abilities that confer more moral value upon them than upon animals. Hence, he would be unwilling to use a severely retarded child, in place of a chimp in basic research on xenotransplantation due to the negative moral impact this would have upon other human beings. This distinction illustrates the special respect we bestow upon the sensibilities and interests of other human beings.

Some argue that if we treat human and non-human animals of equivalent cognitive ability in different ways, we are guilty of 'speciesism': allowing unequal treatment of beings equal in intellect, based solely on the species to which each belongs (Singer 1975). Singer (1992) proposes that we should contemplate using anencephalic and cortically dead human infants as an organ source as opposed to endorsing the use of animals. For Singer, the relevant distinction is one of intellectual potential rather than human relationships.

Whatever one's position on the use of animals in research, we must take their welfare seriously. This prompts us to ask whether there is, underlying the development of xenotransplantation technology, an inevitable attitude of exploitation, and whether there is a substantial difference between rearing animals for spare parts or for food. Most people seem to be willing to use animals sparingly and as a last resort, although the use of primates is rejected by many. The possibility of animal exploitation by xenotransplantation may be diminished by ensuring that those who wish to use animals for such purposes fully justify their position on scientific, clinical, and ethical grounds. Such justification would also serve to allay objections raised on the grounds that vast resources are being committed to xenografting when experimental procedures are inadequate and the outcome uncertain.

Tissue Transplantation

Foetal Motherhood

The shortage of eggs in fertility clinics has opened up a dramatic new possibility—obtaining eggs from foetuses. Inevitably, the foetuses would have been aborted, and in a surreal sense it is the foetuses that would be the biological mothers of any subsequent children. Research to date on experimental animals has shown that it is possible to store foetal germ cells at low temperatures and transplant them to hosts, thereby restoring fertility. This success has led to suggestions that the abundant reserves of germ cells in the ovaries of human abortuses offer opportunities for treating human infertility. The most frequently debated ethical issues have centred around its association with tissue from aborted foetuses, and the likely impact on resulting children of their unusual origin.

The role of abortion in this process raises very similar issues to those already encountered in connection with foetal neural transplantation. One's response to it hinges on an acceptance or rejection of the principle of moral complicity. If this principle is rejected, it is possible to derive benefit from abortion, regardless of the opinion one may hold of abortion *per se*. Provided the conditions laid out with regard to the transplantation of foetal neural tissue are also met in this instance, the link with abortion becomes morally irrelevant.

In 1994, the United Kingdom's Human Fertilisation and Embryology Authority (HFEA) banned the use of foetal oocytes from aborted foetuses in infertility treatment. The authority cited several reasons for the ban, which included: the effects on the recipient mother, the effects on the resulting child, the lack of knowledge regarding the development of foetal eggs, and the strength of underlying public opinion. The authority did, however, support the use of foetal ovarian tissue in research, subject to the controls already in place for research on ovarian tissue taken from live donors and cadavers (Human Fertilisation & Embryology Authority 1995).

Some of these concerns will only be answered when far more scientific information is available, for instance, on the genetic viability, or even the general health, of the foetal oocytes. Other concerns, such as the emotional damage that may or may not be done to resulting children knowing that 'mummy was a foetus' (Berkowitz 1995), also depend on further research, although in this case, on research 'after the event'. To this criticism there is no compelling answer at present. The children will have the same genetic material as mothers who never existed. While they may know their fathers and grandparents, it was the abortion and death of their mothers—and hence existence for no more than a few months of gestation—that were essential preludes to their own existence. Berkowitz (1995) underplays this background, arguing that the element of crucial importance would be acceptance by their families; these children having much in common with those born as a result of IVF or raised by adoptive parents.

Whatever the merits and potential of this procedure, it is not identical to any existing one in the reproductive area. For instance, although the tissue to be taken is gametes, something that occurs in donor procedures, the gametes come from dead foetuses rather than from living adults. The tissue is from foetuses, which again occurs in other situations, such as foetal neural transplantation, but here the difference is between rectifying damaged tissue in existing individuals and producing new individuals. Neither of these considerations constitutes a definitive argument against foetal motherhood, and yet the foetus appears to be doubly disadvantaged. It has died, consent remains problematic, and the subsequent generation who will benefit from this death may find themselves in very unclear ethical territory. Technologically the way ahead may be relatively straightforward; ethically it may be fraught with perplexing uncertainties.

The Potential of Stem Cells

In the latter part of 1998, simultaneously but separately, two sets of researchers isolated and cultured human embryonic stem cells (hES). A third party has also claimed to have used 'cloning' techniques to produce a cell line from which hES cells can be derived. These cells, regardless of their origin, have the potential to divide into any other cell type in the human body and for an indefinite period of time, hence their 'immortality'. They are undifferentiated but, when left within their natural environment, will develop into all the other recognisable cell types in the human body, for example haematopoietic (blood) cells, cardiac (heart) cells, and neural (brain) cells, an ability defined as 'pluripotent'.

Mouse ES cells have been utilised in vast amounts of research, including work on embryogenesis, gene function, and the modelling of human disease (Gearhart 1999). However, until recently, difficulties in isolating and culturing these cells have meant that researchers have been unable to establish and maintain a similar human cell line. This was the situation until November 1998, when two teams of researchers, both funded by the same private company, Geron, isolated the first hES cells. The first group, headed by James Thomson, derived the cells from the inner cell mass of blastocysts acquired from 'leftover' embryos donated to cooperating IVF clinics (Thomson et al. 1998). The second research team hypothesised that primordial germ cells, which are the precursors to egg and sperm cells, should be undifferentiated at the very early stages of development (Shamblott et al. 1998). Embryonic germ (EG) cells were derived from human foetuses at five to nine weeks of age (aborted for therapeutic reasons), when undifferentiated cells are migrating to the developing ovaries and testis. When grown on a specific 'feeder' layer of mouse fibroblasts (which secrete factors that inhibit differentiation), EG cells have properties that parallel those of ES cells. Both sets of stem cells, ES and EG, display pluripotency, including the ability to differentiate into cells derived from all three embryonic germ layers.

An alternative approach is the use of cell nuclear replacement technology to derive human stem cells. With this method, any human somatic cell could be fused with an enucleated donor egg cell that, given the right conditions, would then develop into a blastocyst. If such an embryo could develop to the blastocyst stage, inner cell mass and therefore stem cells could be obtained. These embryonic stem cells would be compatible with the donor of the somatic cell, thereby circumventing any possible graft rejections that may normally arise due to immune incompatibility. This technique does not require the fertilisation of human eggs, and so may bypass bans on embryo research.

The potential of these new cells is profound. Any disorder involving loss of normal cells could be a candidate for replacement therapy, including neural cells for Parkinson's disease, pancreatic cells for diabetes, and cardiac cells for repairing heart damage. A universal bank of graft tissue could be generated for blood, bone marrow, lung, liver, kidney, tendons, ligaments, muscle, skin, bone, teeth, retina, and lens (Wright 1999). There have already been successful examples of the culturing of mouse ES cells to form *in vitro* colonies of neurons, skeletal muscle, and vascular endothelial cells. Besides these, human ES cells could also be used to generate tissue for pharmaceutical testing of new drugs and toxicological agents. They also have the ability to improve our understanding of the complex human events that occur during normal human development with a view to understanding what goes wrong to cause diseases and conditions such as birth defects and cancer.

The pluripotential nature of the stem cells of the inner cell mass demonstrates that these cells cannot be dismissed as nothing more than nondescript cells within the blastocyst. Since they can be manipulated to develop into human tissues, they are of interest in their own right, both legally and ethically. In practice, this means ensuring that early embryonic tissue is only used in research that incorporates substantive values, which may lead to reduction of human suffering. Since the goals of human embryonic stem cell research are seen by some ethics boards and government committees as providing such substantive values, these same boards and committees are prepared to encourage human embryonic stem cell research up to fourteen days gestation.

For example, in the United Kingdom, any research on human embryos must comply with the *Human Fertilisation and Embryology Act 1990*, which is enforced by the HFEA. The 1990 Act permits the creation and use of embryos for research purposes, provided that the research is for a number of purposes specified, and is granted a licence by the HFEA. The HFEA has stated that the derivation of stem cells from early embryos no longer needed for infertility treatment ('spare embryos'), or from embryos created by *in vitro* fertilisation specifically for research, does not raise any new ethical issues, providing that the research is licensed and carried out under the aegis of the 1990 Act (Department of Health 2000). Research using embryos created by cell nuclear replacement will be allowed on the grounds that the HFEA is satisfied that there are no other means of meeting the objectives of the research. In these cases, fully informed consent must be given by individuals whose eggs or sperm are used to create the embryos from which stem cells are later derived. The HFEA also recommends the continuing review of the need for legislation to permit the use of embryo-derived cells in actual treatments.

In a recent discussion paper on stem cell research, the Nuffield Council on Bioethics echoed the recommendations put forth by the HFEA (Nuffield Council on Bioethics 2000). In addition, the Nuffield Council takes the view that as long as there is a sufficient supply of spare embryos from IVF treatments, there are no compelling reasons to permit the creation of additional embryos for use in stem cell research.

These restrictions and controls on stem cell research involving human embryos reflect the special status of the early embryo, but allow this to be weighed against the benefits of the proposed research. This is a compromise position that will not satisfy those for whom any research on human embryos is unacceptable. It may also fail to pay adequate attention to the possibility that taking human embryonic stem cells out of their ordinary reproductive context alters their status. In addition, stem cell technology focuses attention on the blastocyst rather than on the embryo as a whole, and this may prove significant in ethical discussion.

9
The Challenge of AIDS

Ethical responses to AIDS

The 1960s and 1970s seemed to be an age of sexual freedom. Venereal diseases, while still common, were no longer the source of serious harm that they once had been, and public sexual mores were relaxing in most societies under pressure from 'free love' ideologies and post-Freudian theories about sexual repression. By the late 1970s gay sexuality was becoming destigmatised. Then along came AIDS. Thunderous voices raised moral and health-based fears about what was regarded as a gay disease. We have to some extent left these responses behind us and can now take a more careful look at the ethical issues raised by AIDS and HIV infection. The need to do so has become acute as we have watched with mounting horror the epidemic sweeping many African countries. The ethical challenges arising in our response to patients with AIDS include informed consent to investigation and treatment, the public health issues, the politicisation of disease, the problem of stigmatisation, the clinical relationship, confidentiality, and our medical response to terminal disease. It is the unique clinical profile of HIV/AIDS that forms the basis on which the ethical issues must be discussed.

1   AIDS is at present a fatal disease caused by Human Immunodeficiency Virus (HIV).
2   HIV is a virus transmitted in fresh bodily fluids, most commonly during sexual intercourse, particularly anal intercourse, but also through sharing needles in intravenous drug abuse, or through receiving contaminated blood products. It is transmitted to the foetus in 30 to 40 per cent of cases involving HIV-positive mothers.
3   Most cases of HIV infection probably proceed to AIDS, although the rate of progression is variable.
4   It is possible that a range of therapeutic agents may influence progression to clinical disease or the course of the disease.

This combination of features, as well as the existence of vulnerable and already marginalised groups in society—active homosexual men and women in rural Africa—who are the principal victims of AIDS, sets the agenda for our ethical discussion.

Informed Consent and HIV Testing

The clinical profile and natural history of AIDS mean that it is quite traumatic for a person to find out that he or she is infected with HIV. The psychological response to a positive test result varies a great deal (Coxon 1990; Deuchar 1984). Some individuals become severely depressed, even suicidal; some experience a tremendous upsurge of guilt, often associated with feelings of uncleanness; and some cope very well. The typical pattern of shock, guilt, denial, fear, anger, sadness, bargaining, acceptance and resignation, described by Kubler-Ross (1969) for dying patients, is often seen also in those who learn they are HIV positive. This is an understandable pattern of response, in that AIDS ranks with cancer as a feared disease. Some patients enter into a state of irresponsible hedonism in which they determine to 'enjoy' their remaining life with an intensity that sometimes borders on the pathological. In a few others a darker motive appears, and they form the intent to infect others with the 'curse' they see themselves as having fallen under. Yet others become withdrawn, ascetic, and severe in their personal relationships. The more extreme reactions may be associated with the extent to which the individual is unhappy with his or her 'gay identity', but there is no good evidence that this is so.

In any event, it is clear that to learn that one is HIV positive is to undergo a change in life. Sexual relationships, which could once have been seen as a pleasurable aspect of life, have to be regarded as potentially hazardous to one's partner. This poses a dilemma for the patient: whether to be honest and risk sexual rejection, or to be discreet or even deceitful in a close relationship. This problem is not so psychologically taxing in a casual or transient relationship but can be deeply disturbing in an established partnership where there are expectations of fidelity that may have been broken. The implications of one's HIV status are often misinterpreted by the patient or their partner, and the emotional effects can be profound. For this reason it is important to counsel the patient, and to give realistic information and preparatory advice before the test is taken. Because of the implications for one's life and relationships, there is, in fact, widespread consensus that HIV testing should be the subject of informed consent and that people should not be tested surreptitiously, or against their will.

Public Health Issues

Many people argue that HIV testing and the treatment of AIDS are not adequately dealt with under the rubric of autonomy and respect for individual rights, because AIDS is a public health menace; the health of the community, they argue, is of prime importance. In our view, this reaction is excessive. One commentator notes 'this can now be called a panic and demands for extreme draconian measures seen as extreme over-reactions' (Pinching et al. 2000).

The facts on transmission suggest that there is no purpose to be served by mandatory or general HIV testing whose results are linked to specific patients and made available for public health purposes. HIV is unlike tuberculosis, which could be caught by casual contact with an infected person because it is primarily a droplet-borne infection. The fact that direct inoculation by body fluids is necessary to transmit the HIV virus means that the average citizen walking down the street, going into a restaurant, sharing a crowded bus or being served by a shop assistant is at no risk: 'ordinary human intercourse, bar the sexual, is . . . of no risk at all' (Smithurst 1990). Thus the hysteria about quarantine, compulsory notification of particular cases, and informing employers or other social contacts, is both unnecessary and unethical. There are a limited number of relatively avoidable situations where individuals can be infected by the HIV virus, and the risk in these situations can be minimised by taking measures such as the use of a condom.

This reinforces a point repeatedly made by the Australian judge Justice Michael Kirby that the single most effective public health measure to limit the spread of AIDS encompasses education and the encouragement of responsible and caring sexual behaviour (Kirby 1989). Those most at risk have, in fact, realised this: 'the homosexual community, which initially had a very low take-up of testing, has achieved a remarkable slowing of the rate of the spread of HIV; this has been largely effected through behavioural change' (Pinching 1990). 'An emerging solidarity, reinforced by the cumulative personal losses, soon led to action to protect each other through prevention programmes, based on peer-based education and influence' (Pinching et al. 2000). The public cannot be protected by the detection and notification of every new case of AIDS, and the ill-informed, 'knee-jerk' response to the statistics that leads to this kind of measure is only likely to increase the difficulties in achieving effective control, and perhaps eradication, of the disease.

HIV testing for epidemiological purposes is, however, clearly important (Gillett 1989), and indeed, in the light of statistics from around the world, vital to monitoring and mounting an effective response to the disease. The obvious worry is that if informed consent is needed and if, as we know, those who refuse to take the test in a sexually transmitted disease clinic are those most likely to have positive results, then the data derived from a study of HIV status on a sample population will be grossly inaccurate (Skegg 1989). It has been argued that this impasse is resolved once it is realised that the need for consent is based on the linking of information with a particular patient. Since the epidemiologist does not want patient-specific information, tests should be of no concern to patients, provided that the HIV results are derived in such a way that they cannot be traced to individuals. We could even say, provided that a special venipuncture was not performed, that nothing had been done to *that patient* at all. Thus, one can justify taking unidentified blood samples for epidemiological tests of HIV status without the consent of those whose blood has been tested. Privacy legislation in some countries including Australia and New Zealand may, however, limit the form in which—and the purposes for which—such information can be used.

HIV, AIDS, and Societal Injustice

In many of the countries where HIV/AIDS is most prevalent there are social problems that perpetuate the disease, and the very fact that these are Third World countries links HIV with social inequity (Bagasao 1995). Julie Hamblin, a lawyer writing on this topic, remarks:

> For me it was not possible to comprehend the true enormity of the HIV epidemic in the developing world until I visited East Africa. In countries such as Kenya and Uganda, it has pervaded every level of society . . . and it is literally true to say that no family remains untouched [Hamblin 1994].

The aggravating factors include not only poverty *per se*, but also the systematic repression of women and their exclusion from any kind of power over their own life choices. Hamblin comments:

> One of the features that has marked the impact of the HIV epidemic, particularly in the third world but also in some parts of the developed world, has been the way in which it has reflected vulnerabilities and inequalities within communities [Hamblin 1994].

Hamblin also makes the point that the most effective measures against HIV infection and spread may involve a degree of informed and empowered choice about one's sexual behaviour. There are certain settings in which psychological and sociological factors deny people such choices, and this is particularly the case for African women.

> There is nothing more poignant than talking to an African woman who knows all about HIV . . . but who says: I know my husband has other women but what can I do? If I suggest that he use a condom, he will assume that I must have had other lovers and tell me to leave. There is nowhere else for my children and me to go [Hamblin 1994].

This is one of the clearest examples of a situation in which the ethical aspects of medicine and its effectiveness cannot be separated. In order to cut down the rate of HIV in Africa and some other Third World countries, one may need to reform society and begin to do away with the systematic repression and exploitation of women. Fortunately, this type of broad and inclusive thinking is increasingly informing international strategies (Pinching et al. 2000). This will mean that certain traditional mores come under pressure, but by not empowering women to make sexual choices one is, in effect, condemning many thousands of them to death, and their children to being orphaned and living in poverty. Human rights and health in relation to HIV and AIDS are inextricably linked, and here epidemiology and preventive medicine must work hand in hand with ethics, law, and sociology to have any impact on a massive human tragedy that, if it occurred in the Western world, would soon be recognised as being intolerable.

AIDS in the Third World

The situation in the Third World, and Africa in particular, has also given rise to problems of drug research and access to treatment for AIDS, and, more specifically, the ethical conduct of drug-related research, and the availability of expensive drugs to ameliorate the disease.

Placebo-controlled trials of anti-AIDS drugs have been stymied in many Western countries by HIV and AIDS sufferers networks sharing drugs that are thought to be effective (Mirkin 1995). Third World countries have the twin advantages of large numbers of patients and fairly controlled supplies of drugs, such that placebo-treatment separation can be more easily maintained. The question then arises as to whether, on the basis of existing evidence of benefit, such placebo-controlled trials in economically and politically disadvantaged settings are unethical. The debates have raged to and fro since the issue was raised in 1997 (Angell 1997; Lurie & Wolfe 1997). Some ethicists argue that we cannot give patients in the Third World a lower standard of care than we give people in a developed country and then seek to benefit from that deprivation. The thought is that the effects of Zidovudine seem to be beneficial in certain settings, but a subject in the placebo arm of a trial is denied that benefit. Conversely, it is pointed out that by being included in the trial, the people concerned—impoverished and disadvantaged as they are—get much better treatment than they could otherwise hope to access, no matter which group they end up in (Resnick 1998).

We would argue that this issue must be looked at from the point of view of the target population. If one were in a high HIV area in Africa, the thought that a major company was to move into one's area and establish clinics and services for a trial in no way detracts from the resulting improved access to health care services. Even a 50 per cent chance of effective medication, when combined with a 100 per cent improvement in access to better health care services, seems like manna from heaven if one is otherwise doomed to suffer and die from HIV-related diseases without any treatment at all. Consequently, ethical arguments should take account, not of absolute principles in this area, but of a careful understanding of the predicament of those most closely involved, and a compassionate and caring response to this.

A question then arises about whether it is ethically defensible to use a population for experimentation designed to produce treatments that the population itself could never afford. This is an issue of global justice and requires careful consideration (Cochrane 2000). We can lament the glaring evidence of double standards in health care throughout the world (Bayley 2000), and we can also express ethical concern about the pricing and profit-fixing practices of multi-national pharmaceutical companies. At the same time, we should applaud attempts to make effective drugs available to the disadvantaged populations in which they have been developed. Again, from the perspective of a Third World sufferer, the development of a set of services, contingently related to research and development by a major pharmaceutical company, is an unqualified good. The global injustice that allows differences in health status to be perpetuated by corrupt governments, Western greed, and multinational profiteering is a remote concern in the face of the provision of a new venereal health clinic in a village—whether or not the drugs developed from work in that clinic are affordable. It would, of course, be better if the conditions of research and development work guaranteed lasting access to any effective treatments discovered. This ought to be regarded as an obligatory cost imposed on such research programs. The global issues must be addressed and should be of moral concern to all, but if we fail to respond to their plight as a real and present danger we run the risk of sacrificing the lives of HIV and AIDS sufferers on the altar of ethical principles.

HIV Tests and Conflicts Between Patients

We have suggested that ethical considerations make informed consent a pre-requisite to HIV testing of individuals. Grounded in principles of autonomy and respect for individuals, this implies that we cannot force any person to have an HIV test. However, there are situations where more than one individual is con-cerned, and where the possibility of a conflict of interests suggests that we must pay some regard to the principle of justice and the rights of others.

The least troublesome situation concerns blood transfusion. Here the overall aim is to benefit the recipient of the donated blood. But the patient will be harmed rather than benefited if the blood carries live HIV particles. Therefore, the doctor taking the blood for transfusion purposes has to be satisfied that the donor is not infected with HIV. This means that HIV testing can reasonably be required on entry into the blood donation program. It is, of course, a voluntary program so that the tests can be avoided by simply declining to volunteer.

A more difficult problem concerns the procedure to be adopted if there is a needlestick or other penetrating injury in a health care setting. Here the issues can rapidly be clouded beyond the point of reasonable debate. First, the likeli-hood of transmission of HIV is slight even when the patient is HIV positive; second, the status of the patient at the time of the injury is not an infallible guide to the risk to the health care worker; third, there are no recorded cases of patients refusing consent to HIV testing under these circumstances; and, finally, it is unwise to base general policies on difficult cases.

The risk to a health care worker from exposure to body fluids from a patient with HIV infection is something between 0.1 and 0.7 per cent (Marcus & the CDC Cooperative Needlestick Surveillance Group 1988). Thus, most of the time, even if the patient is HIV positive, a health care worker who incurs a penetrating injury with blood or body fluids has nothing to fear. For this reason no momentous decisions ought to be based on the result of a test on the patient. However, the possibility that AZT or similar substances may modify the course of the infection makes it important to ascertain whether the injured person is truly at risk. Thus a case can be made that the injured person has a right to know if the patient whose blood is involved is HIV positive.

However, there is a 'window' between infection and positivity on HIV testing, so that even a negative result is not clear proof that no risk exists. The fact that patients, by and large, appreciate the concerns after needlestick injuries, and feel some obligation to those looking after them, implies that draconian measures designed to license mandatory testing on uncooperative patients are both ill-informed and unnecessary.

It seems, therefore, that a reasonable policy in this difficult situation would be to tell patients that, in the unlikely event of an accident, a test for HIV (and other infectious agents such as hepatitis B) would be required, and that they could indicate whether or not they would wish to know the result. If a patient objected to this procedure, an authorisation for mandatory testing would be ethically justified on the grounds of justice and on a consideration of the interests of all parties concerned. As things stand, it is unclear who could give such authorisation. In any event, recognition of this procedure would probably obviate any difficulties with unreasonable and uncooperative patients. (The patient would be regarded as unreasonable here because of the failure to act out of reasonable or decent consideration for the welfare of others who have provided care, not for any more general reason.)

The Doctor–Patient Relationship

Treating AIDS sufferers as a stigmatised and hostile group whom the 'clean' members of society must detect and isolate is exactly the kind of thing that will threaten the balanced three-way relationship between the doctor, the patient, and the community—a relationship that is required to deal with any health threat. Many doctors are influenced by the stereotypes that prevail in upper-middle-class society, and in the case of AIDS these are potentially disastrous. Doctors and other health care workers who encounter new cases of AIDS need to (and generally do) develop a deep commitment to their patients, and earn the trust of those groups from which most new cases will come. They cannot do this if they subscribe to damaging stereotypes. The doctor should be aware that a person at risk of AIDS is a potential ally in the fight against a life-threatening disease, but one who may feel very insecure. Often the values and lifestyle choices of at-risk patients are quite different from those of their doctors, and they may see doctors as representing many of the attitudes they have come to feel alienated from through rejection by family or 'straight' friends (Coxon 1990). AIDS has in fact led to a rethinking of the doctor–patient relationship as concepts of empowerment become increasingly influential. Patients are required to understand and own difficult decisions about uncertain therapies and life-strategies to cope with the disease and its consequences (Pinching et al. 2000).

The potential problems in the doctor–patient relationship can become serious when someone finds he or she is HIV positive. As the pressures mount and, perhaps, certain unresolved personal tensions surface, the doctor must be sensitive to the thoughts and feelings that often need to be expressed, even if it is only in order that the patient may work through them in an atmosphere that is not charged with suspicion and fear. A doctor can fill the role of counsellor and confidant in this situation and help patients to find the personal resources to meet the crises they will face including threats to personal relationships.

Confidentiality

> Terry is tested for HIV after having been on a Caribbean holiday and is found to be positive. In talking to his doctor about the result, Terry agrees that there is a risk to John, his partner, but refuses to allow him to be told. He claims that John will become very jealous and upset, and may walk out on him. He also resists the idea that he should start using condoms because he believes this will make John suspect that there is something wrong.

The General Medical Council of Britain (GMC) has addressed the difficult conflict between confidentiality and the duty to warn that is potentially raised by finding that a patient is HIV positive. The recently reaffirmed GMC stand to inform at-risk partners has been widely followed elsewhere (e.g. National Medical Council of New Zealand 1990). These groups accept the argument of the following general form. If the patient is in an active sexual relationship, whether in a marriage or with a gay partner, there is a real and identifiable risk posed to the partner. To ignore this risk would be to deny the presumption that, where it is within their power, doctors will keep other people from harm, whether or not those people are their own patients. (It is on this basis that doctors and nurses stop to help at road accidents, and so on.)

It goes without saying that the doctor who has an HIV-positive patient ought first to counsel the patient about the meaning of that result, and discuss its implications for his or her sexual partner. On occasion this may fail, and the doctor may become aware that the partner is being put at risk. What then? The

GMC states: 'there are grounds for disclosing that a patient is HIV positive to a third party, without the consent of the patient only where there is a serious and identifiable risk to a specific individual who, if not so informed, would be exposed to infection' (General Medical Council of Britain 1988). But is this advice ethically sound?

It is clear that the magnitude of the harm resulting from an uninfected person developing AIDS far outweighs the harm done to the individual whose confidences are breached. This is true and, indeed, is given as a justification for infringing the rights of an individual in other areas of conduct. It is, however, a delicate path to tread and it should not be extended beyond this condition without very careful consideration. How much, and when, are we entitled to dismantle a traditional aspect of the relationship between doctor or health professional and patient to protect a third person?

We could claim that abandoning a moral constraint is justified whenever one party to the trust is acting unreasonably or in bad faith. This is the basis for revealing confidential information shared by psychotic patients who do not rightly perceive the consequences and moral import of their intentions, and whose own autonomy or individual rights are suspended until they can again take a responsible place in society. That line of reasoning seems to be at least part of the rationale of the decision in the Tarasoff case, where the court judged that a doctor in the USA should have warned a potential victim on the basis of clinical information obtained from a psychotic patient (see Chapter 10). In that case a great deal of discussion turned on the mental disturbance behind the patient's potential to cause harm, and the view that, because of his mental state, he could not be treated as a normal person would be. However, it is clear that the AIDS patient is not mentally impaired and does not lose his or her right to confidentiality on this score.

We look to be on more promising ground with the concept of 'bad faith', or what has been called 'moral free-loading' (Gillett 1996). This occurs whenever an individual behaves in such a way as to undermine the credibility of his or her appeal to certain principles. Patients who expect confidentiality are appealing to the value that normal and sensitive people attach to the feelings and reactions of others. Because the feelings of others matter to them, they do not wish those others to be told things that might be damaging. Terry's concern for confidentiality, therefore, arises from his desire to remain in the allegedly caring and supportive relationship he shares with John. But his own disregard for John's welfare undermines his claim that the relationship is of the valued sort; indeed, it implies that it is far less.

We could compare this with the situation in which parents negate the presumption that they are acting in the best interests of their children by abusing them (that is, by treating the children in such a way that those interests are jeopardised). In this case we deprive the parents of their normal authority in decisions affecting their children because that authority is based on their claim to be the proper representatives of their children's interests. We reason that the parents' behaviour evinces bad faith, 'moral free-loading', or rational inconsistency with their presumed commitments. By similar reasoning, we would suspend the HIV-positive patient's right to confidentiality because that is based on a presumed sensitivity to and care for a partner that is inconsistent with the intention to expose the partner to harm. The doctor's warning is, of course, a last resort and is meant to be issued 'in a fashion that would preserve the privacy of his patient to the fullest extent compatible with the threatened danger' (General Medical Council of Britain 1993). Doctors cannot be ethically obliged to act as accomplices in immoral and dangerous actions.

It is worth noting that the honesty encouraged by the doctor's intervention might well allow a more constructive, cooperative, and caring management of the patient's need for support and commitment should he or she develop the full manifestations of AIDS. This 'moral free-loading' argument does not, however, undermine our traditional commitments. The argument gives us a reason to weaken our obligation in an area where the values appealed to do not tally with the behaviour shown, and evince bad faith on the part of the one making the moral claim.

A Terminal Illness

The grim prospects of a patient with AIDS have occasioned renewed interest in the relationship between suicide and euthanasia. We have already noted the need for a relationship of empowerment to be cultivated when the patient is suffering from HIV-related disease and the terminal nature of the disease naturally means that debate in this area must include end-of-life decisions. Opinions vary greatly on the correct way to respond to these issues. On the one hand, philosophers are prepared to accept that both suicide and euthanasia can be rational individual choices: 'if there is a right to commit suicide, then, arguably, there is a right to competent medical advice as to how to do this, and to information on obtaining the means, and even perhaps to direct assistance' (Almond 1990). It is noticeable that calls for the legalisation of euthanasia are more muted from AIDS groups than from other quarters, and many commentators have serious reservations about any such move. On the other hand, some feel that AIDS sufferers should be able to decide their own manner of death as many of them will have seen close friends and lovers suffer and die from the disease.

The main worry is that a group already stigmatised to some extent would be particularly vulnerable to any tendency for the awkward situation to be dealt with quietly and conveniently rather than by careful consideration of the deep ethical and personal issues involved. If the normal patient is vulnerable because of the medicalisation of death, how much more so is the patient who is already seen as being slightly marginal? If a young person having all sorts of difficulties in coming to terms with his or her life and identity is liable to make rash and tragic decisions, how much more this might be the case with a person who feels guilty and may well be struggling with emotional problems because of sexual identity, lifestyle, and, perhaps, estrangement from family. Anyone's wishes in this regard are likely to be uncertain and unsettled, as the widely varying reactions to an HIV test result show. All these factors may lead one to feel that the AIDS patient is highly vulnerable to the appeal of a gentle death, and that there are special reasons, therefore, to worry about euthanasia for AIDS.

However, it seems that a number of AIDS patients do choose some means of ending their own life (Coxon 1990), and to deny such people access to sensitive help from a qualified health care professional seems wrong. It is clear that people with AIDS should be able to say that they do not want further treatment to prolong their lives. Thus AIDS remains a challenge until the death of the patient, with a number of issues surrounding life-and-death decisions unable to be resolved simply by a blanket statement one way or the other.

We have so far said little about the ethical impact of drugs to treat AIDS. If AZT, or other drugs like it, come to offer a reasonable prospect of cure or control of the virus, then some of our problems will be lessened and others will intensify. We will have to consider the problem of a life-saving treatment whose availability is limited by expense and opportunity, and deal with the potential problems created by a black market operated by entrepreneurial 'patients'. On the other hand, HIV will no longer be directly linked with death, and therefore some of the emotive and fearful hysteria attached to the disease will be removed. AIDS will occupy the spot once occupied by syphilis, and we will have to reconsider the ethics of detection, notification, and contact-tracing because issues of individual patient welfare and public welfare will coincide; it will be in everybody's best interests to detect those who are HIV positive. We will also have further cause to examine the disparity in treatments available to the rich and the poor in those countries where health care is barely recognised as a public good.

The production of treatments for HIV/AIDS should cause us to reflect on the ways in which doom-criers and flag-wavers produce an overreaction to a historically limited phenomenon, and warn us of the inadvisability of legislation relating to drastic measures such as euthanasia for a disease in which the therapeutic possibilities are evolving.

For the health care professions, the challenge implicit in the unique profile of AIDS fundamentally concerns their role in dispelling the myths and stigmas that attach to the disease.

AIDS victims have been fired from their jobs, driven from their homes by terrified and ashamed families, and abandoned by similarly disposed lovers. The body of one patient was disowned by his family, and funeral directors are declining to handle the bodies of others [Deuchar 1984].

The near-hysteria found in some circles cries out to be met by reasoned ethical discussion that recognises the issues and examines them in an analytical but concerned manner. This is a charge on the health care professions, and a responsibility they ought to accept in accordance with their duties to individuals and communities that look to them for expert help and guidance.

AIDS also presents a challenge to our legislative morality as a caring society. Legislation too often reflects the cynical morality of vote-catching rather than a considered response to a crisis needing careful, compassionate thought. Vote-catching by subscribing to slogans and stereotypes, and feeding off public anxiety, is a notorious tool in the political armoury, and incompatible with a well-ordered set of policies designed to preserve a caring and decent society. We certainly cannot claim that we have a caring society when a minority that risks being marginalised is excluded from our community of care, and made the target of public fear and insecurity. This has happened all too often in history and with well-known results. It is to be hoped that it will not happen again in the case of AIDS.

10
Ethical Issues in Psychiatry

Introduction

Psychiatry and the disorders that it encounters pose special ethical problems that are a little different from those in other areas of medicine. The basic approach we have outlined, which allows us to take account of the relationships between individuals as thinking, socially engaged beings, is not quite applicable to this unique area of discussion, where an emphasis on patient autonomy has some almost intractable problems. However, the strands of ethical theory that emphasise empowerment and the doctor as a trusted and virtuous healer have a great deal to recommend them in this area of ethics.

Patients with psychiatric disorders suffer, in one way or another, from an impairment of the mental and moral faculties that underpin our lives as ethical creatures. The patient's autonomy—the ability to make reasonable decisions about his or her own preferences and interests—rests on just these faculties and is the basis of the medical partnership. Because a psychiatric patient's actions do not fit the pattern of personality and self-regarding interests that constitute autonomy, we cannot treat him or her as we would a physically unwell person whose thoughts and emotions remain more or less intact. The fact that any psychiatric illness affects the character, desires, thoughts, and feelings of the patient makes us unsure whether a person's wishes about treatment can have the same pivotal role that they are given in other clinical situations.

These facts raise ethical problems about psychiatric diagnosis and classification, the nature of the doctor–patient relationship, iatrogenic disease, compulsory treatment, psychosurgery, confidentiality, suicide and its management, and reproductive ethics.

Diagnosis, Classification, and Stigmatisation

The diagnosis that a patient is psychiatrically disordered classifies him or her as 'abnormal' in a very fundamental way. To some extent, a person's physical condition can be defined quite separately from any comment on the kind of person he or she is. But a judgment that one is disordered in the mind is not so easily separable from the gamut of personal and moral attitudes that others take towards oneself. Thus, psychiatric patients are often stigmatised as being some-how tainted in the essence of their identity as persons, and not just as afflicted by an incidental condition. They are called names: 'loonies' (touched by the moon), 'nutcases' (something wrong in the 'nut', the head), 'mentals' (something wrong with the mind), or 'crazies' (unpredictable, dangerous). They are also marginalised, set apart as *defective persons* from the rest of society who are 'normal', and this attitude towards psychiatric patients and ex-patients creates a deep ethical problem for a caring society. There is a legitimate need to take extraordinary measures in order to benefit such a patient, yet patients them-selves may resent being classified as 'disordered' in this way and may not see any need for treatment. As a result, we have to override a person's normal right to refuse medical treatment or to be an empowered partner in the clinical relation-ship. In this way, to intervene and benefit such patients is to treat them as less than individuals with regard to decisions central to their life and well-being. Thus the problem of classification and diagnosis is loaded with ethical signifi-cance even before we consider treatment issues.

> The roots are primitive, powerful, and universal. When we want to do unto others as we would not have them do unto ourselves, we find some way of turning them into others. We usually do that by labelling them, by excluding them from our own group, and by dehuman-izing them (Reich 1999).

The fact that we regard psychiatric patients as radically *other* than normal and to some extent alienated from themselves (Gillett 1999), is based not only on the fact that they must be treated differently from other people, but also on the fact that they often react differently to others. This has been taken, at various times in the history of psychiatry, to legitimise treatments we would never dream of inflicting on others. That such patients are vulnerable to treatments not directly connected to therapeutic knowledge that might benefit them, is a sad comment on the scientific basis of psychiatry (Micale and Porter 1994). What is more, some of the treatment modes are harmful or degrading. Literature is replete with examples of books written about discriminatory and dehumanising attitudes masquerading as care of the insane, books such as *Faces in the Water* (Frame 1982) and *One Flew over the Cuckoo's Nest* (Kesey 1962). In each story the same processes tend to occur: the patient is diagnosed as mentally disor-dered, admitted to an institution, treated as less than a person; the patient objects to that treatment, the objection is regarded as further evidence that he or she is unable to see what is for his or her own good, harsher measures are instituted to overcome the resistance to treatment, and 'treatments' are used that may damage the patient further. The patient is truly dehumanised—in his or her person, not just in his or her *persona* (the way he or she is presented and perceived as being)—and the defects of relationship and conduct that existed at the outset are amplified and fixed so that rehabilitation becomes a more and more remote possibility. One ex-patient has described this as 'the snowball effect' and has graphically portrayed the fear and anxiety in patients who are already unable to cope with life and sometimes tended by less-than-sympathetic custodians (Kocan 1980).

The problems do not start with the process of treatment or institutionalisation that follows the making of a psychiatric diagnosis. They begin within the diagnostic event itself and even, in some cases, long before it. Writers such as Laing (1965) and Szasz (1983) have judged psychiatric diagnosis to be a process of evaluation of the conduct of those whom a society (or micro-society such as a family) finds disturbing. Whatever one may think of the so-called 'anti-psychiatry' of Laing and others, it has made us take careful note of the fact that psychiatric disorders are not only *intrapersonal* but also *interpersonal*. Most psychiatric diagnoses, even where we are persuaded that a disease model is both realistic and compelling, involve a breakdown of interpersonal relationships, and therefore they render patients vulnerable and needy within themselves at the very point where help can often be found to cope with the stress of a major crisis in their life and well-being. Because of this vulnerability, there are special hazards in the therapeutic relationships of psychiatric health care.

When is a Syndrome Not a Syndrome?

The unbalanced relationship between professional and patient and the effect of social stereotypes on all of us, especially those who are vulnerable for other reasons, poses a special problem for psychiatric and psychological treatment. In the midst of a confusing world, we all tend to look for some kind of guidance, and a therapist is the avenue sought by those who find themselves seriously troubled in their minds. The therapist is, therefore, in a privileged position not only to help a person make sense out of his or her life but also to provide a strong lead as to what kind of sense should be made. Some therapists construct a narrative around childhood events and attitudes, usually invoking various subconscious psychic traces of these events to explain current feelings and disorders. Other narratives trade in concepts like the 'authentic self' or 'self-actualisation'. All methods have in common the key role of the therapist as the one who helps the individual to construct a story about himself or herself and, in so doing, reconstruct the self or, as one writer says, 'rewrite the soul' (Hacking 1995). Therefore, we find that in therapy a needy person rebuilds an understanding of his or her life by using two powerful resources: the 'stories of self' accepted in the particular community; and the views of the therapist. This is particularly relevant to Multiple Personality Disorder (DSM IV: Dissociative Identity Disorder (American Psychiatric Association 1994)).

These syndromes are usually diagnosed when a person presents to a therapist with fairly non-specific psychiatric symptoms that may include depression or anxiety. A process of exploration then occurs and at this point the picture becomes slightly confused. In the classic cases the person would complain of missing tracts of time and, if stressed or emotionally challenged during therapy, or if subjected to hypnosis, might revert to another personality that could be quite different from the person he or she seemed to be. Consider the following case:

> Carrie is a rather awkward and slightly rigid young woman who has made a moderately successful career as an accountant but has never married or had children. She has sought therapy for headaches, complaining also of losing track of things as if someone were playing tricks upon her. She claims that her friends have told her that at times she behaves outrageously at parties, flirting shamelessly with men, both eligible and elsewhere attached, and dancing in a provocative and sometimes embarrassing way. She has a reputation for being quite promiscuous in these settings. She cannot understand how she would come to do these things and has no real recollection of having acted in those ways; she says she is sometimes blank for whole periods of time.

Carrie's therapy could go a number of ways, but one would be for her to discover that she has within her two or three separate personalities, one of whom (let's call her Margo) is promiscuous, unconventional, and uninhibited. If this were to happen, it might well be a discovery that explained her periods of absence and changes of behaviour. 'Margo' might not spontaneously emerge, but Carrie might be encouraged to think of her problems in this way by the therapist. This could allow the tendencies she exhibits as her alter self to be handled without the complex conflicts within Carrie's own personality being confronted directly. The problem arises when the personalities so discovered are thought of as being latent within Carrie all the time, having perhaps formed during childhood. While this may be true it is, in many cases, a working theory to frame therapy and counselling. So far, dispute over this theory may seem marginal in terms of ethics and to be of local interest within psychiatric theory, but it has been given a deeply ethical turn with the link between adult syndromes such as Dissociative Identity Disorder and child abuse (Gillett 1999).

A number of clients have 'rediscovered' memories under the guidance of a therapist. Some of these memories are of episodes of emotional, physical, and sexual abuse as children. Such memories, if true, help to make a coherent story of the adult's psychological disturbance by linking it to deeply disturbing events affecting the formation of personality in childhood. No doubt some of the memories and accounts that emerge during therapy represent experiences that a person has not been able to talk about because of their deeply distressing nature, but it seems that some of the 'repressed memories' are in fact false and more or less created in the narrative interaction of the therapeutic encounter, or as a way of sorting out childhood conflicts in the mind of the client. This is understandable when we realise that both therapist and client are struggling to make sense of an intrinsically puzzling psychological picture. And it is probably important to remember that the events carry psychic truth, even if not factual and historical truth as is required in a court of law. It is natural, since Freud, to think that such a picture must have its origins in childhood, but some of the stories of ritual abuse of the most bizarre and gothically melodramatic types occurring in the most mundane of settings strain the credibility of any reasonable person (Mulhern 1994; Putnam 1991).

Given the fierce controversy that rages over dissociative disorders in general and 'repressed memory' in particular, it is important for us to stress that ethical practice has a central relationship with the Hippocratic ethos of detailed observation, cumulative documentation, and cautious epidemiology as the foundation for clinical diagnosis and treatment. It seems that certain therapists have made immodest—even injudicious—claims, and that these have resulted in great harm to families and to their clients. Thus, in psychiatric and counselling practice clinicians need not only to be attentive to clients and to help them tell their story and be heard, but also to abide by well-established procedures of observation, investigation, scientific scrutiny (whether qualitative or positivistic), and validation. Only thus can they assure themselves and the public that they are sound in their practice and will not abuse their position as experts to advance personal opinions and passionately held prejudices where they should be developing a *techne*—skill based on knowledge.

This example in fact represents the general problem of the battleground of psychiatric diagnosis and therapy where different theories have fought each other to a stalemate and clinicians have been encouraged by medical and intellectual politics to take sides. But a *sine qua non* of clinical ethics dictates that patients should not be adversely affected by Olympian struggles among the demigods of the medical pantheon. For this reason, we must again stress the special level of responsibility that attaches to psychiatric care because of the inherent and exaggerated vulnerability of the psychologically disturbed person.

Along with theoretical disputes about the mind and its disorders there are more localised areas of clinical uncertainty; for instance, there is widespread uncertainty about the personality disorders and their nature. Most of these are characterised by an excessive degree of some trait or traits that many normal individuals show to some extent or another, such as impulsiveness and irresponsibility (psychopathy or antisocial personality disorder), distrust and suspicion (paranoid personality disorder), emotional instability and fear of abandonment (borderline personality disorder), or self-centredness (narcissistic personality disorder). If we begin to look at all deviations from some notional norm as indicating a disorder of some type we are in danger of transforming the entire population into a set of not-yet-diagnosed psychiatric patients. Yet it is clear that in some cases the observed deviation is either severely disruptive to the life of the individual or a cause of significant distress and suffering or both. As we contemplate the many ways that the development of such a wide range of unusual human behaviours might arise, we are also led to wonder where medicine ends and social engineering or education begins in attending to the well-being of any person. The ramifications of psychological distress in the lives of those who suffer such things can also put a great deal of pressure on the health care professionals who specialise in such problems.

Clinicians, Patients, and Therapeutic Relationships

The fact that psychiatric illness affects the psyche implies that the threat to the dignity and autonomy of the patient in psychiatric therapy is much greater than in normal clinical care. The theory that there are unconscious and irrational determinants of the attitudes, interests, desires, and beliefs of the psychologically disturbed person intensifies this 'insufficient regard for the patient's intentionality or will' even more. A guiding theme in therapy is that the person should be helped to overcome whatever is distorting his or her beliefs, perception, and action, and thus the therapist is a key figure. Patients are likely to make normalising reference to the therapist by trying to reorder their perception of themselves in terms of the words and reactions of the therapist. Thus, the therapist's ideas have normative force in shaping the personality readjustment of patients and their view of what normal interpersonal life ought to be like. The very nature of the relationship means that the therapist's ideas are of paramount structural importance in the psychiatric process. It is a relationship in which the therapist has the role of discoverer, conceptualiser, judge, and corrector of the patient's problems and thus the patient is put in a role that can hardly help but be dependent, deferential, and, to some extent, worshipful: the therapist must seem to be worthy of respect and admiration.

Many psychotherapists realise that their authority opens the doctor–patient relationship to transference or to the development of intense and potentially transforming relationships, fuelled by unresolved problems of early life or of crucial stages of one's development. The individual therapist is, therefore, in a position of power that is open to abuse. The therapist's role can, however, be taken by a group of people. When the therapeutic medium is a group, the risk of individual therapeutic idiosyncrasy is lessened, although it is sometimes replaced by a no less powerful group influence that may be harder for the patient to question, or to understand and deal with. If we believe that balanced reflection about, and understanding of, oneself as a person are important in overcoming a psychological disorder, these inherent problems of power must be faced and a pattern of practice sketched in which abuses arising from them can be minimised.

There are clear guidelines to ethical practice in any area of medicine, and they include the following:

1   The methods used must be attested to and validated as likely to benefit the patient; that is, they must tend to return the patient to proper functioning as a responsible and self-directed individual.
2   The clinician must refrain from harming or damaging the patient by his or her advice or actions.
3   The professional must always preserve a certain 'distance' from the patient so as to act in accordance with good clinical practice and not on the basis of emotional entanglement.

These cornerstones of care can guard a practitioner against some of the worst breaches of professional conduct within psychiatry. The problems may involve emotional or sexual abuse of patients, affronts to the patient's dignity or autonomy, or ill-considered 'treatments' that not only are of unproven benefit to patients but also carry uncharted risks of harm.

In part, the problems in psychiatric practice and its regulation (as we have already noted with dissociation and repressed memories) stem from the vast array of different methodologies and theories about mental illness. The methodological diversity in particular is staggering, and is exemplified by the opposing camps of talk-therapy (analysis, cognitive behavioural therapy, and so on) and biological therapy (drugs). In fact, many therapists use a mixture of techniques, depending on the problem they are dealing with. But within this broad-brush dichotomy treatments like 'feeling therapy', 'sleep/coma therapy', 'nude therapy', 'screaming cure', and 'orgasm cure' can arise, and these seem to be highly vulnerable to abuse by patient and therapist (Karasu 1981). The breadth and diversity of approaches to, and formulations of, psychiatric disorder make ethical principles difficult to apply to many therapeutic situations. For instance, is it abusive or helpful to be merciless in confronting the patient with his or her inadequacies to the point that he or she 'breaks down' emotionally? The vulnerability of psychiatric therapy to abuse is compounded by the emotional vulnerability and proneness to exploitation of many psychiatric patients. Patients seeking psychiatric help may well have been damaged by interpersonal and social injuries. They enter into a clinical relationship that is necessarily 'private, highly personal, and sometimes intensely emotional' (Karasu 1981). Some patients will look to manipulate the relationship to create an illusion of involvement that is not properly part of professional care, and some therapists will seek, through a succession of relationships with dependent and adoring patients, a source of satisfaction and self-esteem that their non-professional lives may not offer.

The most obvious and widely publicised type of professional misconduct involves sexual entanglement with clients or patients.

Dr H is seeing Dave, a bank manager, for temper tantrums at home and loss of motivation at work. It emerges that Dave, despite an aura of easy-going competence at his job and a very congenial and confident manner with his peers, is actually quite insecure. His lack of motivation at work is related to a fear that he will lose his job, and an inability to complete reports in case they do not reach what he perceives to be the high standards required for success. He is also being distracted by what he sees as a passionate involvement with one of the secretaries in the bank, herself a recent casualty of a relationship break-up. His violence at home is related to an increasing intolerance of any indication that he is less than a fully adequate male. Little things, such as minor repairs on the car or around the house, or any suggestion of financial constraints on family activities, annoy him intensely and lead to sullen, withdrawn moods in which any family member who crosses his path will be chastised for a real or imagined fault. Dr H begins to work with Dave's sense of self-esteem and does some basic assertion training.

Things at work start to improve but problems at home do not, and Dr H arranges to see Dave and his wife, Elaine, together. These sessions are slightly strained, and Elaine asks for some time in counselling by herself. Elaine expresses her fears that Dave is having an affair, and also her worries that the recent deterioration in their relationship might have been based on her reluctance as a sexual partner. She mentions that Dave does not seem very interested any more. Her fears about him having an affair are confirmed by Dr H. She says it must be because she is no longer attractive. She is reassured by Dr H. One thing leads to another over the next few weeks, and she and Dr H develop a sexual liaison. When all these goings-on come to light there is a major scandal and Dave initiates a malpractice suit against Dr H.

The complications of this case not only indicate considerable lack of wisdom in Dr H's conduct but also raise the general problem of defining the bounds of acceptable patient contact in psychotherapy. What if Dr H had not had a sexual relationship with Elaine but had merely conveyed to her, by physical and emotive contact, that she was attractive and could reclaim Dave's attention from his temporary emotional refuge in the woman at work?

Is sexual contact between therapist and patient unequivocally unethical regardless of outcome? If it is unethical, what about 'non-erotic' kissing, hugging, and touching, that, it seems, more than 50 per cent of psychiatrists engage in with patients? [Karasu 1981].

We must surely ask of such practices, admitting our doubts about their validity, whether they preserve 'professional distance' and avoid any harm or damage to the patient (as per Hippocrates). On any view of human relationships, it seems quite unlikely that temporary sexual liaisons with therapists are likely to leave patients more integrated, more balanced, less exploited and more sexually at peace with themselves than they were before such entanglements (Gabbard 1999). Many patients are vulnerable, and have a history of unsatisfactory emotional involvements that readily form a witch's brew of psychological forces when combined with exploitation by a therapist. The sexual relationships that are developed in therapy seem to be just that: 'such ostensibly therapeutic sexual interaction almost always involves a male therapist and a young female patient . . . there is little evidence of the therapist providing such help for the fat or ugly who might receive from it more benefit to their self-esteem' (Bancroft 1981). This astute comment alerts us to the double standards that attach to the kind of rationalisations brought to bear on sexual misconduct by professionals. It emphasises something we tend to forget: that properly validated professional care is a skill to be exercised with care for, but not emotional entanglement with, a patient.

The problem of harm also seems to attend interventions such as aversion therapy, shame therapy, and 'strategic' therapies that demean or humiliate the patient. No doubt there are contexts within which such practices can be used in a restorative, healing way, but the intuitive sense that someone is being harmed by being so treated should be closely heeded, and set aside only where clear indications of benefit are well grounded in reputable clinical literature.

A particularly insidious, widespread, and elusive problem in our general care of patients with psychological disorders is the indiscriminate use of drugs where drug therapy is not proven to be innocuous in its effects. In fact, the pervasiveness of this failure of adequate professional care is evident in the medicalising of life's problems by the use of psychotropic drugs. Many patients have personal and social problems that need positive constructive answers, which someone working in the traditional medical model may or may not be able to supply. This is just as legitimate a demand upon the expertise of health care professionals and a health care system as any other cause of human suffering. We cannot pretend that we are exercising competent professional care if such problems are met with a speedily scribbled note for some drug and a cursory interview that skirts the patient's real needs.

These types of aberration in care seem quite different, and some at least are hard to detect and correct. We have argued that mental health care revolves around clinical skills enabling an informed response to the patient's needs; professional distance; the proper exercise of those skills; and an acute sense of the vulnerability of the patient to the harm caused by psychological abuse, exploitation, or depersonalisation. Validating and adequately funding these skills are both essential if we are to address these problems, and make some impact in mental health. The requisite skills are under threat when we have a scientific establishment that asks for biological bases for every cause of human suffering, and a funding system that prefers neatly packaged remedies to a carefully formulated but often extended plan of care. The skills involved in properly professional mental health care are also essential in protecting professionals from error in dealing with psychiatric patients.

The uncertainties and difficulties of the complex relationship between psychiatric professional and patient mean that professional judgment and wisdom are at a premium. The vulnerability of the patient puts tremendous ethical weight on the clinical decisions made. This is nowhere more evident than in the process of securing involuntary treatment for those we consider to be insane or mentally disordered. These patients not only find themselves in great distress, but also 'may suffer other indignities or punishments in addition to their liberty being curtailed' (Szasz 1983). The indignities include enforced medication, which may have unpleasant or serious side effects; the imposition of a special status for the purposes of employment and other civil entitlements; the administration of the patient's affairs by others; and even submission to invasive and potentially damaging physical treatments in the attempt to alleviate the problem. The alienating nature of these measures, and the context of an area of health care in which compulsory treatment is a possibility, have potentially devastating effects on the therapeutic relationship, effects that go beyond the interpersonal problems we have already discussed.

Compulsory Treatment

The possibility that a close friend, or even we ourselves, might be forcibly restrained and treated by methods that to many would seem barbaric—methods such as intramuscular injections, electroconvulsive therapy (ECT), or isolation—is truly frightening to most people. The fact that it is done to some members of our community seems to contradict many of the emphases of this book. Compulsory treatment 'is, in itself, an evil; it can only be justified by large countervailing gains' (Hare 1991). Compulsory treatment is, of course, required only where the patient will not cooperate with efforts to treat the problem. Compulsory treatment contravenes the requirement to seek informed consent for medical interventions, something that is part of a therapeutic relationship with any reasonable person. The psychiatrist, in fact, has an unenviable task. He or she must pay heed to the overriding value of *beneficence*, or the desire to help the patient, in the face of the patient's (often very persuasive) appeal not to be treated. The only way to override the interpersonal appeal of the patient in this circumstance, and yet keep a firm hold on the ethical principles we have enunciated, is to realise that the patient has 'a mental defect which seriously impairs their judgment' (McGarry & Chodoff 1981). In fact this 'mental defect', along with the considered opinion that the patient may well act to the detriment of his or her own or others' welfare, is a legally required aspect of the justification of compulsory treatment in most jurisdictions.

The mental defect means that one of the foundations of our ethical framework is absent, in that the patient concerned is not thinking and acting as a rational social being would. The opinion that this is so and that there is also a real danger to the patient or others is, of course, a difficult clinical judgment to make, and for that reason it should be made, wherever possible, by a clinician with adequate psychiatric expertise. In most countries this is not a firm requirement, and its neglect, in the absence of a system that ensures careful review of the decisions made and the right of the patient to appeal, can lead to abuse.

The institution of compulsory treatment can be softened somewhat by giving the patient information and cooperation where possible. This avoids the 'prisoner syndrome', whereby the patient's often paranoid fears are in fact realised.

> Albert began talking to his landlady about the fact that people were treating him strangely, and expressed the fear that they were going to lock him up. This became a preoccupation, and he began to tell people that the word was getting around and that the doctors were starting to take an interest so that he would not be surprised if one day they did visit him, take him away, and try to alter his mind with poisonous drugs without telling him what they were doing. This all duly happened, and was justified on the basis that Albert was confused and suffered paranoid delusions, such that he did not really understand what was happening to him and was a danger to himself. The magistrate making out the order for his committal was, not unsurprisingly, a little difficult to convince.

Communicating with patients, so that they are not cut off from developing an understanding of their problems and the strategies that might be used to counteract them, is becoming more and more the norm in psychiatry. It is important that a patient not be kept in ignorance—where that can be avoided (even though the patient may not respond appropriately to the attempt at communication)—because a key factor in continuing psychiatric treatment is going to be the therapeutic relationship that the patient forms. That relationship aims to restore the patient to autonomous functioning as a person, a rational social being. Nothing could be more damaging to such a relationship than the perception that the psychiatrist is an enemy or a repressive figure of authority whose mode of action is to confine, disempower, and override the patient as a person.

Attempts to communicate with patients and include them in decisions (which may involve an element of beneficent coercion) enhance the possibility of safeguarding their dignity in what is necessarily a humiliating situation. When the phase of restoration to something like normal function is reached, the patient must rebuild his or her personality and relationships on whatever shreds of personal dignity and integrity are left, and his or her ally in this process should be the therapist. It is, therefore, intrinsic to good practice, even where it does involve compulsory treatment, that everything possible has been done to preserve the semblance of a normal clinical relationship between health care worker and patient.

Alcohol and Drug Addiction

Where patients become dependent on substances damaging to their well-being, special problems can arise in their management. Patients may not be able to trust their own judgment when it comes to life choices or the use of money. The same problems can arise with gambling and other addictions that seriously impact on the patient's well-being or relationships and commitments. The problem is that the choices seem to be made with a sound mind, in that the person is not demented or clearly insane when the relevant decisions are made, even though later they may deeply regret what has happened. In most jurisdictions the ability to subject a person to compulsory treatment or restraint of some kind depends on a judgment that the person's ability to act in his or her own best interests is disrupted by an abnormal mental state and that serious harm is likely to result from the actions concerned. It strains the usual definitions of an abnormal state of mind to deal with addiction in this manner. Consequently, some therapists find that the way to respect patient autonomy and allow for aberrations that the patient believes on reflection to be truly damaging to themselves, is to forge a strong therapeutic alliance, perhaps bolstered by some kind of a Ulysses bargain.

The concept of a Ulysses bargain arises from Greek mythology when Ulysses both wanted to hear the song of the sirens but not to endanger the lives of himself or his crew by giving in to the lure of their song. He therefore asked to be tied to the mast of his boat, blocked the ears of his crew, and gave them strict instructions not to do anything he said until they were well out of danger. In essence, such an arrangement involves setting in place a mechanism that can be triggered to disempower the person and to neutralise the possibility of doing something that will adversely affect that person's interests and will later be deeply regretted. This may involve a mechanism whereby access to bank accounts or ability to enter into binding legal agreements can be suspended. Such arrangements preserve the patient's overall or long-term autonomy and quality of life at the expense of temporary limitations to their autonomy, but they can only work where the relationship between caregiver and client is a partnership built on trust. Unfortunately, in the psychiatric area, this is often not the case as the patient's ability to engage in such a partnership is either limited or not explored.

Psychosurgery and ECT

Psychosurgery began with an operation on the frontal lobes of the brain by the Portuguese neurologist Egas Moniz and his surgical colleague Almeida Lima. The standard procedure involved cutting the major connections, or a large proportion of them, between the frontal lobe—the seat of personality, higher-order motivations, and socialisation—and the rest of the brain. The effects of the operation are difficult to assess. It undoubtedly helped a number of severely depressed and disturbed patients at a time when little else was available. The state to which many of these patients had been reduced should warn us against making wild claims about the damage produced by the operation itself. However, the operation seems to result in reduced emotional reactions, an impoverishment of personality and character, and a state of motivational destitution that many would regard as inhuman. We must, therefore, recognise that it inflicts serious and irreversible harm as the cost of relief from an identifiable psychological disorder.

Between 1942 and 1954, 10 365 patients were treated by this procedure in England alone. To many contemporary commentators this seems almost incomprehensible, but we ought to recall that little else was available to help those patients at the time.

A further procedure is amygdalotomy, which is used to treat aggressive disorders and some types of hyperactivity. Its use is limited to certain geographical areas, and in some it has been suggested as a means of controlling violent criminals. The effects of this are relatively uncharted but seem to include motivational alteration. Both frontal lobe surgery and amygdalotomy carry a risk of death or permanent alteration of psychological function and, *ex hypothesi*, are being offered to individuals suffering psychological impairments. For these reasons, ethical justification for the procedures is hard to find. Moreover, in the face of anecdotal evidence that less intrusive treatments confer benefits that psychosurgery does not, the use of these more radical procedures may be impossible to defend. The issues should not, however, be obscured by a horrified reaction to the very thought of such things.

Similar shock and horror are often evoked by reports of electroconvulsive therapy (ECT), which undeniably did and still does help certain patients. ECT involves passing an electric current through the brain at a level that, unmodified by anticonvulsant and anaesthetic medication, would cause an epileptic fit. It is claimed that ECT has a dramatic effect on certain patients with severe depression, and that it causes no demonstrable harm if administered properly. We cannot hope to evaluate these claims, but we can outline the ethical principles that go into their assessment.

In both psychotherapy and ECT, procedures have been performed that are not well founded on any scientific understanding of psychological function or psychiatric disorders. In both cases the reason for the popularity of the procedures has been that they served to alleviate, to some extent, the intense suffering of individuals condemned to live in great distress, and often with no hope of release from an institution. There is no doubt that the lack of precise clinical indications for employing the treatments, and feelings of desperation among doctors and patients, led to unwise and overly extensive use of both techniques. In addition, mental health professionals failed to consider seriously the possible long-term risks to personality and brain function posed by these procedures. In both cases we now believe there was serious risk to brain function and a risk of death. Both treatments have been the subject of intensive lobbying by patients and human rights groups, and have drawn the ire of ethicists because of their use without informed consent. But none of these facts give us adequate reason to dismiss the treatments as ethically unacceptable.

We must recall that the treatments were genuinely thought to offer hope to those who had no hope and that, on this basis, they passed the test of beneficence on which we have defended compulsory treatment of other types. That is why a treatment can be ethically acceptable even if it is dangerous, may not have been carried out with the patient's informed consent, and may not be proven to produce a benefit. If it is the only alternative to an unacceptable future for the patient, a reasonable person might well, in spite of all the drawbacks, opt for a slim chance of benefit. If we would allow a reasonable and autonomous patient to make this choice, it seems perverse to deny a mentally impaired patient the same opportunity. Of course we would want to know that the medical evidence really did suggest that the choice was reasonable, and the alternatives truly bleak for the unfortunate person, but given those things, it would be not only permissible but even, to some extent, obligatory to offer the patient the chance of improvement. The need to take account of objective considerations, and not merely patients' choices, in assessing these treatments would also suggest that consent to psychosurgery, though the norm where possible, would not be sufficient justification for undertaking such operations (Kleinig 1985). Desperate and possibly incompetent patients may well make ill-judged choices, and they should not be exposed to harm through those choices.

The fact that such treatments became so widespread for a certain period in psychiatric history reflects not only the desperation that prevailed, but also a pressure that continues to influence psychiatric management. Psychiatric care is always under-resourced and therefore there is a great deal of pressure to limit care and prove its efficacy. Short, sharp, biologically based interventions have the attraction of offering a resolution to an otherwise protracted illness for which other therapies offer uncertain and inconclusive prospects. If psychiatric disorders are seen as problems originating within the individual, then, as with any other diseases, the development of targeted therapies with a quantifiable cost and documented indications becomes a plausible option. However, if psychiatric disorders are a mixture of individual dysfunctions rubbing shoulders with problems that are more complex in their origins, then the neatly packaged illness-and-treatment-options approach is inappropriate. If some disorders are the products of complex forces arising more from an extended process operating throughout the person's life story or in their social context, the resource implications are potentially huge. It has always been easier to exclude psychiatric patients and those who care for them from the main streams of medical funding and service delivery, because once marginalised in this way the importance of the problems can be discounted. More tractable areas of health care can then form the core of health care systems. This recurring problem is only belatedly being addressed, and the waxing and waning of some of the more drastic psychiatric 'remedies' are a cogent historical reminder that the problem is still with us.

Confidentiality

Some psychiatric patients pose dangers to other people, yet not such obvious danger that they can be committed to safe care. Just such a case led to the controversial decision in the Tarasoff case in 1974 (California Supreme Court 1976).

> A young male student, P, who had been in treatment for violent tendencies and paranoid ideas, told his therapist that he intended to kill a female student whom he did not name but who could be identified as T from information he gave about her. The campus police were notified but T's family was not warned. P was detained by the campus police and then released because they thought he was rational. T arrived back from her vacation and P killed her. The family sued the university and the therapists for failure to take proper action which, they claimed, included warning them of the threat to their daughter. The court found in their favour, although it recognised the difficulty of the duty it thereby endorsed, and the conflict between that duty and the duty of confidentiality that forms part of the ethical code for medical practice.

This decision predated guidelines about HIV/AIDS infection, potentially dangerous drivers, and children at risk of abuse. Various bodies have decided in these situations that the magnitude of the harm resulting from an absolute respect for confidentiality outweighs the harm from breach of confidentiality. This is, of course, a very difficult judgment to make, and some psychiatrists would argue that it creates a total distortion in the doctor–patient relationship, because the patient must accept that the doctor is, if a conflict arises, not always in the patient's corner doing the best for him or her as an individual at odds with the world.

We should note that there is also a suspension of the normal terms of the doctor–patient relationship in the compulsory treatment of the insane. Thus, whatever we decide about the aptness or otherwise of the findings in the Tarasoff case concerning the professional judgment of dangerous potential and duty to warn, certain ethical principles emerge. Where the therapist becomes aware that a patient has disclosed information suggesting that an identifiable person is at significant risk of harm, any measures possible should be taken to protect that person. If this involves suspending the therapist's normal duty to respect confidentiality, then so be it. This advice is based on a similar standard and set of considerations to the advice given about HIV infection, and we would expect it to receive similar endorsement from responsible professional bodies.

A difficult problem arises where a patient is known or judged to be dangerous by caregivers but for some reason the decision is taken to release the patient into a situation where he or she might be a danger to others. In such a case there is a conflict, in that we have a responsibility to respect the patient's confidentiality but also to protect the patient and others from harm. The harms are twofold: the actual harm arising from dangerous behaviour and the moral harm to the patient arising from having harmed another. It is often the guilt and remorse over a particular action that blights a psychiatric patient's life as much as anything else that happens during the illness. For this reason, there must be channels for a caregiver or health professional to make a concern known to those arranging for the future management of the patient's problem, and to have a review of any decisions based on an inadequate appraisal of the risks involved in returning the patient to the community.

Suicide and Psychiatric Illness

The accepted practice of the medical profession in relation to suicide has been to take whatever steps are necessary to prevent a suicide attempt from succeeding. This is not just because suicide questions our sense of the sanctity of life (and we have argued that that seems to be a misreading of the values on which most people make health care decisions), but seems rather to have to do with the finality of death, and the realisation that a person must be desperate before he or she attempts to commit suicide. Taken together, these things lead us to doubt whether the decision to take one's own life is generally well reasoned, a doubt that becomes even stronger when we notice the consistent correlation between suicide and psychiatric illness. However, 'the possibility of suicide is considered by almost every human being at some stage of his life' (Heyd & Bloch 1991), despite the fact that most of us turn away from that step. Thus our ethical attitudes in this area are bound to be mixed, and we cannot treat patients as insane merely because they attempt to commit suicide. There is, however, a gamut of cases ranging from those in which suicidal ideation and major psychiatric disorder coincide, to those where it is hard to dispute the reasonable decisions made.

Mark has a diagnosis of bipolar illness predominantly depressive in type. He is initially well maintained on Lithium but when seen in the clinic is noted to have delusional and suicidal ideation. He is extremely difficult to engage in conversation and keeps talking about a black incubus sucking his life force out of his brain. He is advised to come into hospital but refuses, claiming that the hospital will suffocate him because of the malignant gases escaping from the cancer ward. His therapist speaks to his sister, and then arranges for Mark to be committed for compulsory treatment.

Heather is a 23-year-old who lives in a city flat with three others. She has recently lost her job as a teacher because of a reduction in enrolments at her school, and now does relieving work in local schools. She presents to the psychiatric service, having been referred for depression. Her parents are separated and living in different cities from her. She has few local friends. She visits the town where she spent her childhood during most of her holidays but finds fewer and fewer of her old friends there. She expresses little interest in the future, and has no pastimes or plans about which she is enthusiastic. Outpatient care, counselling, and antidepressant medication are of little help to her and, after attending the service for some weeks and having had an inpatient stay of ten days, she says to her therapist that she is going to kill herself. She does not seem mentally impaired and, although the therapist is worried about her, he does not feel he can commit her for compulsory treatment. The police notify the clinic the next morning that she has been found dead and to say that they are seeking information for the coroner.

Edna and Arthur are a well-regarded couple who, in retirement, have enjoyed good health and continued to maintain their contacts with the academic life of the university where Arthur taught for some years. Arthur begins to notice a failing of his memory and general intellect, and a disturbing change in his personality after his seventy-sixth birthday. He recognises in himself the first symptoms of a distressing form of senile dementia to which his family is prone. Two months after this realisation, he and Edna also find out that Edna has a malignant bowel cancer that has spread to her liver and is causing her significant and unremitting pain. They plan and hold a party for their many friends and family over the weekend of Edna's seventy-fourth birthday. Three days later they are found dead in their bed from massive overdoses of her analgesic and cardiac medications.

The undeniable link between suicide and mental disorder means that the last of these three cases is not at all typical. However, it does mean that one might rationally choose to end one's own life, and we have now described a case where that is so. While admitting that there may be cases in which the choice of suicide is rational, we have to take every precaution to reassure ourselves that no features suggesting an underlying psychiatric disorder are evident in a patient. The fact that a number of those who attempt suicide are making their choice while disturbed, and will not choose that way again, justifies life-saving intervention as the policy of an emergency unit. This follows from the fact that, although we can never be certain about the conditions of and rationale for an attempt, we know that if we do not intervene the decision is irreversible. Thus, 'direct responsibility over a potentially irreversible decision under conditions of uncertainty, suggests a policy of postponement' (Heyd & Bloch 1991). This policy is vindicated by the fact that most failed suicides are glad that their lives were saved (British Medical Association 1988). The ethical weight in this area, therefore, seems to fall heavily on the medical policy that runs counter to putting absolute value on patient autonomy. This means, unfortunately, that we will sometimes act inappropriately for the 'Ednas and Arthurs' who fall into our path.

Again we see an intuitive awareness of the realities of human psychology in our policy. People in general are not clear-cut forward planners who have an autonomously formulated and rationally justified agenda to pursue. They feel things and react to things in myriad ways that change over time, and through the vicissitudes of relationships and adverse circumstances. Patients who are psychologically disturbed are particularly vulnerable to instability in their thoughts and intentions, and therefore require special 'parentalistic' concern. Within the shifting sand of the disturbed psyche, some patterns are relatively stable and others are transient, and thus, in clinical practice, we should try to empower patients as best we can to look to their abiding interests and to survive the threats to life and well-being posed by their illness.

Reproduction, Sexuality, and Mental Impairment

Leah is a mentally retarded young woman of twenty-five who has the mental age of a five-year-old. She has irregular heavy periods and gets ill when she is given Depo contraception. She enjoys playing with dolls and babies, and is sexually aware to the extent that she has been observed petting with a young male patient she knows, and has made overtly sexual approaches to other men. Her parents find her periods hard to cope with and do not see hormonal treatment as an answer to her needs. They have asked that she be sterilised by tubal ligation.

The ethical issues in this area are clouded by claims about the human right to reproduce and discrimination against the disabled. To resolve these issues, we need to keep firmly in mind the fact that clinical decisions ought to be made in the best interests of the patient, or with regard to what would be of substantial benefit to the patient, when the patient is not competent to make decisions. Here the patient is clearly not competent, and indeed is regarded in law as being vulnerable in the area of sexuality. This means that someone else must take these highly value-laden decisions for her. This is not always the case, and some patients with mental disabilities are infantilised and discounted by others who are all too happy to take over their lives especially in messy areas like sexuality. Where the patient can take a meaningful part in discussions about the future and about the reproductive choices he or she is facing, the need for decision-making by others would have to be critically assessed.

Common sense dictates that a patient such as Leah could not care for a baby, nor could she understand or prepare herself for childbirth. She should, therefore, be protected from this experience, as her mental age would suggest. For this reason, and because her mental impairment is a permanent condition, it would seem to be in her best interests to sterilise her and others like her, a decision that has been endorsed by courts in the United Kingdom and elsewhere (Skegg 1988b). In fact, in most Commonwealth jurisdictions it is thought appropriate to leave the decision to the doctors and the parents of the patient as long as they are in agreement. In that there is no reason to suspect that most parents are acting contrary to the best interests of their children, and that it seems reasonable to spare a person such as Leah the problems of pregnancy and childbirth, this would seem to be the right stand to take. However, parents are not the final arbiters of reproductive choices made by young people who in other contexts we regard as not fully competent. It is, therefore, important to have an open mind in approaching the issues surrounding sterilisation and disability.

There are, in fact, some arguments for the sterilisation of the mentally infirm that are not ethically acceptable. The idea that the mentally impaired should be denied any rights to sexual expression or reproduction, solely because they are defective and could corrupt the gene pool, is one such argument, based as much in discriminatory and stigmatising beliefs as in any consideration for their real interests and role in society. Similar doubts can be raised about the contention that mentally defective people as a group are generally unfit to be social parents. It would need to be shown that there was real cause to believe that a particular couple were not fit, and would be likely to harm their child or themselves in some way, before the ethical aspects of the decision would be clear. It may well be that, in an appropriate setting and with the right support, a mentally defective couple could provide a standard of parenting that was fair on any offspring they might have, and on others affected by their decision. Thus we cannot ethically justify the sterilisation of the mentally infirm as a general policy. Each case must be considered on the basis of what would be best for the people concerned. Because those affected often include parents or other caregivers of the couple wanting to reproduce, they ought to be involved in the decision. The fact that any child produced will also be a member of our society with his or her own rights means that those interests too are relevant.

Conclusion

We have discussed a number of areas of clinical care in which the psychiatric patient is vulnerable and cannot adequately be covered by the normal ethical considerations governing relations between health care personnel and patients. The difficulties are compounded by deep academic or scientific controversies over a number of issues in psychiatric theory and practice. This means that we have to place special emphasis here on the Hippocratic admonition *primum non nocere*, since special care must be taken to ensure that the patient does not suffer because of the lack of capacity for autonomy and informed decision-making. To this end, there is a presumption in favour of treatment if it offers significant chance of benefit. However, there must also be a constant awareness of the danger of 'locking the patient in' to a stereotype that can lead to disempowerment, loss of dignity, and chronic dependency beyond what is required for an effective therapeutic relationship. As is in other areas of health care, the underlying aim of all psychiatric treatment should be to restore the patient to a state of functioning as fully as possible. In psychiatric practice this may require special skills of judgment and negotiation as the patients may be vulnerable and 'not in their right minds'.

11
Aging, Dementia, and Mortality

Introduction

The limitations imposed upon us by our aging brains bring our mortality home with brutal force. Not only is aging accompanied by limits on our abilities in general, but by the spectre of dementia in particular. The many accompanying problems affect the value we seek to ascribe to the elderly, and in particular to those unable to cope in any meaningful way with the normal exigencies of daily living. This chapter explores the effects of normal aging before proceeding to a discussion of abnormal aging, with special reference to Alzheimer's disease (AD).

Neurobiology of Aging

A brain from an aged individual, regardless of that individual's state of mental health, will exhibit a variety of peculiarities or abnormalities. These may include any one or a combination of the following: a decline in brain weight, neuronal loss in specific brain regions, neuronal shrinkage, and dendritic tree atrophy including loss of spines and synaptic connections. Some areas of the brain, such as the basal forebrain cholinergic system and substantia nigra, are more susceptible to age-related changes. These anatomical changes can be correlated with the slowing of mental and motor functions, with memory deterioration, and changes in mood, sleep, appetite, and other non-cognitive functions frequently observed in the aged.

In addition to these age-related changes, the brains of elderly individuals may also exhibit morphological changes characteristic of AD, such as the deposition of amyloid plaques and neurofibrillary tangles (see Neurobiology of Alzheimer's Disease later in this chapter). This occurs despite the fact that these individuals are considered neurologically intact or register only minimal impairment on psychometric tests. Thus, the exact relationship between the presence of amyloid plaques in aged brains and the subsequent development of AD remains to be determined.

Approaches to Aging

The Blessing of Mortality

Our lives as human beings are limited. A life of three score years and ten is not a totally misleading guide when discussing the biological, ethical, and social dilemmas of aging. Leon Kass has argued that 'the attachment to life—or the fear of death—knows no limits, certainly not for most human beings . . . we want to live and live, and not to wither and not to die' (Kass 1985b, p. 306).

Alternatively, one may simply have the following aim: not to add years to life, but life to years. Not only are ideals such as these far removed from reality, they encompass a problem. Is it possible to conceive of a situation where this illness-free condition would not lull us into a longing for everlasting life in an illness-free body? Within such a scenario, death would seem even more shocking than it does now. Perhaps both aspirations are misleading, since both attempt to escape from the dis-ease that is all-pervading and that permeates every facet of human experience. In the long term they are of little help in sorting out ethical issues of significance in coping with the aged and demented. It is better to start from the premise that mortality is a blessing.

A longing for some form of human immortality is a longing for more of the same: a longing for a prolonged earthly life, which itself has profound limitations. Once we acknowledge and accept our finitude, we can devote our attention to living well and establishing important priorities for the time that remains to us as mortal and finite human beings. Mortality and aging are inseparable. If we accept mortality, we are forced to accept one of its inevitable consequences, namely, aging. It follows that the end result of the decline inherent in aging is death—what may be referred to as *natural death*. Natural death leads us away from the medicalisation of death, and makes possible communication about the needs of spiritual and palliative care. Included in this is an awareness that death makes way for the birth of children, just as the deaths of others made way for us (Jonas 1992). In this manner aging and mortality intertwine, forming a positive whole that is essential to our thinking about the aging body. But this by itself will not resolve a host of dilemmas presented by competition for resources between patients of different ages.

Resources, the Elderly, and Quality Adjusted Life Years (QALYs)

Consider the following example:

> A teacher, Jon Collis (aged forty-seven) and one of his older neighbours, Mr Collins (seventy-five) are both on the waiting list for open heart surgery. A opening arises at relatively short notice and the surgeon planning admissions notices the pair. As he thinks about whom to admit he wonders about the relative value

to the community of the two and decides that, in general, someone young, in otherwise good physical health and in employment ought to be preferred to somebody older and dependent on the community for support. He therefore tells his secretary to send for Mr Jon Collis, even though, according to dates, Mr Collins is the next in line.

This doctor focuses on the patient's age, but he may also be thinking of other things wrong with Mr Collins, all of which make the use of open heart surgery far less likely to yield long-term benefit. How can these complicating factors be placed in perspective? A number of arguments are used in discussing this matter. One of these is Quality Adjusted Life Years (QALYs). The QALYs argument places a value on the outcome of a medical intervention according to the 'quality adjusted life years' that would result. Someone aged 75, and likely to live for a further five to seven years after a medical procedure, is bound to lose out for resources based on QALYs to a 45-year-old expected to live for twenty to thirty years after the same procedure. This is because, if the procedure results in a net gain in health quality of 0.2, the net QALY gain for the 75-year-old works out at 1.5, and at 5 for the 45-year-old.

Even more extreme (and counter-intuitive) is the situation of a competent adult and a procedure such as an operation on a malignant brain tumour, a procedure that is expected to provide one year of good-quality life. The maximum gain in this instance is 1 QALY. Compare this with the alleviation of a minor problem (0.1 QALY points, say) in a young person, with perhaps fifty further years of life (making 5 QALY points in total). For the person who has only one year to live, that gain of one year may be of immeasurable value no matter what his or her age. For this reason, some advocates for the aged reject QALYs as a fair way of allocating health care resources.

A related approach is provided by the *fair innings* argument: the aged have had a fair innings and our health care resources should be used for young people who have not as yet had their chance. This argument is based on fairness, self-interest, and competition. However, there is no fairness about disease and death, and so it is misleading to compare life with a game of cricket. People are not equal in the health lottery, nor in the lottery of life, and hence there is no compulsion on society to smooth over the inequities of blind natural chance (or providence).

It is also noteworthy that older people themselves often use the phrase 'fair (or good) innings' to indicate that there is more to human motivation than the self-interest implied by this narrow model. Many older people feel they have fulfilled their major life projects and that, even though they continue to enjoy life, they are not desperate to hold on to it at all costs. The fair innings argument might, therefore, be interpreted as a disposition to give life and physical well-being to those (the young) who most thirst for it. However, even this interpretation points to no more than a voluntary relinquishing of health care opportunities for the old, and not to a policy of mandatory preference for the young.

Yet another approach is the *we've paid taxes for years* argument, with its basis in righteous indignation. A government or health service could reply that what we buy with our taxes is limited to coverage for a set number of years and services. On this view the correct response is that offered by any insurance agency to clients who have never called on their policy. 'You have not lost anything in that we have provided an agreed and ever-expanding level of cover compared with the things you might have received when you first joined up. It just so happens that, although we have all shared your risk, you have never fallen foul of the health risks we all run.'

This counter-argument based on risk-sharing is interesting, but it raises the question of the sort of health care system people think they are entitled to. Many believe they qualify for all of the health care they will ever need for the whole of their lives. But, as governments change every few years, the only promise a public health care system can make is to provide that standard of health care considered just and fair at any given point in time. This is analogous to taking out an insurance policy where the insurer is able to change the conditions unilaterally. This type of policy places the elderly, in particular, in a position of considerable uncertainty.

Finally, what about health care based on *social worth*? This approach rapidly becomes a tool of a privileged elite and, if transformed into policy, for example by the privatisation of health services, can be used to further disadvantage the already disadvantaged. Once such an elite sets the terms on which social worth is to be judged, the system can enshrine unjust prejudices against minorities, people with alternative lifestyles, or even devalued vocations and professions. Social worth as a criterion is particularly insidious with respect to the aged.

Problems of Aging

Aging is an integral part of what it means to be human and mortal. The aged remind us of the importance of our interdependence within human communities. They confront us with our treatment of those who are our equals and yet are weaker than us and dependent upon us for care and protection. These values are of considerable significance. However, they do not shield us from major dilemmas implicit in weighing up the resources to be placed at the disposal of the aged versus those to be directed towards other groups within any community. Choices are inevitable.

Mortality is a time-dependent phenomenon. The mortal life begins at one point and concludes at another. For the aged, much of that finite life has already been lived; they have had their opportunities to experience what human life means, and to contribute to the welfare of others. As people age they become more dependent on others within the human community; placing on others the moral obligation to care for and protect them in ways not required since their childhood. They are still one with the rest of us, and we continue to have responsibilities for them since they mirror so much of what we are.

They are, therefore, to be valued alongside others within the human community, although the value attributed to them may not entail devoting the same level of resources to them as to those who are younger. This is especially true when there is competition for those resources. On the basis of our mortality, and therefore of the limited time-span allotted to us, it seems reasonable to suggest that in the competition for resources the needs of younger age groups should, as a very general principle, be placed first. This may have few repercussions for most clinical procedures, since care and provision of the basic necessities of existence are unaffected. Its significance stems from its attempt to come to terms with our mortality.

This approach has been developed far more extensively by Daniel Callahan, especially in his pivotal book *Setting Limits* (1987). Here he argues that we should accept aging as a part of life rather than as another medical obstacle to be overcome. We should find a meaningful place for suffering and decline in life, and should not pretend that old age can be turned into some form of endless middle age. Callahan's position is one in which the interests and claims of elderly individuals are to be protected. This protection does not necessarily include such extreme measures as directing unlimited resources towards these individuals, pursuing unlimited life extension, or failing to balance the needs of different age groups. This approach may mean that some claims of autonomy will have to be set aside so that the needs and autonomy of others have a chance to flourish. In other words, the old may have a duty to the young not to make demands that will harm the young, but at the same time the young have duties to sustain the welfare of the old.

Underlying Callahan's position is a rejection of euthanasia for the elderly, since it conveys the wrong symbolism. This is based on what he sees as a need to maintain and substantiate their dignity, and to develop an understanding of the ways in which old age can be filled with meaning and significance. He believes that society should guarantee elderly people greater control over their dying, in the sense that they are provided with the opportunity to refuse life-extending treatment (Callahan 1987).

Not surprisingly, Callahan's proposal is regarded as provocative by some, and has led to numerous rejoinders. These include: setting limits on the elderly is morally wrong, the data behind Callahan's analysis are too pessimistic, the significant differences that exist between individuals rule out viewing the elderly as a group, chronological age is too arbitrary, and treatment decisions should be based on individual need since the notion of a natural life span is vague and unhelpful.

It needs to be recognised that Callahan's proposals were intended simply as general pointers. The emphasis is on freeing the elderly from unnecessary burdens imposed by excessive life-sustaining treatment. It is not his intention to limit their freedom by unnecessarily restricting access to self-evidently beneficial treatment. At present, limits on medical treatment are implicitly, if not explicitly, set on most age and treatment groups in public health care systems. Thus, Callahan's ideas are not as substantial a departure from accepted practice as some allege. We can, however, ask whether Callahan is right to reject legalised euthanasia as an acceptable choice for the elderly on the basis of its symbolic significance.

P. D. James sets her novel *The Children of Men* in a period when the population is aging and there is an institution of 'quietus' or voluntary group suicide for those who think they may be a burden on others. One passage relates directly to the question of public policy on euthanasia:

> His gaze at Theo was one of fear almost amounting to terror. And then Theo recognized him. He was Digby Yule, a retired Classics don from Merton.
>
> Theo introduced himself. 'It's good to see you, sir. How are you?'
>
> The question seemed to increase Yule's nervousness. His right hand began an apparently uncontrolled drumming of the table-top. He said: 'Oh, very well, yes, very well, thank you, Faron. I'm managing all right. I do for myself, you know. I live in lodgings off the Iffley Road but I manage very well. I do everything for myself. The landlady isn't an easy woman—well, she has her own problems—but I'm no trouble to her. I'm no trouble to anyone.'

We are moved to ask why Digby Yule was so anxious, given that the only provision in his society was for *voluntary* suicide. To understand this we need to consider the wider impact of such social decisions.

A dominant concern for many people, especially when they are ill, is to do what is expected of them. The legalisation of euthanasia sends a signal about death and dying that is subtle but nevertheless real. It tells us that there is a time when death might be the right choice, and that for some it is a reasonable step to choose death. This prompts the question 'Am I one of those? Am I the kind of person who ought to be dead?' These questions, implicitly posed by the possibility of voluntary euthanasia for the aged, discomfort people when their need is to be cared for. Economically they may make sense, but as a symbol of our social attitudes they send another kind of message. Do we want a society in which the 'Digby Yule' response is a further burden of aging? Voluntary euthanasia could well convert aging from being a time of dignity and respect, and a fitting conclusion to human life, into a time of anxiety and stress. Nevertheless this does not preclude setting limits regarding the kinds of care that seem to be compatible with the situation of the aging patient.

The basic ethical principles underlying the care of the aged have been summarised as *justice, beneficence, autonomy*, and *privacy* (Oakley 1992). The justice principle does not entitle an individual patient to every potentially beneficial treatment. Consequently, in the aging domain, expensive medical procedures should not be performed on those with a relatively small chance of deriving worthwhile benefit from them. Beneficence, while promoting the interests and well-being of a patient, may entail conflict between the quantity and the quality of life: the quality of a life can vary regardless of the number of years remaining in it. In what way, therefore, might a person whose life is bereft of meaning be helped by having it prolonged? With regard to patient autonomy, a distinction has been made between autonomous choice and autonomous action, on the ground that any diminution of autonomous action necessitates increased dependence on others. Consequently changes occurring with age diminish autonomy, partly because they interfere with an individual's capacity for action, but also because they undermine both a sense of self and the concept of the meaning of life. It is inevitable that privacy ranks highly in care of the aged, since respect for privacy plays a crucial role in helping elderly people maintain a sense of individuality. In institutionalised care of the aged, respect by caregivers for the private realm of each patient may prove crucial in helping to avoid depersonalisation.

The elderly are 'one of us', and this must be appropriately acknowledged in all our dealings with them: in matters of privacy, in considering their wishes, welcoming them as equal partners in the human endeavour, and forwarding their cause. Nevertheless their time as 'one of us' is limited, and while this in no way invalidates basic values, it does restrict the measures that are appropriate for extending this time-span.

Independence and the Impairments of Age

The potential loss of privacy and independence is a concern for many older folk. This may lead some of them to belittle their handicaps so as not to have to 'go to a home'. The desire of an older person to retain his or her independence is an expression of personal autonomy and identity. This, for some, entails certain risks to health and well-being, such as forgetfulness or absent-mindedness, falls or collapse from a stroke. Consider the following case:

> Sarah had always been a strong and independent person even when her husband, George, was alive. The family had to some extent lived in her shadow and she had encouraged her daughters and their families to be independent. She has, however, begun to be absent-minded, losing her keys or purse, and forgetting to provide food for her meals. She has also fallen on a few occasions. Her daughters are getting worried, but her son argues that he still enjoys mountaineering and that he

is running risks just as great as those his mother runs by her wish to remain in her own home. Sarah's daughters gently point out that it is not he who gets called when their mother runs into strife.

How many risks can a person take in pursuit of a life project, such as being independent when old? We must avoid the Scylla of over-protectiveness towards the elderly, and the Charybdis of turning a blind eye to a real need with a real impact on both the person and others. If Sarah can be helped to maintain independent living, that seems the best outcome for her even though she may have to agree to certain compromises to avoid the worst risks to herself and others. The fact that there is a risk to her life or well-being no more provides a reason for denying her that choice than it does for forbidding people to go mountaineering. Often systems can be set in place, such as timers on the oven and heaters, to avert major dangers. However, if Sarah's lifestyle choices significantly impinge on the lives of her children or create a hazard for her local community, there will be a certain point at which it becomes unjust to prefer her independence over the independence and safety of others. We draw this line at different points at different times. For instance, in many countries it is unacceptable to drive without a seatbelt or ride a cycle without a helmet, limitations involving an intuitive weighting of personal freedom against unreasonable risk-taking. Care should be taken that we do not become so averse to the idea of death in an older person, that we deny that person the right to take risks. By this we mean the sort of risks that younger people take purely for pleasure, the sort of risks most of us find acceptable.

Neurobiology of Alzheimer's Disease

As mentioned previously, the key neuropathological features of Alzheimer's disease (AD) are amyloid plaques and neurofibrillary tangles. Amyloid plaques have been classified into two groups: those with and those without abnormal neuronal processes, *neuritic* (or *senile*) *plaques* and *diffuse plaques* respectively. Both plaques consist of various arrangements of β-amyloid protein. Neurofibrillary tangles are found within the cell body of a neuron, adjacent to the nucleus. The tangles are made up of paired helical filaments, the major component of which is the microtubule-associated protein, tau. Various other neuronal abnormalities exist in AD. These include the depletion of specific neurotransmitter systems, abnormal neuronal metabolism, dendritic regression, and unequivocal synaptic loss.

AD is predominantly a disease manifesting itself in later life, although it occasionally occurs as early as the fourth decade. The median duration of the disease is seven to ten years from the time of diagnosis. Up to 50 per cent of patients have a family history of the disease, although true autosomal-dominant AD affects only around 10 per cent of sufferers. The etiology of AD in the remainder of cases is unclear. Causal pointers are to be found in the increasing prevalence of the disorder with increasing age, the high number of sufferers with a history of traumatic head injury, the possibility of an inflammatory origin, a suggested role for environmental aluminium, and an association with substandard education.

The initial symptoms of AD present as amnesia, subtle personality changes, attention difficulties, depression, hallucinations, and delusions. As the disease progresses patients suffer from further cognitive decline, aphasia, and motor difficulties. Activities integral to everyday life, such as bathing, toileting, and feeding, become impossible. Manifestations of the late stages of AD are poignantly severe and sufferers die unable to recognise spouses and caregivers, incontinent and completely dependent upon others.

Approaches to Alzheimer's Disease

The Personal Experience of Dementia

Dementia more than any other illness confronts us with realities that affect our view of ourselves as human beings. It is one thing to be aware that I have a terminal illness and that my time is very limited, but it is something quite different to know that I will, in all probability, continue to live for some years, but that I will no longer be 'me' and that I will make increasingly unreasonable demands on those very close to me. Instead of caring for others as I am used to doing, I will have to be cared for in a way that has not been required since my early childhood.

A remarkably tender account of coping with someone suffering from AD is provided by John Bayley in his account of the illness of his wife, the famous English novelist Iris Murdoch. He writes:

> But Iris remains her old self in many ways. The power of concentration has gone, along with the ability to form coherent sentences, and to remember where she is, or has been. She does not know she has written twenty-seven remarkable novels, as well as her books on philosophy . . . If an admirer or friend asks her to sign a copy of one of her novels she looks at it with pleasure and surprise before laboriously writing her name and, if she can, theirs . . . She is always anxious to oblige. And her old gentleness remains [Bayley 1998, p. 41].

A number of generalisations can be made about what the demented person thinks and feels. Many sufferers have a full awareness that something is wrong with their intellectual capacities, and this awareness is preserved to some extent throughout the course of the disease. The opposite situation (that is, no awareness of any deficiency) also occurs with some sufferers, and this situation may persist even while the patient's world disintegrates. In between these two extremes are those who are aware that something is wrong but actively deny it, and others who initially have good insight but lose it as the disease progresses, becoming totally unaware of their predicament later on. In the light of these considerations, AD patients should not be denied input into their care on the basis of the misconception that dementia necessarily robs its victims of the ability to participate in decisions regarding their care and their life.

A graphic and intensely personal account of AD is provided by Robert Davis in his autobiography: *My Journey into Alzheimer's Disease* (1989). At the age of fifty-three Davis was diagnosed as suffering from AD, and with some assistance he recorded his thoughts as the dementia progressed. Davis did not drift into dementia; rather, he worked through it and strove to control it as his own brain mechanisms were failing. With muted and tragic eloquence, he sums up the predicament of this condition:

> I am still human. I laugh at the ridiculous disease that steals the most obvious things from my thoughts and leaves me spouting some of the most obscure, irrelevant information when the right button is pushed. I want to participate in life to my utmost limit. The reduced capacity, however, leaves me barely able to take care of my basic living needs, and there is nothing left over for being a productive member of society. This leaves me in a terrible dilemma. When I go out into society I look whole. There is no wheelchair, no bandage, or missing part to remind people of my loss [Davis 1989, p. 114].

Davis was able eventually to come to terms with the appalling losses of his present state, and the even more devastating destruction that he knew awaited him in the near future. This case provides one example, but how do other AD patients cope with their illness? In the relatively few studies that have been carried out it has been found that AD patients use a variety of coping mechanisms, high among which is partial or complete denial of the disease. For instance, some patients avoid naming the illness, or do not seek information about it. Sometimes they are vague in discussing their situation, blame themselves for their limitations, or minimise the severity of their impairment. Of those patients who demonstrate an awareness of the illness afflicting them, a process of mourning for the loss of the previous self is common (Bahro et al. 1995). Dementia is closely associated with a loss of dignity in the eyes of others, as these others adapt to the situation, become accustomed to the patient's incompetence, and often finally come to consider the patient less than a person (Moody 1992). The dementia victim may be likened to an infrahuman being who lives among human beings but is no longer able to share their world.

In dementia the body organ for which compensation is required is not an arm or leg, but the brain. As a result, the caregiver with responsibility for another's brain is in a position of great power, performing functions of judgment and self-control, besides those of memory and language. The difficulties in this caring relationship are immense in view of the lack of reciprocity in the relationship with the patient. Success in this form of relationship, then, is marked by criteria such as the accident prevented, the nutrition maintained, and the cleanliness obtained (Martin & Post 1992).

Personhood and Dementia

The behavioural and personality changes associated with AD raise fundamental questions about personhood. How does the patient respond to personality and behavioural changes of which he or she may initially be aware, and what consequence does this have for self-image? Does the loss of the personality traits that once characterised a person have consequences for the value we, as a society, ascribe to that person? Should any medical resources be devoted to a person with advanced dementia, beyond that of basic care? Underlying every aspect of the dementia debate is this question: *how much do demented people matter?* One way of answering this question is to consider whether Alzheimer patients are persons.

If individuals are classified as persons when they are self-conscious, rational, and in possession of a minimal moral sense (Engelhardt 1986), an AD patient will count less than the rest of us as dementia advances. Any diminution of responsibility will be accompanied by a diminished form of moral status, and even at some point a possible end to being regarded as a moral agent altogether. This could mean that such a patient no longer has a claim on our respect, our love, or our resources. This perspective may lead not only to a great deal of insensitivity, but it may also contradict important moral sentiments (Smith 1992).

In arguments against this perspective, it has been suggested that, although Alzheimer sufferers may have ceased to be persons, they have not lost their human dignity. Consequently, even as life becomes undignified, human dignity is retained since the series of relationships foundational to identity remain. The Alzheimer patient is still Edith, regardless of the changes that have taken place over the years and especially since the onset of the dementia. She is still a wife, mother, and grandmother, no matter how frail some of these realities have become. Consequently, because the dignity of the demented arises from their identifications and involvements, dementia sufferers make full claims on justice as members of the human community. They continue to be part of our family and community (Smith 1992).

Despite these assertions, severe dementia leads to loss of a recognisable personality and of all that we considered inseparable from the person we knew. Even though Edith's body is still here, Edith may no longer be with us as Edith, even bearing in mind that she makes a plethora of demands on her caregivers.

This brings us face to face with the tragedy of the human condition, in which someone we knew and loved has to all appearances died and gone. The tragedy is that the death is a prolonged one (perhaps a very prolonged one) and the interregnum may be devastating for those left behind with the onerous task of caring for the personality-depleted person. In one sense, of course, Edith remains a wife, mother, and grandmother, but this is true for *our* memories and not for hers. It is we who recall who and what she once was; she herself is unable to live out these relationships in the present, and she may even be unable to comprehend what they mean. Any perception must be our perception, not that of the demented. We ourselves have to make the decision regarding the extent of care to be given. The interrelatedness of the human community should force us to deflect some of our attention away from the demented person to those left behind, to those who are caring and possibly being destroyed in the process. It is they who are now our neighbours in the foremost sense, and it is them that we should look to help and support. They tend to be forgotten, but they are humans whose value we are to undergird and protect.

In summary, we are to do our best to bestow as much value as we can upon all humans, whatever their circumstances. Sadly, this value is always limited and in some conditions it is more restricted than in others. Such is the case in aging when it gradually becomes narrower still. But caution is called for here, since chronological aging frequently bears little relationship to psychological aging. When there is very severe brain damage the value we are able to place on human beings becomes ever more circumscribed, although it does not cease to exist, even at death.

Appropriate Care in Alzheimer's Disease

Of the many millions of people worldwide suffering from dementia, at least half are sufficiently severely incapacitated to require continuous care. The prevalence of dementia increases with age: fewer than 1 per cent of the population under the age of sixty-five years, to 1 per cent between the ages of sixty-five and seventy-four, up to 7 per cent between seventy-five and eighty-four years, with a devastating increase to at least 25 per cent of those above the age of eighty-five years. With the increasing number of people in the higher age groups, one estimate proposes a quadrupling of the number of severely and moderately demented patients by the year 2040.

The dilemmas implicit in such figures are obvious: there is no end to the potential cost of combating the inevitable biological decline and death inherent in aging. The consequence of this approach would be to place the highest priority on averting death, thus distorting the distribution of resources to the detriment of all other groups within the community. If this is to be avoided, and if adequate attention is to be given to the needs of AD patients, a change of priorities is essential—from curing to caring. The central question, then, is: what efforts should be expended in keeping a patient with advanced dementia alive?

The first place to look for guidance may be in the ethical principles of beneficence, autonomy, and justice. However, as Moody (1992) has pointed out, these may prove deceptive when confronted by AD. For instance, he writes about the temptations of beneficence, stemming from the powerful attractions of killing people in the face of overburdened caregivers who think of the patient as already dead, or at least as no longer a person. Moody advocates *communicative ethics*, placing stress on the primacy of communication, negotiated consent, and the centrality of family decision-making. Using this analysis, he considers that empowerment in the face of dementia does not mean finding a cure, but recovering dignity, hope, and a sense of meaning in the midst of tragedy.

Callahan (1992) starts from the premise that in old age, and especially in demented old age, there should be a policy bias in favour of caring, rather than acute-care, life-extending medicine. He argues against the invariable use of the latter in advanced dementia, since the goal of this form of medicine is to extend the life of the patient and enhance the patient's appreciation of his or her circumstances. Where personhood has been severely compromised, this goal is no longer reasonable, since its only objective is maintenance of bodily organs, and additional time for a demented existence (Callahan 1992). An emphasis on care ensures that the patient is protected by the positive dimensions of caring medicine, mainly comfort and palliation. Callahan argues that it is possible to treat patients with dignity while acknowledging that high-technology acute care would be out of place. In other words, our moral horizons should not be determined solely by the availability of high-technology medicine.

Thomasma (1992) takes this matter further with what he describes as clinical ethical principles in the treatment of severely demented and other highly vulnerable people. According to the first of these 'the greater the degree of the patient's incompetence, and the less the invasiveness of medical procedure, the more formal the quality of the individual's preferences which should be required' (Thomasma 1992, p. 114). In practice, the withholding of fluids and nutrition is considered less invasive than the use of, say, respirators, and so it requires a very explicit form of evidence to allow it to proceed. This might be in the form of a living will or written advance directive. A second principle is concerned with the other end of the spectrum, that is, protecting incompetent patients from the enthusiasm of those who would employ life-prolonging technology to keep them alive:

> The greater the permanent assault on the quality of personal, interactive human life, the less formal the quality of consent required in order to withhold and withdraw medical treatment that might prolong life in such uncertain conditions, and the greater might be reliance on the patient's preferences as expressed informally to the family or as constructed by the family from the patient's value history [Thomasma 1992, p. 115].

The essence of this second principle is again the protection of vulnerable patients. The two principles together are aimed at treating demented patients in ways that maintain the dignity of those whose personhood has almost entirely vanished. They also need to be seen within a context that recognises no place for active euthanasia (Thomasma 1992).

Would the Demented be Better Off Dead?

Active euthanasia is a hotly debated issue in advanced dementia. One writer has concluded that permitting active euthanasia in conjunction with an antecedently executed living will or personal directive is probably the best policy compromise. Implicit within this position is the issue of justice and the distribution of considerable resources to Alzheimer patients. Do these patients want resources allocated to them, in the sense that they might benefit from the resources in some way? Do they want the ongoing life that medical treatment might bring, even though they no longer have any conception of what the continuation of life signifies for them?

Many of the features generally considered to make life worth living are absent in advanced dementia. Such patients are unable to enjoy human interaction, or to plan ahead and devise new projects; they are excluded from religious and aesthetic experiences, and can no longer act in a rational fashion. If a patient has no sense of self, it has to be asked whether the continuation of life is an enduring good. If it is not, making allocations towards its continuation must be questioned. Nevertheless, this in itself does not lead to the conclusion that active euthanasia is a desirable policy goal, although it does open up resource issues, and hence health care policy. What might be in the best interests of the severely demented? Do such individuals *have* interests?

It is sometimes argued that such patients do not benefit from their continued existence, although the opposite may also be the case since they have no preferences. Given the lack of knowledge of the patient's *present* values, we cannot be sure what is in his or her best interests, beyond possibly alleviation of pain. When dealing with patients unable to recognise family or caregivers, it has been suggested that most reasonable people would rather die than continue to live in such a physically, emotionally, and socially impoverished state. If this is the case, a patient's real interests are not served by the use of technologies that do nothing more than prolong biological existence.

Can we go further than this, and propose that severely demented individuals should be put to death? Since severely demented elderly patients lack potential, all that remains for others are memories of these people. Post (1990) contends that they are more than 'mere' shells, since an affective core remains; neither can we be certain of the extent of the cognitive devastation. Since they are neither brain-dead nor in a persistent vegetative state, some aspects of biographical life continue, with the possibility that their lives may embody redeeming experiences. Post (1990) also wishes to protect and care for the demented because we should maintain the general prohibition against killing, even if nothing remains that could be harmed by killing. Such people are retained within the circle of protection because we remember what they once achieved, and we honour their biographical past.

From this it follows that the severely demented elderly are to be provided with basic care, but seldom with life-sustaining technologies such as respirators, cardiopulmonary resuscitation, dialysis, or artificial feeding. Alongside this, custodial care, minimisation of anxiety and distress, and emotional support are always to be provided, in order to ensure that the severely demented do not suffer from indignities. The emphasis here is on what the severely demented once were and what they once represented. The dignity they once had and elicited undergirds how they are to be treated in the present. Basic care also builds on the recognisable elements that remain.

Genetic Counselling

A discussion of counselling possibilities appears premature, since genetic knowledge is fragmentary at present. Any discussion has to be tentative. Post (1994), in his analysis of AD genetics and ethics, has highlighted the following areas for discussion: justice and allocation, presymptomatic screening and disclosure, and prenatal screening and selective abortion.

The magnitude of the justice and allocation question depends on whether more AD cases are familial than has previously been thought. If this proves to be the case, the demand for testing could come from a very wide section of the population, which in itself throws doubt on the extent to which genetic testing could be seriously contemplated, given that no effective treatment is yet available. However, were this situation to change, the pressure to screen early and widely for AD would increase and would have to be considered a legitimate competitor for resources. Any procedures capable of slowing the death of neurons and synapses would prove revolutionary in AD management, and would have to figure in both ethical and biomedical analyses.

The question of testing also raises the possibility of presymptomatic screening. Depending on the age at which the screening is carried out, it could be many decades before the first symptoms manifested themselves. Given the lack of any effective preventative or treatment measures there would appear to be no justification for carrying out such testing in early adulthood.

Prenatal screening takes these considerations even further. Quite apart from the time that would elapse (possibly a period between fifty and eighty years) from the initial screening to the manifestation of symptoms, the disabling nature of the disease has to be seen alongside a life (frequently a long life) of health and fulfilment. One also has to ask whether a disease that appears to be an aggravation of normal aging is sufficient reason for preventing those who might develop this condition from coming into the world in the first place. There is no justification for this on the ground of suffering for the offspring. While the suffering of AD is real, there is no suffering for most of these patients for up to eighty years. Even with early-onset AD, the individual will not show signs of dementia for around fifty years. Additionally, the suffering of AD should be viewed alongside the many other grounds of suffering in the lives of all ordinary people, only some of which are related to our genetic constitutions.

Brain Death

Significance of the Brain

In 1968 the Harvard criteria for a permanently non-functioning brain were developed. The major feature of these criteria was the total and *irreversible* loss of functioning of the *whole* brain, with total unawareness and unresponsiveness to external stimuli (including noxious stimuli), no spontaneous respiration, and no reflexes. Additional criteria were recommended as confirmatory tests. These included the presence of a flat electroencephalogram (EEG) and the absence of circulation to the brain.

The reasons for identifying the brain as the one organ that can be equated with death of the individual, include the following (McCullagh 1993, p.13):

- after irreversible cessation of brain function, all other organ systems will inevitably cease to function;
- unlike other organ systems, brain function, once lost, is irreplaceable;
- irreversible loss of brain function is synonymous with permanent loss of consciousness;
- loss of sentience is a feature of loss of brain function;
- the integrative function of the brain is lost if the brain ceases to function;
- death on the basis of loss of brain function is doing no more than recognising overtly the reason underlying the traditional diagnosis of death following cessation of the blood circulation.

Eventually, brain death came to be accepted as an indicator of death. Along with this came the realisation that brain death was associated with the permanent loss of cognitive functions such as consciousness, memory, thought, or any of the senses. Thus, the loss of such higher brain functions may be the basis for the whole brain definition of death. An opposing view stresses that brain function and other body functions are inextricably linked, and that brain death marks the disintegration of all organ systems, and hence the body.

Discussions of this nature invariably introduce the concepts of 'personal life' and 'bodily life'. This distinction between these two concepts is difficult to grasp. Medicine allows the body of a brain-dead patient to be sustained on an artificial ventilator. The various systems of the body continue with their biological processes, consuming oxygen, creating heat, and reacting to noxious stimuli. This is not a 'dead body' but a body that is kept alive even after the patient as a person is categorised as dead. If this distinction is accepted, any disadvantages in viewing a brain-dead person as dead have to be weighed against the disadvantage of regarding a brain-dead patient as a 'ventilated corpse' or a 'beating-heart cadaver' (Skegg 1988a). When spontaneous respiration and circulation have ceased, any suggestion that a cadaver is in some way alive is misleading.

For many death is nothing less than brain death, since the critical locus of the life of the person dwells within the brain; once the brain has died the person has died. While this assumption has its dissenters, its acceptance leads to the conclusion that death is marked by the permanent cessation of the functioning of the organism as a whole, rather than of the whole organism (Pallis 1983).

Definitions of Death and Brain Death

The preceding discussion has alluded to the validity of equating brain death with death. However, this viewpoint is not universally accepted and vigorous debate continues to be the hallmark of the academic literature. One of the main critics of equating 'brain death' with death is McCullagh (1993), who feels that brain death occurs subsequent to the cessation of integrated organ functions, and therefore, cannot be equated with bodily death. Along similar lines he contends that the loss of both sentience and consciousness are *consequences* of death: neither establishes that it is the loss of function that denotes death. He has various other concerns including the possibility that subconscious activity may still be present despite severe brain damage. It would be difficult to satisfy his requirements for establishing the centrality of the brain for a diagnosis of death, especially when he contends that the loss of sentience and consciousness are no more than consequences of death.

These arguments reflect the pressures that have led to brain-based definitions of death. There is little about this move that is neat and tidy, whether in neurological or ethical terms. As a society that has the ability to sustain individuals with dead brains on life-support, we are faced with the quandary of which is the most appropriate path to take. What is the most rigorous indicator of death: the traditional cardio-respiratory definition or brain death? Jones (2000) and Lamb (1985) are of a common mind with regard to this dilemma. These authors consider that brain death indicates permanent cessation of functioning of the organism as a whole and hence, by no means does it embody some form of intermediate stage between life, on one hand, and death on the other. For them, the traditional cardio-respiratory criteria of death merely indicate that brain death is imminent, regardless of the time that has elapsed between brain death and cardio-respiratory death.

Up to this point the term 'brain death' has been used to refer to the irreversible cessation of function of both the brainstem and higher parts of the brain, including the cerebral hemispheres. This is the definition that holds sway in the United States, whereas the United Kingdom has adopted a different stance. In the United Kingdom, brain death refers to loss of brainstem function alone, on the grounds that this is predictive of the rapid cessation of function of the higher parts of the brain.

The categorisation of brain death can be extended further to include cerebral (neocortical) death, in which the cerebral hemispheres are obliterated but brainstem functions retained. Confusion may arise on the rare occasion when the terms 'brain death' and 'cerebral death' are used interchangeably. Brain death signifies an irreversible loss of bodily integration. In contrast, cerebral death entails an irreversible loss of the capacities characteristic of our personal lives as human beings, such as cognition, consciousness, rationality, planning for the future, and our hopes and fears.

More recently there has been a move towards two new terms: *whole brain definition of death* and *higher brain definition of death*. The whole brain definition equates with brain death. The higher brain definition shares similarities with cerebral death, yet it places far greater emphasis on *functional* losses. The choice between these two terms is a choice between two definitions of death, entailing radically divergent concepts.

Whole Brain Definition of Death

The journey towards an acceptance of a whole brain definition of death was initiated in 1981 by the President's Commission in the United States when they asserted that death may be accepted on the grounds of 'irreversible cessation of all brain functioning'. In these terms, death of the brain is both a necessary and sufficient indicator of death of the individual, while death of the brainstem is crucial to brain death. In other words, brainstem death is synonymous with death of the individual.

What is being advocated here is a *biological* concept of death (Lamb 1985). This concept entails the cessation of functioning of a biological unit, in the sense that there is no difference between the deaths of any biological life, be it a dog, a cat, or a human being. This approach places an emphasis on the inability to integrate functions within a biological system once brainstem death has occurred. For Lamb, irreversible loss of essential integrative functions occurs at a point in the dying process *beyond* the loss of the criteria indicative of self-consciousness or personhood. The brainstem concept of death means that death does not occur until both the brain as a whole and the body as a whole are irreversibly dysfunctional.

Early accounts of the whole brain definition had assumed complete loss of all vital functions—that is, spontaneous breathing, autonomic control of circulation, homeostatic control mechanisms and consciousness (Bernat 1998)—and devastation of all structures in the brainstem and cerebral hemispheres. However, this is an over-simplification as studies have revealed that cellular activity may be present in isolated brain regions (Grigg et al. 1987). Bernat (1998) contends that 'such purposeless and random cellular activity has no bearing on the status of the organism as a whole', and so does not invalidate the concept of whole brain death, which must be seen as destruction at the macro level. Consequently, the whole brain definition should not be interpreted as an exhaustive, or all-inclusive, description, and it has to live with the contention that some cellular activity at least is purposeless (Jones 2000). For other writers, this whole brain definition fails to recognise the difference between what death is and what causes it (Bartlett & Youngner 1988). These authors feel that the life remaining after destruction of the cerebral cortex represents solely metabolic activity. For them personhood is lost with the destruction of the cortex, and the subsequent death of what remains represents the death of a 'mindless organism' or a 'thing', not a human being.

McMahan (1995) rejects the whole brain definition along similar lines: the body has biological life, whereas the self has a biography; it is the death of the person and not of the body that is morally significant. For McMahan a body does not have interests, and so brain death is the death of the person.

This dualistic approach serves to amplify the contrast between biological and personhood conceptions of death, and forces us to confront just exactly what it is we consider a biological conception to be. Is it possible to think of a brain-dead individual as being 'more dead' than one with higher brain death? If individuals with intact integrative functions (signifying an intact brainstem), but without the marks of personhood (due to damage to the cerebral hemispheres) are said to be alive, are they alive in any meaningful sense?

Higher Brain Definition of Death

For this definition, the significance lies in the destruction of the cerebral hemispheres and the consequent absence of higher brain functions, such as the capacity for consciousness and the ability to think, feel, and be aware of others. According to Bartlett and Youngner (1988), a human being is a 'person', not merely a body, so that destruction of the cerebral hemispheres, the centre of all that makes us persons, constitutes death. These authors propose that we grieve for the loss of a loved one in a manner incompatible with the way in which we would grieve for the demise of a mere 'breathing body'. Veatch (1988) echoes these sentiments when he argues that persons with dead brains are 'individuals who are dead', rather than persons who are 'brain dead'.

As the pursuit of a brain-based definition of death continues to gather momentum, increasing stress is placed upon the irreversible loss of functions seen as characteristic of human existence and of our meaning as human persons. These include our individual personalities, conscious life and uniqueness, and the capacity for remembering, judging, reasoning, acting, enjoying, and worrying. Veatch (1993) believes that these functions are of more consequence for the definition of brain death than are isolated brainstem reflexes following destruction of the cerebral hemispheres.

The emphasis given to higher brain functions in a higher brain definition of death might give the impression that some functions are treated as more significant than others. Criticisms of this nature gain force against the backdrop of a non-arbitrary whole brain definition, according to which all functions must be lost before a pronouncement of death is made. However, we have already seen that this distinction is far from unambiguous.

Objections to this higher brain definition revolve around biological and personalist concepts of death (Jones 2000). Proponents of a biological concept will not accept a personalist one, nor a higher brain definition. This difference of opinion seems irreconcilable. For instance, Lamb (1985) writes that 'life without conscious experience may be meaningless, possibly futile, but it does not amount to death . . . the concept of "death" can only be applied to organisms, not persons . . . a person in a PVS is just that: alive in the most basic biological sense'. PVS or Persistent Vegetative State, is the clinical manifestation of the higher brain definition of death (see Chapter 12).

Lamb's arguments are alleged criticisms of a higher brain definition, yet they also point to its fundamental ideology. The centrality of the person lies at the heart of the higher brain definition, focusing attention onto our humanness and onto the responsibilities lying at the core of human community (Jones 2000).

In the final analysis, personalist and biological definitions of death in their purist forms fail to resolve the issues at stake. As we saw in Chapter 4, the relationship between human cadavers and the persons they once were is an intimate one. Someone's cadaver serves as an ever-present reminder of all that they were when they were alive, their likes and dislikes, attitudes, and relationships. They may be dead but the memory of who they once were lives on, perpetuating their personhood.

Does this help in resolving the issue of brain death? A whole brain definition, with its emphasis on death of the body, is of limited help in the face of a patient who is little more than a breathing cadaver. In this situation, higher brain or whole brain destruction ultimately amount to the same thing: the person we once knew is now alien to us and their body does nothing more than remind us of the person who once was. A higher brain definition concedes this loss even in the presence of lingering biological life. It may be, then, that the 'person' occupies a more central place in discussions of death than some ardent proponents of the whole brain definition are prepared to admit. Conversely, a living body presents immense challenges to our ethical decision-making, since we generally assume that human beings are more than simply thinking machines.

12
Ending Human Lives

Introduction

Human beings have a deep-seated belief that a person's mode of dying is an important part of the totality that is his or her life. This is quite explicit in the practices and beliefs of some ethnic groups, but is present to a certain extent in all human cultures. The moment of passing on from this world is, therefore, a very important point in the human life story. However, advances in medicine have made the determination of the time of a person's death less simple than it used to be. In the past a doctor would have visited the dying patient during his or her last illness, and then been called to certify that the patient had died. At times there would have been a sudden death and the doctor would have elicited the story of the events leading to death, then examined the body and tried to diagnose the cause of death. In either case, the cessation of breathing and heart-beat would be taken as definitive signs that death had occurred. This is sometimes, but not always, still the way things happen.

For some people death is stayed by, or follows, a period of intense medical intervention in the attempt to rescue the patient from a life-threatening injury or illness. This raises questions about when a human being is dead. If we have a human body being ventilated on a respirator, but in which there is no sign of brain activity, ought we to regard that person as dead or alive? As soon as we face the responsibility for such choices, a host of other issues are raised. How should we regard a person in permanent coma? When should we cease to persist with life-prolonging treatment? Under what circumstances can patients decline life-saving measures? Should we ever offer a patient euthanasia or active help to die?

The Death of a Person

Most Western countries now accept the brain-death criteria as criteria by which we determine that a person has died (see Chapter 11). These criteria involve absence of eye-opening, absence of verbal or motor response to pain, and loss of brainstem reflexes (such as pupil responses, corneal reflexes, caloric response to vestibular stimulation, cough reflex, and hypercapnia). These indicate not only that the person concerned has no mental or conscious activity, but also that there is loss of significant function at all levels of brain activity. Total unresponsiveness to these tests, combined with good evidence that it is caused by irreversible structural damage to the brain, means that the person will never regain consciousness. We have taken the view that the purpose of medical intervention and life-saving treatment is to benefit the patient (to effect changes in the patient's condition that now or in the future he or she would regard as worthwhile). It is clear that an individual in the state we are discussing can no longer be benefited by anything that happens to the body. In fact, keeping such a person alive seems to imply that there is no significant difference between beheading (or the loss of the functioning brain) and the amputation of a limb (or the loss of any other organ), which none of us believe. It follows that we can cease our medical efforts to keep alive someone who is brain dead. However, clinical situations are not always as clear-cut as those in which we diagnose brain death.

> Horace is a 22-year-old student who has been injured in a road accident. It is now three months from his time of injury and Horace is in the condition we call 'Persistent Vegetative State' (PVS). He swallows, breathes, absorbs nutrients from his gut and blinks, and sometimes his eyes open and rove around in his head without direction or focus. He is being kept alive by a nasogastric tube and occasional courses of antibiotics for chest infections. There are no electrical or clinical signs of activity in his cerebral cortex.

PVS is the clinical manifestation of the higher brain definition of death (see Chapter 11). Patients in this state do not have any mental activity, they do not dream, think, or experience sensations because they lack the neurological equipment to do so (President's Commission for the Study of Ethical Problems in Medicine and Biomedical and Behavioral Research 1983; Gillett 1990); that is, they are cut off from others and the world around them. They are literally 'vacant'. What is more, there is good evidence that recovery never occurs in those patients in whom the diagnosis is properly made. It is, therefore, important to make sure that the diagnosis is secure because a number of patients where due care was not taken to make a careful diagnosis have responded to intense rehabilitation and have 'woken up' after weeks, months or years.

The Multi-Society Task Force on PVS (1994) put forward the following as criteria for the diagnosis of the vegetative state:

- no evidence of awareness of self or environment and an inability to interact with others;
- no evidence of sustained, reproducible, purposeful, or voluntary behavioural responses to visual, auditory, tactile, or noxious stimuli;

- no evidence of language comprehension or expression;
- intermittent wakefulness manifested by the presence of sleep–wake cycles;
- sufficiently preserved hypothalamic and brainstem autonomic functions to permit survival with medical and nursing care;
- bowel and bladder incontinence;
- variably preserved cranial-nerve and spinal reflexes.

Despite the gravity of these criteria, PVS patients may move their trunk or limbs in meaningless ways, and may occasionally smile, or shed tears. They may even utter grunts or scream. There is however, no psychological awareness behind these motor activities. Most vegetative patients retain good to normal reflexive visual regulation, as well as retention of the gag, cough, suck and swallow reflexes and gastrointestinal function. Preservation of the latter function allows in many cases long-term survival of PVS patients. Survival for five, ten or twenty years is common, with the longest reported survival without recovery being over thirty-seven years.

PVS is quite different from 'coma vigilante' or 'locked in syndrome' in which the patient's cortex is intact; these patients experience things around them and understand what is said, but have lost all voluntary control of motor function (except, usually, upward movements of the eyes). In the 'locked in' state the EEG is active, as it is in the waking state, indicating active cortical processing of incoming information, and the patient can sometimes establish effective communication with others by using eye movements. A victim of this condition, Jean-Dominique Bauby, graphically described his experience in *The Diving Bell and the Butterfly*, a book dictated entirely by eye movements:

> Paralysed from head to toe, the patient, his mind intact, is imprisoned inside his own body, but unable to move or speak. In my case blinking my left eyelid is my only means of communication . . . My heels hurt, my head weighs a ton, and something like a giant invisible diving-bell holds my whole body prisoner [Bauby 1997].

Clearly, the 'locked in' patient must be regarded as a person who is tragically incapacitated, as distinct from PVS, in which it is hard to defend the idea that the person (as distinct from a mere biological human organism) is still there. In fact, relatives of patients in PVS will often say something like, 'It's weird, he's not really there any more, is he?' It would, therefore, seem that we are not morally bound to prolong the life of a patient in PVS, because only a biological remnant of a person remains alive, and there is no longer a person who can benefit from our care. It is now a widely held legal position that where the diagnosis is certain, it is not illegal to withdraw artificial means of life support, including tube feeding, from patients in PVS. This follows the decision of the House of Lords, in the case of Anthony Bland, who was left in a PVS following the

Hillsborough football stadium disaster on April 15 1989. Three and a half years later, the House of Lords found that it was not in Bland's best interests to continue nutrition and hydration, and they authorised their withdrawal in his case. It should be noted, however, that all similar cases in the future are required to be taken to court for a judgment.

Cases like that of Anthony Bland have lent force to the view that we should have a neocortical rather than brainstem definition of death (see Chapter 11). Under this definition, the death of a person is said to happen when the cortex is destroyed in such a way that the person will never recover from profound coma, such as that seen in PVS (Gillett 1986; 1987). It is argued that we can say a person's life has ended when that person enters irreversible coma, even though the illusion that he or she is still alive might persist, and indeed, be sustained for a while.

In a landmark case (that of 'Mr L') a court in New Zealand ruled that the same lack-of-benefit argument applying in PVS might be appropriate in a case in which the patient was conscious and probably able to see things, even though he was permanently and totally unable to interact in any way with others and could not live without an artificial ventilator (Gillett et al. 1995). On the basis of certain remarks the patient had made while still capable, the judge ruled that it would not be unlawful for the team looking after the patient to withdraw his ventilator and let him die. This has greatly widened the scope of withdrawal-of-treatment decisions although it has still, on one interpretation, allowed an assessment of substantial benefit to the person concerned to be the key factor.

In a further New Zealand decision a man, Mr G, was allowed to die after withdrawal of nasogastric feeding and fluid on the basis that life—in the near PVS state into which he had fallen as a result of a severe head injury and loss of oxygen—was no longer of benefit to him (Peart & Gillett 1998). The reasoning behind the decision revolved around three facts:

1   expert neurological and neurosurgical testimony was unanimous that he had no chance of significant recovery and discontinuation of treatment would be reasonable (the reasonable practice consideration);
2   it would be reasonable for any person not to want to live in the state he was in (the objective assessment of best interests);
3   it seemed most consistent with his wishes and attitudes prior to his injury that he would not be kept alive in that state (a subjective consideration of best interests).

These seem to be entirely consistent with what we have suggested as the standard of substantial benefit that any medical intervention should meet: that it would most likely produce 'an outcome that now or in the future the patient would regard as worthwhile'.

The problem of outcomes has provoked the concept of the RUB or the Risk of Unacceptable Badness. This refers to the fact that the result of an intervention designed to rescue a patient who has suffered a dire insult might be to leave that patient in a state that if having had the choice, they would never have chosen. The RUB comes from Hamlet, who contemplates suicide to escape his moral dilemma about his father's murder and his uncle's subsequent marriage to Hamlet's mother and ascension to the throne. However, he realises that this might not result in the oblivion he desires but rather a state of tormented dreaming sleep in which his dilemma will continually haunt him. For a patient unable through incompetence to make a choice between healthy life, life in an intolerable state, and death, the RUB reminds us of the false dichotomy between life and death that otherwise tends to provoke the thought that 'any chance of life is better than none at all'. For many patients it may seem that the risk of unacceptable badness makes the hazardous course through attempts at rescue look much less attractive than one might think at first pass.

These issues are subject to intense debate in many advanced countries that are grappling with the problems created by modern intensive care treatment. Many commentators believe that the authorisation to withdraw food and liquid in the above cases represents a dangerous crossing of the line between withdrawing treatment and active euthanasia.

Facing Death

Cases of PVS and severe brain damage make it clear that there are states in which a reasonable person may well not want to be kept alive. The very fact that many are prepared to heed this wish means that we cannot settle for simplistic interpretations of a principle like the sanctity of life when we are discussing end-of-life decisions. But, whatever we think about the appropriateness of death in certain situations, for many people, death is an unknown and its approach is feared. This means that the caring duties of doctors and other health care workers do not cease when patients reach a point at which pills, potions, and procedures can no longer benefit them.

We need to prepare our patients for the ending of their lives by being honest about what the future holds. Elisabeth Kubler-Ross (1969, p. 29) remarks: 'If a doctor can speak freely with his patients about the diagnosis of malignancy without equating it necessarily with impending death, he will do the patient a great service.' There is no worse situation in clinical practice than the terrible web of deceit that is often woven around a dying patient. This is allegedly done for reasons of kindness but, if we were honest, most clinical staff would probably admit that their reluctance to give people bad news is more often the motive. This reluctance is evident in the case of a little boy dying of leukemia.

John's mother and father had always insisted that he should never be told his diagnosis. He was only eight, and they did not think he could cope with the knowledge that he was to die. One weekend it was arranged that John would have a relief stay in the children's hospice where he had often been cared for. On this occasion he said that he would be all right on his own and that his mother and father could have a little holiday. They delivered him to the nurses at the hospice and drove off. After their car had left, John turned to the sister and said, 'Right, this weekend we are going to get a few things straight. I know that I am dying of leukemia, and that mum and dad don't want me to know about it, but I have a whole lot of questions I want to ask.' Needless to say, it was a humbling and enriching experience for all concerned.

It is unpleasant to have to tell people that soon they are going to die, and it leaves one feeling helpless because no more medical 'magic' is available to combat the process that is killing them. But the honesty required to deal with this challenge is part of a character that addresses itself to the real needs of people, and does not seek to avoid them or bury them under mind-dulling medications.

The need for honesty does not mean that we should be stark and brutal in our communications to patients. Honesty and gentleness are congenial companions in terminal care. We should remember that patients need some hope, however slight, to sustain them through terminal illness, and that hope should never be totally destroyed. In fact, such hope is sometimes well grounded, even though the chance of surviving or the illness resolving may be slight. Every newspaper carries stories of people who proved their doctors wrong, which almost certainly implies that there are a number of doctors who make overly confident prognoses. However, this does not justify deceit or evasion (Kubler-Ross 1969, p. 140), which almost always have bad effects.

Myra presents herself to the surgeon with tests that are almost conclusive of a malignant tumour of the bowel. He talks to her about her symptoms and the tests that have been done, and tells her that there is a cyst or growth of some kind. The possibility of a tumour is raised in the context of a general discussion of the need for an operation and possible follow-up care. Myra has her operation, which relieves her symptoms but fails to remove all the tumour, which is found to have metastasised to her liver. She is told that the operation has gone well, and that the growth was some kind of tumour but could not be completely removed. She asks and is told that this will need further treatment. The fact that it is cancer, and that she may well not benefit from radiotherapy or chemotherapy, are then discussed a few days later.

Patients in Myra's situation often express profound gratitude for being told the truth in a way they can gradually digest. When directly asked whether they should have been told more at an earlier stage, they will often say that having the news broken slowly (but within a reasonable time of it being known) enabled them to cope with it much better. This has the added advantage of making sure that the doctor sticks to proven fact rather than acting on partial information. A series of conflicting, half-baked, or uncertain opinions about what might be going on, before the evidence is in, can be worse than a policy of restraint and progressive disclosure that is accompanied by explanations about the illness and its effects. Our aim after all is to allow people to hear the truth, not just to announce it in their presence. Sometimes a concern with honesty can mean that we do not deliver the truth to a receptive ear, but rather find it bouncing off the walls that the patient has hastily erected around a confused and fearful mind.

Treating people as reasonable, and encouraging them to make major decisions for themselves, is part of our respect for patients as persons. But most people also need and want support in facing unknown challenges. This implies that we ought to create a climate of care in which terminal illness and the fear of death can be confronted and dealt with: 'It is the one who is beyond medical help who needs as much if not more care than the one who can look forward to another discharge' (Kubler-Ross 1969, p. 141).

Suicide

Suicide is a traditional dilemma for ethics. Seneca (1920 ed.) remarked that 'the wise man will live as long as he ought, not as long as he can', and that 'dying well means escape from the danger of living ill'. However, other philosophers have strongly disagreed. Kant (1963, p. 151) remarks that 'suicide is in no circumstances permissible. Humanity in one's own person is inviolable; it is a holy trust; man is master of all else but he must not lay hands upon himself'. Kant's argument shares common ground with the almost universal rejection of suicide by the great world religions. For Kant, the rejection was based on the irrationality of a rational will that sought its own destruction, but for the great religions such as Judaism, Christianity, and Islam, the opposition to suicide was on the basis that God has given life and human beings should not presume to destroy that gift. A moment's reflection reveals, however, that this is not straightforward, as the problems of martyrdom and the forgoing of life-saving treatment under certain circumstances both illustrate. In each case a certain amount of reasoned interpretation by the believer is required as to when the circumstances permit or even commend giving one's life. However, we live in an age where secular reason rules for many people, and thus ethicists must find other grounds if they wish to oppose the arguments for suicide.

Kant expresses a common intuition when he argues that we treat a human life as in some sense worthless if we are prepared to take it into our own hands to destroy it at the behest of a human will. Thus, there is an impasse in our moral thought. On the one hand, it goes against our intuitions that a rational person should seek to end his or her life. On the other hand, we find ourselves in agreement with the choice people make in certain desperate situations where the only alternative is to 'live ill'.

The first intuition leads us to conclude that people cannot be in their right mind to attempt suicide and, on this basis, our laws empower other individuals to prevent them from succeeding. This implies that, even though you do not commit a crime when you commit suicide, you do not have any right to do so. It is obvious that you do not have a right to do anything that people in general are entitled to stop you doing. We have some support for this stance from the fact that most people who are rescued will later not seek to repeat their attempt (Suokas & Lonnqvist 1991). It seems, too, that many people who attempt suicide are in a state of mind that, at their best, they would not endorse; they are depressed, hurt, or emotionally unstable (Barraclough et al. 1974; Gethin Morgan et al. 1975). Therefore, our law enables us to respect what we believe to be their more enduring wishes as autonomous rational beings by blocking their more unstable intentions (as empathically and statistically assessed). This is not to say that all potential suicide victims are irrational, but rather to reflect the probability that suicide is associated with an irrational and usually unsustained wish to die. We also recognise that a completed suicide is irrevocable; one does not have a chance to reconsider, and we know that often people do think differently about things as a result of hindsight, and having actually experienced the sought-after event. One cannot, of course, actually experience death and reconsider (not, at least, for the purposes of secular clinical ethics), but one can, and indeed many seem to, come close enough to be dissuaded from repeating the experience—a fact suggesting that 'the "right" to suicide is a "right" desired only temporarily' (Murphy 1973).

Aside from these things, we realise that a decision to quit life is sensitive to the way life is for the person who makes it, and that this depends a great deal on how we treat such a person. Thus we realise that we all, implicitly, have played a part in the genesis of a suicide and that condoning the rescue is, in effect, asking for a chance to do better. This is probably why the suicide of any person has such an emotional and moral impact on close relatives, family, and friends who are 'left behind'. Their most common comment is 'If only we had known'. It seems, however, that for some individuals, such as victims of HIV/AIDS, the decision is seen in a more constructive light, somewhat akin to Seneca's injunction to 'live as long as one ought'.

However, there remains the point that a person can elect to sacrifice his or her life for others, or elect not to have it prolonged by medical means. To level against these actions, an absolute stance based on suicide seems illogical because it seems possible that 'some suicide decisions are quite rational, being taken by people with a very clear assessment of their future lives, so that interference is unjustified' (Glover 1977, p. 180).

> Irene had realised that she was developing the first signs of the cognitive deterioration that had led to her sister's slow and degrading slide into terminal dementia. She had watched her sister lose control over her bladder and bowel, descend from confused speech to animal-like cries and whimpers when her arthritis was plaguing her, and become unable to feed herself or even swallow her food without being tended like a baby. At the end she had been an apathetic remnant of her once vigorous and engaging self. Irene waited for some months until it was clear that the course of her illness was to be similar and then, one morning, early on the day her home-help was due, she took a lethal overdose of sleeping tablets. She recorded her reasons and her fears, and when she was discovered, although she was still faintly breathing, her doctor elected not to initiate resuscitation.

There is clearly a point beyond which we regard it as immoral and unjust to interfere with the lives of autonomous beings because of our own moral convictions; and it is debatable where this point is reached in dealing with the diverse reality of suicide. Suicide has already been considered in the context of psychiatric ethics (see Chapter 10), but in general we seem to have good reasons to intervene in suicide even when this may seem to be against the wishes of the victim. In many cases a suicide is an act of desperation, and our intervention buys time for reconsideration and reconstruction of those things needed to make the individual's life worthwhile.

Euthanasia

The question of whether we should allow patients to be offered active aid in dying raises a number of complex issues. The most straightforward and compelling argument here is the argument for patient autonomy: if human beings are allowed to make other major decisions about their medical care, even where those decisions concern their living or dying, why should they not be able to request that a doctor help them to die if living becomes so burdensome that their situation is intolerable?

We need first to make certain basic distinctions. *Active euthanasia* occurs when the doctor kills the patient, and is the only meaning with which we will use the term. Such an action can be at the patient's request—*voluntary* euthanasia—or without such a request. The latter could involve either a patient who could meaningfully consent but did not do so before his or her life was ended—*involuntary* euthanasia—or a patient who was incapable of giving meaningful consent—*non-voluntary* euthanasia.

There is also *passive euthanasia* or letting die, which involves bringing about the death of another by inaction (declining to perform a life-saving act or withdrawing medical treatment). Because most philosophers do not recognise a moral difference between acts and omissions, they deny the intuitive distinction that many doctors make between killing and letting die. This is the first major question to be faced in a discussion of active euthanasia. James Rachels (1975) asks us to consider the following case.

> Smith and Jones both have six-year-old nephews and stand to gain if they should die. Both determine to drown their nephews in the bath. Smith sneaks into the bathroom and drowns his nephew. Jones sneaks in with the same intent but before he does anything he sees his nephew slip under the water; he watches him drown.

Rachels asks 'Did either man behave better, from a moral point of view?' The answer is clearly 'No'. Rachels claims that this shows that there is no moral difference between killing and letting die, but his conclusion seems too strong. In his case we are so horrified by the moral dereliction of both Smith and Jones that details seem irrelevant. One might rather conclude that the difference between killing and letting die cannot rest on whether or not one performs certain active bodily movements. Indeed it has been argued that a society comprising people who are prepared to kill for selfish ends is more morally desperate than one in which people will not act to save the lives of others. One can construct a scenario in which a rich colonialist will not donate money to save starving children in the next village but would be horrified at the thought of driving through the village shooting children dead. Arguably this person is less evil than the psychopathic gunman, even though we may feel uncomfortable with both positions.

In the medical situation we might also have to look further for reasons to believe that there is a difference between health professionals who will kill and those who are prepared to withdraw futile and burdensome treatment. In its 1988 report on the topic, the British Medical Association stressed the difference between active euthanasia and withdrawal of treatment, which may lead to death. Even though its overall stance was roundly criticised by some commentators (Nowell Smith 1989), and although the association has revisited the topic on a number of occasions since that date, its position on the issue remains essentially the same. The most recent report from the association (British Medical Association 1999) establishes guidelines for withholding or withdrawing treatment from patients whose wishes cannot be ascertained. They stress that this is *not* active euthanasia, but simply acceptance that the aims of medicine, which are to restore or maintain health, cannot in these circumstances be achieved. The earlier report gave a number of reasons for maintaining the distinction (1988 pp. 23–24):

1 Medical knowledge is limited and it is presumptuous, even arrogant, for a doctor to determine the moment a person will die. We ought, however, to notice that this loses some of its force if it is the patient who chooses the time to die.
2 The pressure for active euthanasia can often be met adequately and more creatively by suitable and sympathetic terminal care.
3 There is some connection between euthanasia and suicide and most who are rescued from suicide attempts are unlikely to make the same choice again (see also Suokas & Lonnqvist 1991).
4 There is a danger in making the intent to actively hasten death part of our medical ethos.

The British Medical Association's discussion made certain distinctions. The first is between dehumanising and intrusive treatment solely for the purpose of prolonging life, and 'true' medical care or 'rescue' (this is a bit like the distinction between 'ordinary' and 'extraordinary' treatment).

> Alfred is an elderly man with metastatic cancer of the lung. He is admitted with an acute episode of breathlessness and is found to be emaciated, anorexic, and exhausted. He claims that he has had enough and that he does not want any treatment. His wife and daughter remark that they have expected this for some time, and they agree that he ought not to have extensive medical tests and treatment. The admitting doctor notes that he has a swollen left leg, and a chest examination reveals an area of decreased air entry. She records a diagnosis of deep venous thrombosis with pulmonary embolus and orders a chest X-ray to confirm it. She then charts morphine 10–20 mg as required for pain relief and a nocturnal dose of amitriptyline. She discusses the management with the patient and his family and writes a 'Do not resuscitate' order in Alfred's notes.

This doctor is prepared to let her patient die because there is no available course of medical management that will restore him to a satisfactory state of living. The treatments and tests that might have been arranged—venography, VQ lung scan, anticoagulants, possible cardio-pulmonary resuscitation, and so on—are intrusive, costly, and offer little potential benefit. In such cases many doctors, having discussed the situation with the patient and his or her relatives, may decline to offer certain medical treatments even though they stand a chance of prolonging life. A cardio-pulmonary resuscitation, in the circumstances described, is just such an intervention and would not be indicated because it could not substantially benefit the patient. It would be a further step if the doctor concerned had decided to chart sufficient morphine to bring about Alfred's death earlier rather than later, but her orders make it clear that her purpose is pain relief and not the hastening of death.

This, in effect, is a decision to let Alfred die, but it is not quite the same as acceding to a request to help him to die here and now. The withholding or withdrawal of medical treatment from someone who cannot benefit from it does not open the door to medical killing, because it is based on compassion for the sufferer and wisdom in our use of medical technology. An active decision to kill or help to die could, however, be based on motives that vary widely from kindness and the wish to spare suffering, to a policy of expedient eradication of those who cannot be helped by medical science. In Germany, for instance, the very mention of euthanasia provokes howls of public protest because of the history of abuse associated with the term. One of us recently asked a conference audience whether they saw any difference between giving patients with a terminal condition enough drugs to take away their pain and going a step further to give a lethal dose where this had been requested. The audience was unanimous in claiming that the two acts were very different. But these reactions do not amount to a clear set of reasons why killing patients (even with their consent) is not the right thing to do.

One commonly cited difference is the matter of *intent*, which is often confused with motive. There are, of course, well-intentioned motives for voluntary euthanasia. Doctors may wish to be kind and spare their patients terminal distress and agony. They may wish to show respect for people by letting them end their lives at a point where they are threatened by the possibility of becoming infrahuman with no remaining dignity or integrity. They may wish to accede to patients' wishes about their modes of death; after all, if patients are autonomous why should they not make this final choice? One might see the choice of ways of living as naturally extending to a choice about one's mode of dying.

Many doctors would agree with some of these motives. There are, however, a number of ways of serving them that do not involve an act intended to bring about death. Patients can almost always be given a judicious mix of anxiolytic and analgesic medications (such as morphine and amitriptyline) to ensure that they will not suffer even where, with their full knowledge, the drugs may weaken their biological urge to live and so shorten their lives. According to the doctrine of 'double effect', such acts are legal and morally acceptable, even though the death of the patient may be foreseen. The doctrine focuses on the intent with which the health care worker acts. Where the intent is solely to relieve distress, the act can be countenanced by any professional; but, where the act is to kill, there is a significant difference, at least in the eyes of the law. Moreover, the intent can easily be discerned from the medication used. A dose commensurate with the intent of decreasing anxiety, and relieving pain or respiratory distress, will clearly be different to an overdose designed to kill. In making this point, we are not claiming any special status for medical decisions. There is, in fact, a clear moral and legal distinction between murder and manslaughter, and the crucial difference hinges entirely on the prior malign intent of the murderer. But why do we reason this way in both medical and legal argument?

We can probably trace this reasoning to the settled 'habits of the heart' that form the character of human beings. For health care workers, such habits are part of the healing ethos. It takes a certain kind of character to detect and respond to the real (sometimes concealed) needs of dying patients. However, in clinical practice, subtle and careful sensitivity to such needs is often diminished where a problem can be solved by purely technical means. Some professionals enjoy such interventions, and therefore avoid the personal and emotive aspects of patient care that are bound to be central in clinical disciplines such as palliative or terminal care, and psychiatry. Active euthanasia is, of course, an intervention to be used when a dying patient's problems become too difficult to cope with. But many hospice workers volunteer the information that even their patients who are suffering unbearably on admission to hospice care almost never need purely technical interventions, such as increased levels of pain relief. The answer does not lie with 'panalgesia' but with caring human counsel; 'where humane care and a positive affirmation of the value of each person (no matter what their condition) is the prevailing clinical attitude (hospices are a good example) euthanasia requests are rare' (British Medical Association 1988, p. 24). What is more, most patients in terminal care do not want their death hastened and of those who do, most are found to have a diagnosable psychiatric disorder likely to contribute to such a request (Brown et al. 1986) Thus, we are toying with a potentially tragic cocktail when we mix a soupçon of the intent to kill into the attitudes of those who care for the dying. It is too tempting to put an end to difficult problems in clinical practice. Therefore, terminal care workers, even more than others, must guard their sensitive and caring intuitions.

There are other reasons for this stand. First, there is some evidence that a proportion of people dying from an incurable disease are asking the question 'Am I still worthwhile?' To answer this question with euthanasia is perhaps something about which we ought to have reservations.

Second, human death is a very individual thing, and medical knowledge is limited. There are unpredictable and unknown aspects to an individual's death that, for many, make their last moments of inestimable worth. Many palliative care workers feel it is not right to intervene so irrevocably at such a time. It is, however, clear from conversations with doctors from the Netherlands that complying with a euthanasia request is just as demanding as any other response to the dying patient and genuinely requires all those concerned to face this crisis as persons of depth. Because people differ in ways directly relevant to how they choose to live and to end their lives, it is very hard to develop general indications for human euthanasia similar to those we have for animals. When we consider the needs that bring people to hospice care, and the relative unimportance of pure pain relief in that context, this becomes quite evident.

Third, it is unclear to what extent hospice care of the type practised in, say, the United Kingdom, is available where there are strong demands for euthanasia. When the alternatives are limited, doctors are sometimes forced into desperate measures.

Despite all these worries, active euthanasia by doctors is available to patients in the Netherlands, and seems to answer a very real set of needs. A doctor can administer euthanasia when certain clear conditions have been met and, although technically guilty of murder, he or she will not be prosecuted for it under these conditions (Leenen 1987). Even there, however, many feel very uneasy about the whole practice. Some of their worries have been discussed already, and similar worries have been voiced by doctors in countries other than the Netherlands. It is worth listening to their worries even though some of them rely on intuitions rather than clear evidence.

1 Some feel that the fear of death, particularly death from AIDS or cancer, has been exploited by those who advocate euthanasia, and argue that most patients can be managed without this desperate expedient.
2 Some worry that the active termination of life will be extended to cases where the clear conditions of voluntariness and a settled, carefully considered choice do not apply.
3 Some worry that the practice of euthanasia will create pressure on elderly and vulnerable patients to comply, which might affect particularly those individuals most in need of support and care from others.
4 Some fear that if the doctor is seen as being prepared not only to cure but also to kill, the ethos of medical practice and the confidence patients can have in their doctors will be eroded.

It does seem that there has been a significant extension of the indications for active euthanasia since it was originally introduced in the Netherlands (Keown 1992; Griffiths 1995). In the Chabot case (Griffiths 1995), a distressed and lonely woman who had recently lost a well-loved son (following a marriage break-up and a previous suicide by her first son) was given active euthanasia because her psychiatric adviser thought her situation intolerable and incurable. In fact, the judge in this case found that the psychotherapist concerned had not followed the guidelines for active voluntary euthanasia, although he discharged the therapist without penalty. This course of action would not be taken in most Western countries, nor would the indications be regarded as being so desperate as this adviser made them out to be. Given that the slippery slope that many fear in relation to euthanasia is, in the light of this case, an actuality not just a conjecture, it illustrates the fact that the law has a symbolic and not merely a permissive effect on our actions in crucial areas (Gillett et al. 1995). We tend to take the law as showing what is acceptable or reasonable, not just as telling us what is legally permissible, and thus it changes our morals as well as reflecting them.

The situation is clearly not simple. There is a powerful argument that people should be able to make their own decisions about the significant passages that mark human life, and death is surely one of those: we may regard the decision to end one's life as a moral decision belonging to the individual patient, and as being grounded in the patient's right to moral autonomy (Charlesworth 1993, p. 53). It is hard to deny the powerful force of this argument and still claim that one is serious about safeguarding the central position of the patient in health care decision-making. The arguments against active voluntary euthanasia are much less clear-cut than the argument from autonomy except where they appeal to a fundamental value such as the sanctity of life. But we have already shown that such a value is by no means absolute, either in theory or in practice. The question as to whether we should endorse active euthanasia is therefore delicately balanced, with well-respected ethicists having opposite opinions on the issue.

Death is, in one sense, not an event in human life (Wittgenstein 1922). Human death is an unknown, surrounded by myth, dreams, fears, uncertainties, and distress of all kinds, and its dynamic is not the kind of thing that is amenable to a model that encourages decisive medical interventions. It is true that, where euthanasia is considered acceptable, the request for that intervention and the decision as to when it will be used should be made by the patient. We have already noted the vulnerability of the patient in the face of a medical establishment. Thus we must move cautiously and with due consideration when we contemplate legal changes to allow doctors to intervene to end the life of a patient, even at the patient's request. We should, however, always remember the other side of the coin: the vulnerability of the patient to situations where our high-technology medicine has extended his or her life, quite possibly far beyond a point at which the patient or any reasonable person would regard life as being a benefit and where the patient's right to say 'enough' seems unassailable. Doctors and other health care professionals must remember that the criterion for treatment is that it offers a benefit to the patient and that that benefit, as we have stressed, is to be measured in terms of what the patient would find worthwhile—not what we as health care workers are inclined to do. If it seems undeniable that a competent patient can refuse medical treatment to prolong life, then there is a very powerful case for the right of a competent patient to request a compassionate death even where that would involve active euthanasia. It remains unclear whether the needs of a small number of patients for whom that is the only acceptable way of managing a distressing terminal condition warrant a change in the law of such significance. This issue is currently being debated in a number of settings. The arguments for and against do not mandate either a pro-euthanasia or an anti-euthanasia decision, and most commentators endorse a view that expresses a deep personal commitment to one or the other stance.

Quite apart from the particularities of the dying patient, there is a great temptation in modern medicine to develop powerful technologies and efficient interventions that obscure the fact that our patients are increasingly turning to health professionals as people. When faced with a problem that may seem insoluble, it will often emerge that the real issue concerns communication and relationships. (In fact, a great majority of the ethical problems in contemporary clinical practice have to do with such issues.) Closer attention to the humane art that is medicine, rather than the technical discipline it threatens to become in a cut-and-dried, cost-effective world, would almost certainly avoid many of these problems. One contemplates with horror the kind of society where death and its mysteries are seen as a fleeting problem; where expediency and general contentment are all. Where we have ready answers for all human dilemmas, we seem to end up with a type of life that is subhuman (which is probably why most people regard *Brave New World* as the opposite of Utopia). Therefore, we would argue that compassionate, restrained care and the judicious use of those resources that have a proven beneficial role in terms of pain relief, comfort, and dignity are the best response to the needs of people with tragic and terminal diseases. The modern hospital or any health care institution must, as far as is compatible with delivering genuinely beneficial treatment, strive to become 'sensitive to the autonomy of the individual patient, particularly in the delicate but momentous area of patients making decisions about the manner of their dying' (Charlesworth 1993, p. 60).

PART III

Medicine and Society

13
Research Ethics

Introduction

At the end of the Second World War the full horrors of life in institutions for the intellectually handicapped and in the concentration camps of the Third Reich were disclosed to the public. The Nuremberg Trials revealed that (among other atrocities) doctors had performed mutilating and totally experimental gynaecological operations on female inmates, and had tested the limits of human survival at low temperatures by immersing prisoners in baths of icy water. Recently evidence has emerged of similar atrocities carried out by the Japanese during the Second World War, but the perpetrators of these crimes were never brought to trial because of a deal struck by the US occupying forces at the conclusion of the war in the Pacific. The philosophy underlying such actions appeared to be that certain classes of human being were totally expendable and of no individual worth, but merely the means to some alleged 'common good', such as the advancement of science.

No one seriously supports such a viewpoint today. Indeed, among the many topics of medical ethics, this is one in which the ethical issues seem now to be clear and unambiguous. Whatever the benefits that might be gained from the use of human beings as participants in experiments, there cannot be any justification for treating people as mere means to an end. The rights of the individual remain paramount, and no scientific advance can outweigh the harm done by unethical research. Yet, even after all these years, there are still areas where some uncertainty remains (though not at the barbarous level of the Nazi experiments), in terms of the balance to be achieved between worthy social goals and individual rights. (An example of this is the debate concerning the individual's right to privacy with regard to health information.)

The basic principles guiding research with human participants were firmly enunciated in the Nuremberg Code, drawn up at the conclusion of the War Crime Trials. The code stressed the necessity of gaining fully informed consent from participants, with the obligation on the researcher to ensure that there were no undue risks, and that any minimal risks were clearly outweighed by the benefits to be gained. Although the code was promulgated in 1947, its application to biomedical research was not always perceived. There was no repetition of the Nazi atrocities among the medical and scientific community, though certainly in subsequent wars and conflicts 'crimes against humanity' did continue. However, some medical research was carried out in the postwar era that did entail substantial risks to research participants, risks of which they had no knowledge. In the early 1960s awareness of this lack of ethical supervision in medical research was growing, particularly as a result of the writings of Pappworth (1967) and Beecher (1970)—see McNeill, 1993. The World Medical Association prepared a draft code of ethics relating to human experimentation in 1962, which after wide circulation and comment was adopted by the WMA Assembly meeting in Helsinki in 1964. The Declaration of Helsinki, which has subsequently gone through several revisions (the latest one being in 1989), forms the basis for the ethical monitoring and control of medical research worldwide (see Appendix). The examples of unethical research that follow will demonstrate why a clear enunciation of principles and guidelines was needed.

> In 1957 an experimental program was introduced in the Willowbrook Hospital, an institution for intellectually handicapped children in New York State. Numerous infections were rife in the hospital, including viral hepatitis. The researchers set up a special unit in which selected children were deliberately infected with the virus in order to study the course of the disease. The researchers argued that, since the children would probably be infected anyway, they were better off in the special unit than in the general wards of the hospital.

But this calculation of harm versus benefit would be sustainable only if no attempt were made to improve the hygiene and level of infection in the hospital as a whole. Moreover, parents giving consent to the admission of their children to the unit were, in effect, coerced into their decision by being warned that the alternative was likely infection without sustained medical attention. Thus, a vulnerable group was induced to participate in a research program that under normal circumstances might not attract any volunteers. (On the other hand, there may be something to be said for allowing a child to suffer a perhaps inevitable infection in circumstances where the treatment would be optimal.)

In the next example the intention to benefit the participants was much clearer, but there was no proper assessment of their risks, and a complete failure to gain informed consent to participation.

> In 1966 a research proposal was instituted in National Women's Hospital, Auckland, that was designed to demonstrate that carcinoma *in situ*, a symptomless lesion in the cervix, was not (as had been hitherto thought) a precursor to invasive carcinoma. The proposal entailed taking no action to excise the abnormal area, but rather following up the women at regular intervals to determine whether there were any signs of progression. As the subsequent judicial inquiry (the Cartwright Inquiry) showed, this was a risky, poorly designed experiment that led to unnecessary disease (in some cases fatal) in a number of participants.

Moreover, none of the women involved were ever made aware that they were participating in an unusual and experimental treatment; the need for frequent return visits for checking was both an inconvenience for them, and—in those cases in which invasive cancer developed—a false reassurance.

These two examples illustrate how important it is for medical researchers to be aware of the fundamental ethical principles governing research with human beings, and to establish proper procedures for assessing and monitoring the ethical aspects of research projects. We shall look at the application of the basic principles under the following headings: scientific validity; risks and benefits; information and consent; and procedures.

Scientific Validity

A research proposal cannot be ethical if it lacks scientific validity. Poorly designed research entails putting participants at risk, or at least to some inconvenience, for no clear benefit. This means that every proposal to undertake research must be subjected to scientific assessment, to determine whether there is a clear and *prima facie* useful hypothesis to be tested and to make sure that the research design will yield the result sought after. When research is supported by major funding bodies this assessment will be carried out as a matter of course before any grant is awarded. When research is commercially funded (by pharmaceutical companies, for example) an independent assessment of the research proposal must be made to determine whether any useful and *new* information will be gained, or whether what is claimed to be 'research' is in fact a marketing exercise (designed to draw the attention of general practitioners to a particular brand of drug, for example). If a research project is carried out by an individual without reference to any external funding body, scientific assessment will be an integral part of the decision about whether there are ethical objections to its implementation. At best poorly designed research wastes the time of research participants, and at worst it subjects people to unnecessary risk. We may say, without doubt, that bad science is also bad ethics.

Even if a research project is scientifically valid, it may not be justifiable. In some instances the research may merely be going over old ground. In other instances, the information to be gained may be of little obvious use or benefit to anyone. Thus, the question should be asked of every proposed piece of research, would anything be lost if this project did *not* proceed? This question need not be answered in too narrowly a pragmatic sense. Much research is contributing to fundamental scientific understanding of processes without any practical advantage being immediately evident. It is, however, on such well-researched foundations that future practical applications of science will be based. But whenever human participants are involved, it is essential to avoid what can be seen as trivial or permanently insignificant and pointless research. Once again, a proper scientific assessment can establish the relationship of the proposed research to other work in the field and to promising lines of development.

One area where scientific validity is particularly difficult to establish is where qualitative research is being undertaken. In such research there may be no hypothesis as such. Nevertheless there is a large literature on the nature of the qualitative approach, which can be used to lay down principles for assessing the validity of the proposed research.

Risks and Benefits

Once the general scientific viability of the project has been established, the balance of risks and benefits must be assessed. The Declaration of Helsinki has drawn a basic distinction between therapeutic and non-therapeutic research. The former may be of direct or indirect benefit to the participants since it consists of improving knowledge about either the diseased condition of the participants or possible improvements in therapy for their condition. For example, a surgeon may wish to try out a new operative technique, or a physician may wish to test a new drug, using as research participants a group of patients under his or her care.

In therapeutic research the main guideline to be followed is that, without the research, there can be no certainty about which of the interventions being tested will be of greater benefit to the patient. This is sometimes referred to as the principle of equipoise. In these circumstances it is justifiable to direct patients to one treatment or another in a random way since, until the research is complete, one cannot tell whether the patients being given the new treatment, or the patients not being given it, will benefit more. Of course, if there is reasonable evidence that harm could be caused to one group, the research should never begin. The basic principle in medical care is that each patient should be given the best treatment available for that particular condition, and that harm should never be knowingly caused (*primum non nocere*). One cannot justify withholding a treatment of known benefit to patients merely in the interests of research.

It is obvious that in some therapeutic trials there will be an element of risk for participants. For example, in order to test a new drug for hypertension, there would have to be a weaning-off period in which a placebo is administered, prior to the administration of the drug to the experimental group. To ensure validity, this would have to be 'blinded' to both researchers and research participants. Risks of this kind, created by the design of the trial itself, can be dealt with only by very thorough procedures for monitoring the medical condition of participants, in order to give immediate warning of the need to break the code and give appropriate treatment to the person affected. A research design is acceptable only when the safety of participants throughout the trial period is the paramount concern.

In non-therapeutic research, when there is no anticipated advantage to the participants (apart perhaps from the satisfaction of assisting in the advance of medical knowledge), the protection of the rights of participants must again be of paramount importance. For example, researchers might wish to improve their understanding of the mechanisms of conception by obtaining samples of uterine tissue from post-menopausal women. The procedure involved (biopsy) has a very low risk, but could cause some discomfort and might be embarrassing for some women. Yet participation in such a project could only be from purely altruistic motives, since reproductive capacity is no longer relevant to that group. We must, therefore, be sure that participants are fully informed of the nature of the research, especially of the precise nature of the sampling procedures, so that they are not in any way coerced into taking part.

When people are enlisted as controls in a therapeutic trial, that aspect of the trial is non-therapeutic research. For example, research into children with behavioural problems might include as controls a group of children who were known not to have such problems. Since there is no benefit to such children, risks that might otherwise be thought to be quite minor (for example, inconvenience or the causing of embarrassment or transient anxiety) assume greater importance. Some writers believe that individuals who are incapable of giving informed consent (such as very young children) should never be enlisted in non-therapeutic research, because proxy decisions are not justifiable for procedures of no clear benefit to them (see the fuller discussion of this issue in Chapter 7). But this rigorous standard would in effect bring to a halt all research in paediatrics, and much research in psychiatry and geriatrics. The alternative to this absolutist view is to insist that the risk must be so minimal as to be negligible in all circumstances where the consent of the participant cannot be obtained. In assessing risk, account must be taken not only of possible physical injury but of levels of discomfort, inconvenience, anxiety, or invasion of privacy. The more intrusive the research, the less justification can be offered for enlisting individuals who cannot assess the risks for themselves.

Information and Consent

In all types of research, whether therapeutic or non-therapeutic, the provision of comprehensive and accurate information to participants, or their proxy decision-makers, is crucial. Without such information, the consent granted will not be valid. Giving informed consent is not to be confused with the signing of a consent form. This should merely be the formal acknowledgment of a process whereby the person giving consent has come to a full understanding of what is entailed, and has been made aware that there is complete freedom either to grant or withhold consent, and that the consent may be withdrawn at any stage in the research. To achieve this fully valid form of consent, great attention must be paid to the quality of the communication about the project. All explanations must be in non-technical and readily understood language, and (except in the most trivial circumstances) be provided in a written as well as a spoken form. The information should include a clear description of any risks and an assurance that refusal to participate will in no way alter the health care the person is receiving.

In addition to adequate information, valid consent requires that participants are not coerced or induced into participation. Participants in a special relationship to the researcher (as patients or students, for example) can be protected from coercion by the use of independent third parties (such as nurses not connected with the ward or department) to seek consent. Payments to participants that are substantial enough to constitute an inducement invalidate consent. In practice, it may be hard to distinguish between payments that are in effect a bribe, and those described as a refund of expenses and recompense for the inconvenience. A total ban on payments, on the other hand, may prevent much useful research taking place. Certainly, where there is any risk to participants or where the participants themselves are vulnerable because of their impoverished condition, the ethical justification of paying them is very dubious. The volunteer relationship in medical research seems much more securely based ethically, since it gives the research subject a sense of partnership in the project. A serious danger in all research is that the person may be treated merely as a means to an end, rather than as a freely participating moral agent.

It is because of this emphasis on respect for the person of the research participant that only in exceptional circumstances is it justifiable to omit to gain consent. An absence of risk to the subject is not a justification in itself.

> Two researchers in a medical school want to do a study on the placentas of primigravida women. They submit a proposal to an ethical committee that outlines what they are intending to do but contains no consent form, since (they claim) consent is unnecessary in view of the fact that the placentas would be incinerated anyway. What harm then would there be in a few tests on them first?

Consent is necessary in such a case because, although the tissue is of no further use to the individual, it is that person's right to determine how it shall be used. Failure to give full information and to gain consent betrays a lack of respect for the women concerned; they are being treated as sources of useful research material, rather than as potential partners in a project whose value they could appreciate. (For this reason the word 'participant' rather than 'subject' is to be preferred in describing any research involving people. Human beings should actively participate in, not be subjected to, research.) Moreover, there is a possibility of harm in the use of the placenta, in the case of those women who, for cultural or religious reasons, would regard such a use of the products of birth as disrespectful or distasteful. The same strictures must apply to the use of any tissue removed at operation. A particularly sensitive area is the use of tissues or other human material removed at autopsy for research purposes. It is not acceptable to retain such material for teaching or research use, unless specific consent has been obtained from the relatives of the deceased (see Central Office of Information 2000, and Chapter 4).

We can see, then, that consent is important, not only because it signifies that the participants in research have been given the opportunity to make their own assessment of the risks and benefits, but because the consent process recognises that the research participant is a person in his or her own right, with a set of personal values that must be respected. Research without consent constitutes an invasion of the personal integrity of the research participants, even if no physical harm is caused to them.

The situations in which the omission of consent (or proxy consent) is permissible are those in which totally non-invasive procedures are proposed, and the obtaining of consent would be impractical or possibly even alarming or harmful to the participants. These conditions sometimes arise in epidemiological research. For example, the following arguments have been put forward for responsible accessing of medical records. Research into the incidence of cancer in certain groups (such as those in specific occupations) may entail following up hospital records over a number of years to identify risk factors. It would not be possible to contact all the participants to obtain consent for access to their records, because of changes of address and so on. Moreover, to contact people with an explanation of the possible correlations with the onset of cancer could cause unnecessary anxiety, since the research could yield a negative result. Thus a less than honest explanation would have to be given. If this is the case, would it not be more acceptable to access the records without seeking consent, and then contact at-risk participants if the hypotheses were established?

Not everyone would agree that the above arguments are convincing enough to permit the omission of consent to access health records, which can contain much personal detail given by the individual solely for the purposes of obtaining appropriate treatment. In practice, requests of this kind are considered on their merits by individual ethics committees, which will investigate whether the omission of consent is justified in each case. There is certainly no automatic right of access to medical records by researchers, and in the future it may be appropriate to document in a person's record specific consent (or refusal of consent) for its use in research.

When research is relatively non-intrusive (as in the administration of questionnaires that do not contain highly personal material), verbal consent may be sufficient. However, adequate information must still be presented to participants first, and the opportunity offered for them to consider whether or not they wish to participate. An advantage of printed consent forms is that they can specify clearly the nature of the project and the freedom of the participant to withdraw at any stage. Verbal consent can be more coercive of participants, and may appear to be an 'all or nothing' commitment.

Procedures

In order to ensure that the guidelines for research ethics are followed in practice, it is essential to institute adequate procedures for protocols to be assessed by properly constituted committees. The composition, function, and procedures of these committees vary widely from country to country (see McNeill 1993), and there are no agreed international guidelines. Even the names of such committees are different; for example, in the USA they are called Institutional Review Boards (IRBs); in the United Kingdom they are called Research Ethics Committees (RECs) and there are both local (LRECs) and multicentre committees (MRECs); in New Zealand they are known simply as Ethics Committees (although they deal with ethical issues in treatment as well as research); in Australia they are called Institutional Ethics Committees, and are under the supervision of the Australian Health Ethics Committee. These differences are less significant than other variations, including the scope of membership, the rules of procedure, and the accountability of the committees to other bodies such as hospital boards or area health boards.

We can identify a number of principles that should ensure that, whatever the national variations, the interests of research participants and researchers are protected: they are the principle of independence and impartiality, the principle of due process, and the principle of accountability.

Independence and Impartiality

The best safeguard for the first principle is found in appropriate criteria for membership of the committee. Clearly a committee composed entirely of researchers could not be regarded as sufficiently distant from the research community, or sufficiently close to the community at large, to make impartial judgments about such matters as degrees of risk and discomfort, or the adequacy of information and consent procedures. On the other hand, a committee lacking the necessary scientific expertise could never make accurate assessments of either the scientific validity and usefulness of the project or the possible risks entailed. It is, therefore, essential to have a balanced membership, representing a wide range of perspectives on research, including the various social or cultural milieux of the research participants. Particular attention must be paid to minority and other vulnerable groups; and the perspectives of patients who are involved in research concurrently with treatment must be properly represented. It is also important to have other forms of expertise on the committee, in addition to the relevant scientific knowledge—notably expertise in law and in religious or philosophical ethics.

Token 'lay' membership is never sufficient to ensure the proper independence of the committee from the scientific community it is assessing, since the technical nature of much of the material discussed can easily put the non-scientific members at a psychological disadvantage and may lead to a dominance of decision-making by those with expertise in the research area (Campbell 1987). For instance, in some countries there is a requirement that the committee consist of an equal number of lay members and health professional/scientific members, and that the chairperson be elected from the lay members. Other devices to avoid bias include requiring the presence of at least two lay members to constitute a quorum and/or requiring that all decisions of the committee be unanimous. Clearly, whatever measures are introduced, they should not have the effect of polarising the lay and scientific members into two separate camps, nor is it desirable that the lay members feel themselves to be always spokespersons for specific sectional or community interests. The committees that function best are those in which the division between lay and scientific/professional is not noticeable. This can be achieved by procedures that give all members of the committee the assurance that their voices will be heard and their opinions respected.

Due Process

The assessment of research protocols is a complex matter that cannot be adequately carried out unless committees have clear methods for dealing with the mass of material presented to them. In order to achieve consistency, each protocol must be subjected to the same scrutiny with regard to scientific validity, ratio of risks to benefits, adequacy of information, and consent procedures. Standardised application forms are a prerequisite. The range and phrasing of questions on these forms is best defined after some experience of the information that a committee will find relevant in order to reach a decision, but at the very minimum questions should elicit the following information: design of study; qualifications of researchers; source of research participants and their relationship to the researchers; funding of project, including any payments to participants, and financial or other advantage to researchers; procedures to be carried out and their attendant risks; methods for monitoring and detecting adverse outcomes; safety procedures; compensation arrangements in the event of injury; method of obtaining consent; use of results, including safeguarding of confidentiality and communication of results to participants. All applications should include copies of information sheets, consent forms, and full information about compensation arrangements for participants.

Due process should protect researchers as well as participants. This entails providing full information about the membership, constitution and procedures of the committee, and guidance about appeal procedures in the event of a project being rejected. Researchers should, in the first instance, be given the opportunity to attend the committee in person to explain the justification for their project, before any final rejection. It should also be open to the committee to seek expert advice from outside the committee membership in order to clarify and, if need be, correct their assessment of the acceptability of the project. If the outcome is still a negative one, there should exist some other body (such as a national ethics of research committee) to whom reference can be made by either the applicant or the committee in order to get a second opinion. Alternatively, an external assessor can be used in the appeal process. It is a serious matter for researchers if their project is totally blocked because of ethical objections, but if the full procedures described above are followed, one can be assured that the reasons will be sufficiently grave to justify such a step in order to protect the interests of research participants. In all health research, the interests of the participants must remain paramount.

Accountability

An ethics committee functioning without reference to any other body is always in danger of idiosyncrasy in its judgments, or liable to come under the influence of partisan groups of one kind or another. The accountability of the committee should first be ensured by a declaration that its decisions are taken in accordance with an internationally recognised set of guidelines. Most commonly, normative principles will be derived from the Declaration of Helsinki of the World Medical Association, including its subsequent revisions, or from guidelines issued by the Council for International Organizations of Medical Sciences (CIOMS; both documents are reproduced in the Appendix). In addition, each nation will have its modifications and elaborations, produced by government agencies or professional bodies, or incorporated in statutes. In New Zealand there is a National Standard for Ethics Committees, promulgated jointly by the Health Research Council and the National Advisory Committee on Health and Disability Service Ethics. In Australia the National Health and Medical Research Council has published a set of national guidelines for institutional ethics committees.

Another form of accountability is derived from the relationship of the committee to the health authority or organisation within which it functions. This relationship is necessarily a subtle one. If the committee is too closely allied to the health care institution or authority, it may lack the essential independence of judgment and critical role that is its *raison d'être*, but at the same time the committee must be answerable in a democratic fashion to those responsible for the health care of the community, or for the good administration of the health care facility within which the research is carried out. The required blend of independence and accountability can be achieved by a careful system of seeking nominations to the committee, which is recognised as a fair method by both the research community and the public at large; a rotational system of membership to prevent the entrenchment of particular viewpoints or sectional interests; and a system of reporting that allows both the health authorities and the public to be aware of the activities of the committee, without allowing either breaches of confidentiality or undue influence on its decision-making. Decisions about whether committee meetings are closed or open to the public must be made by assessing the relative strength of requirements for confidentiality and of the need to be publicly accountable.

In the last analysis, the worth of such a thorough system of ethical monitoring of research must be seen in the quality of the research work itself. A system that unduly impedes research and constantly frustrates researchers could never be regarded as ethically justified, since much of the ethical justification of medical care rests on the fact that it is under constant scrutiny and improvement by active and well-designed research into its efficacy. However, since medicine is primarily concerned with the well-being of individuals and of the community as a whole, no research should override the human values medicine seeks to serve.

International Research Ethics

We have already noted that most research ethics committees and funding bodies refer to international standards in research ethics, notably the Declaration of Helsinki (and subsequent revisions) from the World Medical Association. It is evident, however, that the declaration has only persuasive force and that it leaves some problems insufficiently defined and resolved (Schüklenk & Ashcroft 2000). Attention has recently been directed to these difficulties by the controversy over trials of HIV/AIDS therapies and vaccines in developing countries (see Chapter 9). Among the issues that have surfaced are questions of whether a placebo trial of a substance already known to have therapeutic benefit can ever be justified; whether the 'best standard of care' criterion in the declaration can be taken to mean the best standard relative to the country in which the research is being conducted, rather than a universal standard; and whether it is right to trial medicines in a country whose health budget is so meagre that they could never become a standard means of therapy. Debate on these issues continues, as a further revision of the declaration is being discussed not only by the World Medical Association, but also by many other interested organisations, including the World Health Organization and the United Kingdom Nuffield Council on Bioethics. One major outcome of these discussions may be a more reliable and consistent method of assessing and monitoring research carried out in countries that do not themselves have an effective ethics committee structure.

The Use of Animals in Medical Research

The Declaration of Helsinki (1989 revision) states that any health research involving human participants 'should be based on adequately performed laboratory and animal experimentation'. Earlier in the same code it is stated that 'the welfare of animals used for research must be respected'.

A number of writers have questioned the ethical justification of such an approach, claiming that the use of animals to check on the safety of products or procedures prior to their experimental use is an infringement of the rights of animals. Such writers would view the phrase 'respect for the welfare of animals' as much too weak, since it allows humans to disregard animal welfare when they regard it as justified for the 'higher' principle of respect for the welfare of humans. This, it is claimed, is merely speciesism, a discrimination as reprehensible as sexism, agism or racism. The philosopher Peter Singer introduces his book *Animal Liberation* in the following terms:

> This book is about the tyranny of human over non-human animals. This tyranny has caused today and is still causing an amount of pain and suffering that can only be compared with that which resulted from centuries of tyranny by white humans over black humans [Singer 1975].

Arguments of this kind depend upon the view that the only relevant ethical issue is the amount of suffering an animal experiences. It makes no difference, it is asserted, what species the animal belongs to, only how much it suffers. According to the animal rights activist Ingrid Newkirk: 'there is no rational basis for saying that a human being has special rights. A rat is a pig is a dog is a boy. They're all mammals' (Newkirk 1986). It is obvious that if such a view were to prevail, medical research involving human participants would become a much more hazardous and painful pursuit, or would have to be radically curtailed. At the present time, no new drug can be introduced for human use until its effects on animals have been fully studied. This frequently uncovers dangerous or even lethal propensities in the drug that preclude its further development. Similarly, animal experimentation has been necessary to develop and refine surgical techniques, and to further knowledge of physiological and biochemical processes and of anatomical structures.

It is frequently claimed by animal rights advocates that much of this research is either unnecessary or irrelevant, because the difference between humans and other animals precludes accurate comparisons, or because computer modelling or the use of tissues rather than whole animals would be an adequate substitute for the testing required. These claims are not accepted by those involved in bio-medical research, although it is accepted that the *numbers* of animals used could be reduced, and that some tests used in the past were unnecessarily destructive of experimental animals (for example the LD 50 test, which required the establishment of a drug dosage that would cause the death of 50 per cent of the experimental animals). Reduction in numbers or types of test, however, is far removed from the total abolition sought by the advocates of animal rights. Such an abolition would, in the judgment of the medical research community, put an end to whole areas of research that could never proceed using only computer modelling, or by experimenting on tissues rather than whole animals.

The crux of the issue, however, is to be found not simply in assertion and counter-assertion about whether animal research is a necessary precursor to research on humans, but in a difference in moral assumptions about the status of non-human animals. If it is true that animals have rights in the same sense as humans, then all the requirements controlling research on humans would have to be applied equally to the use of animals. This would put animals in the same category as human infants (or other human participants incapable of giving consent), and so would permit their use only in experiments of direct therapeutic benefit to them or in experiments in which there was minimal risk of any harm. But is it correct to say that non-human animals have rights?

Clearly, many species of animal are capable of suffering, not only in the sense of physical pain, but in terms of psychological distress caused by fear, deprivation, being in an alien environment, or being isolated from members of their own species. But we can assert that humans have a *prima facie* obligation not to inflict such suffering on animals, without recourse to the claim that animals are the possessors of rights. This is evident when we consider whether we would put the same obligation upon animals, either in terms of aggression against their own species, or against members of other species. We see no such obligation because we do not regard non-human animals as moral agents who have such constraints on their behaviour. Predators are not morally reprehensible in the sense that violently aggressive humans are. And, although it is true that 'man is the most destructive by far of all mammals' (Storr 1970), it is only in humans that such destructiveness is blameworthy.

If only moral agents have rights (and corresponding obligations), what are we to say of human infants or of the severely intellectually handicapped, who are also incapable of fulfilling an active role in moral behaviour? Should we treat them as we would experimental animals? The argument must be different in each case. So far as infants are concerned, we have an overriding obligation to nurture them in order to allow their eventual development as full members of the community of moral agents (see Chapter 7). To deny this absolute obligation is to undercut the whole ethical basis of human parenting and of the provision of universal education; and it would sanction the abuse of the vulnerability of infants for adult ends. Such considerations prohibit the sale of children and the use of child labour, restrictions that even the animal rights activists do not place on our use of animals. In the case of the intellectually handicapped, their right to absolute protection is based upon the crucial nature of their relationships with fellow humans. We now know that the potential of these individuals for development and a sense of fulfilment can be realised only when they are given every opportunity to become active and cared-for members of the human community. Therefore, we have special obligations to them that far exceed our obligations not to harm non-human animals.

In light of these considerations, we can reject accusations of 'speciesism' as they are not founded upon rational argument. The basis of racial and sexual discrimination is either that *falsely alleged* differences (for example in intelligence or moral capacity) are used to justify unfair treatment, or that *real but irrelevant* differences (as in appearance or physical characteristics) are used in a similar way. The differences between humans and other animals are both real and relevant to treating them as having unequal moral status. Humans alone are capable of that moral agency that commands absolute respect. Humans alone carry the responsibility for determining how the welfare of their own species is to be balanced against the welfare of other living creatures. Only humans must decide when it is right to experiment or to desist from experiment: rats, pigs, dogs, and other mammals depend upon the morality of those decisions.

It is clear from the above argument that denying that non-human animals have rights does not in any way justify the unrestricted use of animals in research. On the contrary, since animals themselves have no voice with which to defend themselves, there are powerful moral obligations upon the human community to protect them from unnecessary harm. This obligation is clearly expressed in international and national guidelines on the use of animals in research. The fundamental principles are stated in CIOMS, *International Guiding Principles for Biomedical Research Involving Animals*:

> Investigators and other personnel should never fail to treat animals as sentient, and should regard their proper care and use and the avoidance or minimization of discomfort, distress, or pain as ethical imperatives.

Increasingly it is being recognised that the suffering of animals is often overlooked or regarded as somehow less than that of humans simply because it is expressed differently (see Rollin 1989). Thus the CIOMS guidelines emphasise the need to assume the presence of pain rather than its absence, unless proven: 'Investigators should assume that procedures that would cause pain in human beings cause pain in other vertebrate species.'

Another area of concern is the excessive use of animals in some sorts of research. A recent estimate stated that 40 million animals are used in one year alone in the USA. There is now an emphasis on the minimum number necessary for the validity of any given experiment, and in every case the number used must be justified by application to an independent ethics committee.

Finally, the infliction of pain or distress on animals as part of an experimental protocol is now regarded as quite unjustifiable, and it is the role of animal ethics committees to ensure that alternative methods of research are devised. All invasive and painful procedures must be carried out with appropriate sedation, analgesics, or total anaesthesia, and if the animal will subsequently suffer severe or chronic pain, distress, discomfort, or disablement that cannot be relieved, it must be painlessly killed. The death of animals, but not the infliction of suffering, is thus regarded as morally acceptable (as it is in their use as food).

Like research with human participants, research involving animals is now the subject of regulation worldwide, though standards vary even more widely than they do for research on human subjects. When there are properly constituted committees for authorising and monitoring research, the inhumane practices of some research with animals, rightly condemned by animal activist groups, may be eliminated from both commercial and scientific research on animals. This will not be enough to satisfy the abolitionists, since such procedures do not accord rights, and so research will continue to be used as mere means to human ends (or, in the case of veterinary research, to benefit other animals). Codes that allow experimentation on animals within specified limits (see Appendix for the full texts of relevant codes) give expression to a 'minimal harm' ethic in relation to our treatment of species other than our own. This is far less than the proponents of animal rights believe to be required, and is of course a standard much lower than those applied to the use of humans in research.

Whether we have the balance of values right is a matter for each individual to decide, but for a person planning a career in science or medicine there is really no possibility of opting out of involvement in the manipulation of animals for the purposes of both teaching and research. In the development of medical science to the present time (and for the foreseeable future), it is not possible to subscribe to the ideals of scientifically grounded medical care without accepting that humans must come first in our scale of values. Cruelty or the gratuitous and unjustified infliction of pain of any kind is alien to the spirit of medicine, but equally it makes no sense to a person seeking to protect or restore human health to assert that 'a rat is a pig is a dog is a boy'.

14
Trying New and Unusual Things

Introduction

Medicine prides itself on being a science-based practice that investigates and intervenes to relieve human suffering caused by disease. Just as for any other science, there are two elements: the investigation of important questions, and the formulation of new theories and ways of interpreting the data. The first part of the enterprise requires the accumulation and careful analysis of data, an activity for which scientific methodology prepares us well. The second is not at all of the same ilk. As we have inherited it, medicine is based on a fairly narrow view of science, which succeeds at explaining the workings of mechanistic devices, and to some extent the biological workings of the human body where relationships of cause and effect can be discerned with relative ease. For medicine to succeed in the latter case, the operation of the cause must be fairly uniform in all individuals studied and the effects that they each show must be measurable in comparable terms. These two assumptions inform the practice of evidence-based medicine.

Even when the system we are studying is complex and not fully understood, we can reduce the degree of uncertainty by understanding how parts of the system work. However, what is difficult to understand is a system with an individual and holistically interconnected set of causes, where the same cause may not always produce the same effect. This arises when there is an interactive confounding factor or factors related to the place of the changes under investigation in the system as a whole. What is more, some malfunctions of the system may be 'cross-grained', that is, the system may be incapable of detecting patterns evident to other ways of thinking. For instance, the categories of sociology cannot discern differences between inflammatory and neoplastic conditions. Interesting problems develop when two types of theorising about the world arise in relation to something like health and disease. In such a case, settling on a clear method for judging the merits of competing theoretical approaches can be problematic.

Medicine is wedded to biomedical science as its knowledge base, and biomedicine embraces the causal model of changes in nature. As a result, clinical practice works under an imperative to treat disease when it occurs, and to protect individuals and communities from its ravages. Both of these commitments are part of medical orthodoxy, whereby we identify a malfunction in a system, isolate the causes of that malfunction, and then proceed to intervene to reverse or counteract the malfunction. Implicit in this process is the idea that a human being is a physical system prone to various physical malfunctions, and that these can be dealt with piecemeal. The orderly march of medical science based on this model and the knowledge generated by it, come into tension with two sets of forces at work in clinical care. The first is the need for innovation, and the second is the possibility of a radically different approach such as that underpinning alternative healing systems. Before we discuss these two areas, we need to examine the status of medicine as both a theoretical and a therapeutic science.

Medicine and the Rationality of Science

When asked, most doctors would align their scientific thinking with Popper's approach to truth in science; where hypotheses are formulated, evidence is gathered, and the hypotheses are disproven or rendered more likely to be true by the results of the analysis of that evidence (Popper 1959). For instance Saunders (1996, p. 111) remarks of medical treatments: 'all form part of an articulate system of thought, all are subject to criticism as to their place in that system, all could in principle be tested and falsified'. Newton-Smith (1981, p. 1) summarises as follows: 'The scientific community sees itself as the very paradigm of institutionalised rationality. It is taken to be in the possession of something, the scientific method, which generates a "logic of justification". That is, it provides a technique for the objective appraisal of scientific theories.'

In fact, many within medicine are of the opinion that we work with facts and not theories at all, even though it is clear that most conditions are investigated and treated on the basis of a theoretical location in our classification systems (infective, inflammatory, neoplastic, and degenerative). But sometimes we get things wrong; for instance, gastric ulceration was thought to be caused by an inflammatory non-infective disease until it was discovered that campylobacter have a crucial role in its pathogenesis. This reminds us that what might be considered false at one stage in medical history, may be regarded as true at another. This should encourage us to be open to some of the critical thinking that is current in the philosophy of science.

The history of science is a tale of numerous shifts of allegiance from one theory to another. Popper himself exhibits a certain modesty in relation to the knowledge claims of science:

The old scientific ideal of *episteme*, of absolutely certain, demonstrable knowledge, has proved to be an idol. The demand for scientific objectivity makes it inevitable that every statement must remain tentative for ever. It may indeed be corroborated, but every corroboration is relative to other statements which, again, are tentative [Popper 1959, p. 280].

But how do we avoid the Scylla of dogmatic thinking—that science yields certainty about factual truth—and the Charybdis of a descent into arguments about subjective opinions in relation to clinical practice?

It is interesting to apply contemporary critical voices to the practice of orthodox medicine and its investigation of disease. The most radical forms of (postmodern) criticism rest on the premise that all knowledge claims arise from the power of certain groups that legitimate some claims as being true, and regard their associated methods as being the correct way to arrive at the truth. Three possible arguments might contribute to a postmodern attack on the idea that medical science reveals the truth about human disease.

1   Medical scientific knowledge is not true because there are many competing truths appropriate to complex human function.
2   Medical scientific knowledge is no more true than its rivals in alternative and traditional medicine.
3   Medical science does not capture the whole truth about human disease and suffering.

Limitations of Medical Scientific Discourse

The opponents of scientific truth who appeal to the complexities of human life say something like 'Orthodox medicine is not true in the way it claims to be, because that kind of truth is not available for complex dynamic systems like human beings'. To examine this claim we will need to look briefly at knowledge, medicine, and the state of contemporary orthodox medical science. Consider the following:

J visits his doctor. He feels out of sorts and is worried that something bad is going to happen to him. He has gone off his pre-dinner drink, and in fact alcohol in general, he has headaches or a heavy head, he sometimes feels as if he is losing his balance, he finds it hard to get to sleep, he has episodes of rhinitis, and episodes of diarrhoea, and an almost constant stiff neck. J's doctor examines him and can find nothing that looks too alarming. A set of standard blood tests shows no major abnormalities. She reassures him that nothing is wrong but he says he is tired of living this way, and can see no sign of things getting better.

Although there is no orthodox medical category into which J can be fitted, a homeopath seeing him might classify him as a gelsemium patient. The problems start when we try to go beyond these opinions based in different healing systems and formulate exclusive claims to truth. One then strikes the problem of the single privileged description that counts as 'the truth'. It is clear that if the homeopathist is correct, there is something going on that falls into a pattern of categories that is cross-grained with respect to biomedicine. Thus, the simple view that there is one right or true description of every human situation, however complex, could be misleading.

Philosophers now realise that there is a problem in the simple idea of truth. Facts are constructed and organised according to the concepts used by the cognitive system of the subject. The ability to select and change one's focus and the way that one describes things to oneself are basic to the flexible and creative properties of human thought. This is not to say that we only see what we expect to see, but it implies that the evidence available to us is dependent to a very large extent on the kinds of concepts and skills we bring to the experiences where that evidence is to be had.

Any discursive context validates certain ways of looking at things and, outside this range, a person will struggle to articulate their experience (Foucault 1981). The ways of thinking that are considered to be valid within a discourse depend on the things considered to be significant in that discourse, and on whoever holds power in that domain of human activity.

For instance, if we place a subject in a scientific medical discourse, the level of serum sodium would be far more important than the fact that the subject is feeling isolated from their family and cultural context, or that there is a pattern of associated symptoms of the type shown by J. But both of these could be important clues to the patient's illness. Medical scientific discourse validates discussions of such things as serum sodium levels, but not those concerning cultural and familial estrangement or more subtle concepts of balance and attunement in the body, which many doctors find deeply mysterious.

Once we understand why the originally simple relation between knowledge and the world is problematic, we begin to realise how knowledge is tied to praxis—doing things. Ways of thinking allow some ways of acting, and obscure others so as to confer certain powers on the agents within the discourse. But why do some discourses become dominant in a domain of human knowledge and others get sidelined?

The concept of *power* helps us answer this complex question. Power is exercised in medical scholarship by authoritative bodies who create an atmosphere whereby any views that significantly depart from statistical methodologies based in the natural sciences are regarded as inferior or suspect. This means that students imbibe the attitude that the basis of real medical knowledge lies in anatomy, physiology, biochemistry, and statistical method. But this picture is very much located within biomedical science and stands or falls with the adequacy of the causal picture in the understanding of complex human function.

Values Intrinsic to Medicine

There are a number of values intrinsic to the study and practice of medicine; they include such things as caring for people and wanting to do one's best for them, being open to new knowledge that might improve our understanding of disease, and what one might call a Hippocratic attitude towards practice and theory. We find the following passage in the Hippocratic writings.

> In all previous attempts to speak or to write about medicine the authors have introduced certain arbitrary hypotheses into their arguments, and have reduced the causes of death and the maladies that affect mankind to a narrow compass [Lloyd 1978, p. 70].

Instead of such hypotheses, postulates, assumptions, or theories, the method espoused by the Hippocratics was the treatment of cases and the accumulation of commonsense observations about those cases. This is practical or clinical knowledge rather than a theory-driven corpus of beliefs, which demands that the questions be narrowed to fit the dominant paradigm. We have noted that the dominant paradigm works with identifiable causes and their identifiable effects, and tries to link cause and effect in a way that lends itself to external impersonal intervention that can be understood without involving oneself in the variations and complexities of individual functioning. This kind of intervention is beloved of companies that want to mass-produce medical substances and devices that can be applied to a wide range of people and produce uniform results. There is a great deal of money to be made out of such inventions (pharmaceutical and mechanical), and therefore there is considerable money available to fund research that falls within this model. However, before we accept the model implicit in this approach to clinical medicine, we ought to reflect for a moment on our Hippocratic roots. Hippocrates warned us about becoming captured by grand theoretical systems, which would narrow our thinking about the problems we actually face in real practice. He asked that we substitute reflective intervention and documentation for such theory-driven ideologies. Indeed, if we pursue the thought that medicine comprises a systematic and reflective practice, we can begin to understand why orthodox medicine has certain failings and the attitude we ought to have when we examine innovative and unconventional medicine.

We will examine surgical innovation, in order to look at problems arising in medical orthodoxy, and then alternative medicine, to scrutinise more radical challenges to the dominant paradigm. These areas illustrate two ways in which the failings of the dominant model may come to light.

Surgical Innovation

The practical side of medical knowledge is nowhere more evident than in surgery, and this means that surgeons are often not well served by the framework provided by the *statistically valid, prospective, double blind, randomised, controlled study*. Although surgeons are oriented towards evidence-based medicine, this practical orientation allies them with other skill-based areas of medicine such as general practice, psychotherapy, and even traditional systems of healing explicitly informed by a holistic assessment of an ailing human being.

Surgeons are both craftspeople and scientists, and this can produce conflicts in their thinking. Like all scientists, they wish to proceed only on the basis of secure evidence, but, like all manual or technical artisans, they fashion techniques to intervene in situations requiring a skilful, hands-on approach to care, based on accumulated experience. The development of surgery as a craft can, however, be seen as a weakness when we look at the paradigm of scientific (or evidence-based) medicine, with its rigorously controlled methods of comparative analysis. Some of the requirements of that methodology become hard to meet when faced with the realities of clinical surgery.

First, every patient presents a unique challenge that may, in the surgeon's opinion, require an individually tailored surgical solution. Second, the surgeon uses tried and well-tested techniques learnt painstakingly from mentors. This constitutes a body of received know-how or expertise, but one that may not have ever been subjected to rigorous scientific investigation. Third, the surgeon may know that if he or she does not treat a patient in the approved manner, despite its lack of scientific backing, he or she may be the subject of a negligence claim because of a departure from the reasonable standard of care. What is more, the surgeon may also be aware that, in the early stages of development of a new surgical technique, the results may compare very unfavourably with more established methods, even though the long-term potential is for a greatly improved way of solving a surgical problem. Finally, surgery is simple-minded. Tubes need unblocking, pressure needs relieving, bones need straightening, and so forth. Thus, a method that produces better and more sustained improvement according to these simple mechanistic conceptions is inherently attractive and, a surgeon feels, more likely to be a good way of doing things. This is how most of the advances in surgery and surgical devices come about—it seems a better way of solving a particular practical problem. But this is not science; this is the craftsmanship of an artisan, which is, in part, what finding practical solutions for complex integrated systems comes to.

There are several scenarios involving surgical innovations or advances, each of which poses its own ethical problems for surgeons. The first is where a tried and tested treatment is introduced to a new clinical setting. The second is where the surgeon adopts a novel use for an established treatment or technique. The third is where a health care professional invents a new approach to a problem. And the fourth is where a serendipitous discovery in relation to the treatment of one or more patients culminates in the development of an innovative treatment.

The first situation is very common. It does not cause any special concern and, in fact, goes on all the time as a result of technical notes in the surgical literature and conference presentations of new techniques in surgery. Because surgeons do simple things—unblocking tubes, removing lumps, and so on—it would take an obtuse observer not to see the good that was being done. Sometimes, however, it is not so simple; the good being done rests on an interpretation or theory about what is going on (it is better to provide a more stable vertebral column where there is pain) or a careful appraisal of the non-obvious or long-term effects of what has been done (what is the long-term effect of fusing stretches of the vertebral column?). In such cases, questions of benefit become more difficult to answer.

The remaining three situations all involve something being tried for the first time and raise a series of common issues that can be applied to conventional, alternative, or non-orthodox medical treatments. In each case we want to know if the health outcomes for this new or adapted technique are better than for existing alternatives. And when we ask this question we are brought face-to-face with the difficulties for a comprehensive science of surgery conceived according to the narrow (biomedical and statistical) conception of clinical knowledge.

At this point we ought to remind ourselves of the Hippocratic injunctions about medicine, which were somewhat less rigid than the current fundamentalism of the prospective, randomised, controlled, double-blind trial. Hippocrates, as we have noted, stressed the need for careful investigation of what nature throws up in the course of clinical practice, with a refusal to be biased by preformed theories. 'Physicians', the Hippocratic writings claim, 'compare the present symptoms with similar cases they have seen in the past, so that they can say how cures were affected then' (Lloyd 1978, p. 142). The texts then go on to recommend the accumulation of careful observations of clinical practice until conclusions can be drawn as to which methods are effective, and which are not. This is obviously important, but it does not meet the rigorous requirements of the dominant paradigm. It is almost as if the Hippocratic corpus appreciated the problem because it enjoins us to reason about a course of clinical management, by reasoning approximate to full knowledge of what we are doing (Lloyd 1978, p. 77).

For surgery—which is a causal intervention in the human body—we could, and should, interpret this within the biomedical context. Saunders (1996) alludes to this when he describes 'an articulate system of thought' within which a new departure either makes sense or has no discernible rationale. But shared reasoning grounded on accepted foundations in basic science (for instance, fluid dynamics, turbulence, and the layering of platelets at points of thrombogenesis) is not available to many of those who have a radically different theory of health and disease. For them, something like a pattern of reasoning that, even if unorthodox, leads to a cumulative understanding of health and disease allowing broader and broader competency in the conditions successfully treated would be the best that can be done. Such a system should make some kind of sense in the light of what we do know about the human organism, but may not be commensurable with orthodox biomedicine at certain points.

In this context questions of honesty, power, and shared decision-making become extremely important in an ethical appraisal of a doctor's advice. We could say that patients must know their options and how the advice they are being given by an innovative orthodox practitioner relates to a representative body of medical opinion. Many clinicians, and surgeons in particular, are bad at this, in that they will make up their mind about a preferred mode of therapy without informing the patient about uncertainties or options for treatment. In the end, where clinical certainty is not to be had, or even where clinical facts are relatively clear but do not unequivocally point to one outcome, patients must be empowered to make their own decisions—for instance mastectomy versus lumpectomy in breast cancer, and the use of holistic therapy for troubling problems like allergic rhinitis, myalgic encephalomyopathy, or any complex immune-related diseases.

Once empowerment begins to happen, patients become participants in designing their own treatment regime and monitoring their own outcomes. Such a partnership allows medical innovation to proceed in a very fruitful way, because the patients feel permitted to contribute their own observations no matter how odd or unusual these seem to be. The Hippocratic enjoinder to develop such an open and exploratory approach is vital here, and any researcher who does not avail him- or herself of this rich source of truly Hippocratic data is cutting off the branch on which advances in medicine have hung for over 2000 years.

However, the possible weakness of this position is the vulnerability of patients and the unequal power relationships in the clinical encounter. Obviously, a partnership model in which patients feel empowered to contribute to the planning of their care tends to counteract this effect but it means that certain further questions must be asked. One question arises from the difficulties of deriving clear evidence for or against the treatments involved. It is not likely that there are vast differences in morbidity and mortality between different ways of doing similar surgical operations, or different ways of treating the kinds of multifaceted problems dealt with by holistic means, and therefore the results of treatment are open to all kinds of influences. For instance, the problem of interpretation is a very significant potential source of bias, which would slant the assessment of outcomes in ways that are related to the beliefs of practitioner and patient.

In fact, there are competing tendencies evident here, as in many areas of clinical care. The first, arising from the concentration on tried and true clinical methods, is a relatively reactionary tendency to revert to received wisdom in areas where innovation may offer new possibilities at the expense of established theory; the infective basis for gastric ulceration springs to mind in conventional medicine but other areas of initially revolutionary thinking are easy to find. There is, for instance, a new operation for Tic douloureux, a painful condition affecting the face. This involves operating on the nerve going to the face as it leaves the brain to try to identify and move a small blood vessel that may be compressing the nerve and causing the pain. This was revolutionary when it was first proposed, and has transformed the lives of many sufferers, for an otherwise intractable condition. For a long time, however, the operation and its rationale were pilloried by reactionary figures in the surgical neurosurgical establishment.

The second competing tendency is a rather bullish enthusiasm for new or fashion-driven methods, which may be costly and relatively untried in their proposed applications. Some doctors like to try the new thing—and are encouraged to do so by aggressive marketing. The marketing strategy usually involves a plausible biomedical rationale for why the proposed innovative treatment ought to work better than any alternative, with some figures based on retrospective data that seem to show that it does. On this basis, many innovations become widely used without being considered tried and true, or ever being subject to evidential scrutiny of the type that is required to establish the efficacy of any new drug treatment. There is a fine conceptual line between such a widely accepted, but innovative, technique, and a tried and true surgical method.

When we contemplate innovation and advance in an empirical enterprise that faces difficult and complex problems such as surgery or alternative medicine, we must sometimes exercise our critical faculties to work towards filling in the areas of uncertainty and ignorance that abound in the messy world of clinical practice. We can be guided in our attempts to do this by returning to the ancient sources of medical wisdom, and relearning the value of Hippocrates' advice and reflections.

> I contend that the science of medicine must not be rejected as non-existent or ill-investigated because it may sometimes fail in exactness. Even if it is not always accurate in every respect, the fact that it is able to approach close to a standard of infallibility as a result of reasoning, where before there was great ignorance, should commend respect for the discoveries of medical science. Such discoveries are the product of good and true investigation, not chance happenings [Lloyd 1978, p. 77].

Our next task is to explore the ways in which the medical gaze (as restricted by conventional medical science according to the biomedical and statistical model), may prevent us from seeing important features of alternative approaches that only become evident to a richer epistemology of health and disease.

Other systems of healing

It is salutary that large numbers of people are turning to alternative, complementary, and holistic healing systems to find what they cannot find in orthodox medicine (Smith 1983; Pietroni 1992). When we look at most of the traditional and alternative healing systems currently vying for a place within orthodox medicine, we find that they tend to share a core belief in the holistic function of the organism as the basis of health, and that it is disorders in this integrated and balanced property that allow disease to occur. Thus, rather than seeing a disease as an alien event that attacks the organism, and which can itself be independently addressed, they see the ailing organism as a system that is failing to deal with a challenge to its proper function. Foucault (1987) contrasts the two conceptions as follows:

1   illness is an essence, a specific entity that can be mapped by the symptoms that manifest it, but that is anterior to them, and to a certain extent independent of them;
2   whether its first designations are organic or psychological, the illness concerns the overall situation of the individual in the world; instead of being a physiological or psychological essence, the illness is a general reaction of the individual taken in his psychological and physiological totality.

From the latter view it follows that the job of a healing method is to restore the individual to the non-disordered or harmonious state of being that combats illness and constitutes health. We can illustrate the general view by borrowing from homeopathic theory.

Hahnemann, the founder of homeopathy, states 'no external malady . . . can arise, persist or even grow worse without some internal cause, without the cooperation of the whole organism, which must consequently be in a diseased state' (Hahnemann 1993, p. 234). He enjoins his followers to learn to work with 'the vital force', which, in response to a minute dose of homeopathic medicine appropriately tailored to mimic the disease causing alteration to the person, will then 'suffice to effect complete recovery' of the affected individual. One might take a very mystical or a more down-to-earth approach, and depending on which view one takes, one might be open to various criticisms. In general, homeopathy is not alone in seeing the cause of illness as a disturbance of the inner harmony or ordering principle of life, which produces health, and it shares this view with many older systems of healing. But this kind of view has certain corollaries, which should occasion appropriate methods of scientific validation.

1   An accurate diagnosis not just of symptoms but of the deeper derangement of health must be made.
2   A remedy must be exhibited that addresses the deeper problem.

3 The healing systems of the ill person must be mobilised to restore the person to health.

4 A successful remedy, once exhibited, will have altered (in an enduring way) the capacity of the person to deal with a certain kind of derangement.

5 A remedy evaluated according to its effect on surface signs or symptoms of the inner derangement may show no effect.

This last point is crucial in considering the scientific claims of holistic healing systems. Consider for instance the case of Dr K.

> Dr K is both an orthodox and homeopathic practitioner. She has a growing clientele because she seems to offer help where orthodox practitioners cannot even identify a disease state. In her practice, she keeps a well-indexed record of signs and symptoms and the morbid conditions (according to her homeopathic classification) in which they arise. She notices in one of her cases, Mr L, whom she diagnoses as a Hepar, that the patient's return to health coincided with a resolution of his mild hypertension that she had thought she would monitor and treat in the orthodox way once she had addressed his presenting problem (which did not fit any orthodox disease category). She returns to her records and finds that she has had a number of patients who have had their hypertension resolve along with their homeopathically treated illness but they have several different homeopathically defined conditions and only some of them are Hepars. She realises the difficulties in taking this Hippocratic observation any further.

The problem Dr K sees is that her patients come from four different disease groups and therefore a double blind, prospective, placebo-controlled trial of any of her homeopathic regimes would only be expected to have an effect in about 25 per cent of cases and therefore to be indiscernible from a placebo. If, however, we look beneath the symptoms, we no longer have recognisable and objectively validated disease types in terms of the orthodox model and its classification system. She must, therefore, resign herself to the fact that her observation, when seen in orthodox terms, is regarded merely as an anecdotal and unscientific report. What is more, there is no way to advance its scientific claims in the limited terms accepted by the (biomedically dominated) evidence-based literature.

This is a problem completely overlooked by most critics, but evident to anyone after considering the thoughts on philosophy of medical science with which we began this chapter. Saunders (1996) argues that alternative medicine has often arisen in systems of scientific thought that have been abandoned (like vitalism, mesmerism, animism, and botanicals). Boozang (1998, p. 204) goes further and argues that some of these systems are implausible because 'implied mechanisms or putative effects contradict well-established laws, principles, or empirical findings in physics, chemistry, and biology'. Second, there is no evidence that most alternative medicine works (which by implication involves 'adequately controlled outcome research': Boozang 1998). Third, there is no scientific theory to support the practices concerned. Fourth, there are no widely acknowledged tests by which alternative medicine can be assessed. Fifth, there is a view in alternative systems that individuals are responsible for their own health. Sixth, there is no reason to think that reductive medical science will not find answers for malfunctions in a complex integrated system without resorting to holism. Finally, people can be put off effective therapy for their ills.

These are all good points and, as both Boozang (1998) and Saunders (1996) are quick to mention, bogus remedies, fakes, and charlatanism abound in the areas broadly considered under alternative, holistic, and complementary medicine. Boozang suggests that orthodox practitioners have a role in this confused situation. Patients encounter numerous alternative treatment offerings that basically fall into four categories: 'spiritual and psychological; nutritional; drug and biologic; and physical forces and devices ... Whatever their nature, physicians are bound to aid their patients in sorting through their various promises of cure and relief' (p. 199). Boozang concludes that 'in the case of non-validated treatment, physicians should start with a strong presumption against acceding to the patient's demands' (p. 210). However, alongside the rogues, there do seem to be healing traditions that are dedicated to ideals very similar to those that hold in the Hippocratic tradition. Indeed, the corollaries of the holistic view are independently admirable—diagnosis of the deeper derangement, a remedy directed to the deeper problem, working with the healing systems of the ill person, altering the capacity the person has for dealing with illness, and lack of effect for superficial remedies.

We have noted that such systems may be cross-grained with respect to orthodox medicine and that, therefore, they may be bound to fail the kind of evidence-based tests we impose using orthodox medical categories. We can also concur with a general suspicion of those who hide behind mysticism to defuse any systematic investigation of their claims. However, we are not bereft of guidance in this situation because we have at hand the sound advice Hippocrates gave to his students. The way forward would seem to lie in the careful documentation of cases and outcomes and an audit of regimes by an independent licensing body, which should be able to certify whether practice is being conducted systematically, and with due attention to reflective and critical scrutiny within the understanding fundamental to the healing system itself. To some extent this helps us meet the more cogent of the criticisms levelled by Saunders and Boozang.

We can argue that the lack of evidence for the efficacy of most alternative medicine is an artifact of the kind of trials that are insisted on and then considered publishable. These involve 'adequately controlled outcome research' suited to the cause–effect reasoning of the biomedical model. This is akin to using the science of acoustics to do musicology; we are looking in a cross-grained way.

The argument that there is a lack of a scientific theory or rationale to support the practices concerned is only made in terms of recognised biomedical thinking, although in some cases the ideas of alternative medicine sound like complete nonsense. We need, as Hippocrates observed, to retain some critical stance towards what we are being asked to believe, but we should be aware of the extent to which that stance is affected by biomedical training and what it considers scientific.

There are no widely acknowledged tests by which alternative medicine can be assessed, but within each system the evidence of systematism and reflective practice may or may not be found. Where it is found, we need to take note of what emerges. We ought to insist that something beyond anecdotal impression is essential to any healing system that strives for credibility.

The view in alternative systems that individuals are responsible for their own health is also not uncommon in orthodox medicine, as most doctors who practise ethically will regard the patient as a partner in managing the disease. This does not mean that the occurrence of disease can be tied to a moral or spiritual failing in the patient, but it does imply that there may be lifestyle and other psychological factors that influence the course and tractability of an illness.

There is reason to think that reductive medical science will not find answers for malfunctions in a complex integrated system, because it is possible that a delicate and holistic balance of competing and complementary factors in the individual may play a role in the manifestations of different illnesses. These may not be able to be affected by simplistic and externally imposed remedies, but may rather require practitioners to work responsively with the patient as a whole being. If anything like this is true, it is equally true that we understand very little about it, and that only a diligent application of the Hippocratic method will teach us more.

Sadly, it is often true that people can be put off effective therapy for their ills by adopting and persisting with inappropriate treatment in the belief that it will work. However, this is a failure engendered by a poor diagnostician and an opinionated rather than reflective practitioner. This should not be seen as a reason to reject a whole school of thought to which such a practitioner might happen to belong.

A Clinical Modus Operandi

We seem to have a 'stand-off' between narrow and inclusive conceptions of clinical knowledge. But at least it is clear that the narrow conception (underlying the prospective, randomised, controlled, clinical trial type of evidence) is unsuitable to a practice that aims at careful attunement of remedy to the response system being treated. This throws us back to the care and systematism of the observations and understandings that define the practice, and the possibility within the practice of there being significant participation by the sufferer, which we have called the Hippocratic method. Consider the following experience.

> A neurosurgeon who was deeply convinced of the doctrine of informed consent used to take the time to discuss his findings and recommendations with his patients when they were seen in his outpatient clinic. However, every clinic finished with him having a tension headache. He gradually drifted into the practice of showing his patients their X-ray investigations and thereby inviting comment and question about the evidence on which he based his recommendations, and indeed, on the kinds of decisions that flowed from the interpretation of those tests. As this practice became settled, he noticed that his tendency to get headaches on clinic afternoons had virtually vanished. He also noted that his ability to predict exactly what decision a given patient would make prior to meeting them in the clinic had diminished.

This is an interesting (and true) story. The reflective interpretation that recommends itself is that the simple act of engaging the patient with the evidence on which their treatment is planned encourages real participation in any decisions about what should happen to them. The responsibility for treatment and outcome then becomes shared in a way that goes beyond the formal requirements of consent. The moral of the story is that we often systematically deprive ourselves of the most important perspective on patient care by effectively discouraging the patient from taking an intelligent part in the regimen that aims to treat their illness, and by refusing to think outside the square of accepted medical categories. The same realisation has been endorsed by a study on community-based research in developing countries (Ofosu-Amaah 1982). The local situation and its local knowledge might be important in designing effective health care interventions.

The reason why the neurosurgeon in the story succeeded in his attempt to encourage participant decision-making is related in an interesting way to the Hippocratic approach. The problems involved were relatively simple although they lie within one of the most complex surgical disciplines. Lay people can understand the critical concepts like compression, blocking of transmission in nerves, bleeding from a thin-walled blood vessel, and so on. In the example described, the theory was plausible and surveyable according to common sense understandings of the workings of the body. Unfortunately, many different codes of knowledge in contemporary health care and alternative healing make appeal to theories (about immune surveillance, selective receptors for hormones and other physiologically active substances, vital force, and yin and yang) that are opaque to many patients and even to relatively well-informed professionals. Where this is the case, the relevant practice can be both disempowering and exclusive in its claims to right understanding. Disempowerment, when it appears, is a feature of a strain of healing practice of which we have to be suspicious.

In general, alternative methods of healing often emphasise the art of clinical practice more than a rigid science-like approach to medical truth. This is a great strength because it allows the practitioner to deal with the particular patient rather than straight-jacketing the clinical interaction by preconceptions based in an exclusive theoretical framework. Where one is attempting to responsively treat an evolving condition in light of the patient's reaction to various measures, such particularity is important. But in orthodox medical science we often disbelieve or discount a patient's reports and observations, because we tend to emphasise narrow, theory-based conceptions of what counts as real data or genuine truth about a clinical problem. It is probably this attention to the individualities of the case, and the responsive management that goes along with it, that attract many people to alternative practitioners. It is also true that we almost certainly lose many valuable Hippocratic insights by the arrogance we inherit from narrow scientific medicine.

The art of clinical medicine is to meld the general and sketchy fragments of well-grounded theory into a useful and illuminating analysis of a particular episode in health care practice. That art depends as much on a case-based and creative collection of observations and documented interventions as it does on mastery of the 'facts' that are validated by those who impose orthodox medical theory on practitioners. What is more, we need to be careful about the extent to which theory (and the categories we identify through orthodox theory) prejudges what will count as evidence and as a well-designed study. Ideally, we will strive to balance openness with theoretical reflection, and thus moderate any generalisations we make by attending to the particularities of the unique situations of individual patients.

Contemporary Orthodox Medical Science

Orthodox medical science has, in spirit at least, tried to follow the Hippocratic model of science and gain its knowledge from a careful and cumulative experience of the phenomena that make up the domain of clinical practice. However, given the intrinsic power that has become attached to academic and institutional medicine, it has become theory bound and a paradigm dominated by a highly depersonalised and scientific approach to practice, which on the one hand removes bias, but on the other cuts out considerations based on holistic and individual factors. In innumerable areas medicine has succeeded by imposing the scientific model on those ideas that it accepts as true, but it has also ruled out as being deviant ideas that have later proved to be important in understanding a given problem. A good example already mentioned is the theory of gastric ulcer formation and numerous others exist in the area of immunologically informed theory, and spinal disorders.

These facts seem to point to a need for renewed Hippocratic openness to clinical experience. We would extend that view beyond the accumulation of the type of data traditionally legitimated by the natural sciences, such as physiology and pathology. The understanding of disease has to be firmly allied to the understanding of suffering if we are going to gather knowledge that will serve our patients well. The suffering of any patient is a unique pattern that incorporates to varying degrees that patient's individual and complex physiology and pathology, life situation, psychosomatic condition, and relationship with the health system. The rigour attached to knowledge about this complex and convoluted phenomenon cannot possibly be a result of double-blind, controlled trials, because its aim is to grasp the wholeness of a specific and perhaps unique problem. Such problems arise at the micro level between individual patient and care team, and at the macro level between communities and researchers trying to understand patterns of disease and illness in those communities. Experiments that tell us all we need to know about which factors may be important and how they interact cannot be done, although the results of certain experiments may be useful in deciding which questions should be asked and what initial moves should be made. Reflection on the particular case (be it a societal or an individual patient case) is indispensable and needs to be informed by critical thinking about biology, culture, value, social structure, and individual narrative.

It does not help the growth of this kind of inclusive knowledge if we insist that all new ideas and their method of investigation must be procedurally sound according to a narrow scientific conception that has come to displace the Hippocratic method. However, despite this problem, we cannot just give up and allow anything at all to count as a valid way of proceeding. The tests we should apply are intrinsic to the values inherent in the health care enterprise. We need the researchers to be self-critical, sensitive, caring, systematic, and open to the multiple subjective realities that constitute any clinical situation. To encompass this diverse set of virtues we might need a research team, including people who are conversant with the discourses informing the participants and not just the highly abstract discourse of contemporary medical orthodoxy. We also need to be able to develop patterns of thought that allow insight into health and disease from perhaps radically different perspectives.

Conclusion

Health care in all of its guises addresses the experience of human suffering as a result of disease and injury. To understand this problem we need to make use of knowledge gained by treating human beings not simply as dynamic biological systems, but as individuals with their own resources and understandings of disease. Each type of knowledge illuminates the suffering and allows us to attempt a meaningful response to it. The interplay of general and unique features of particular illnesses is itself subject to multiple constructions by the professionals and patients caught up in a health care situation. It is vital for us to appreciate this complexity as we look for something like truth in our understandings of health care. If we obscure or discount aspects of the reality in which we are engaged, we are guilty of falsifying not a theory but a problem and, not surprisingly, we tend to find that the solutions we propose are infected by that falsity. On the other hand, if we abandon exclusive constructions of the problems with which we grapple, we are far more likely to conceptualise or signify a problem in a way that shows not only a truth-like quality, but also a caring quality. On this basis we can offer solutions that inherit those virtues as part of our healing praxis. To achieve this in our clinical practice is, arguably, the art of good health care at any level of intervention.

15
Justice and Health Care

Introduction

There is a danger of excessive individualism in medical ethics, at least in its traditional form. The Hippocratic Oath stresses the responsibility of the doctor for the individual patient, but fails to mention whether the health of the society in which the doctor practises should also be a matter of ethical concern. In similar fashion, the Geneva Declaration, a modernised version of the Oath (see Appendix for both), states: 'The health of my patient will be my first consideration', but makes no mention of the worldwide problem of the lack of facilities for ensuring health, or of inappropriate social factors, for example racial or gender discrimination, that impinge upon health care. This emphasis on the individual character of the doctor–patient relationship ignores totally the communal dimension of health care. We all depend upon the capacity of our society to provide adequate health care, and when that provision is shown to be inadequate in any given case, we must each be affected either directly or indirectly.

The communal dimension of health care ethics is deeper than just the threat posed to each individual by an inadequate health care system. Not only is our own sense of security affected by the possibility that the neglected person could be us or someone close to us; we can also feel a sense of moral outrage that we live in a society where the sick or disabled are inadequately cared for, even though those who are neglected are total strangers to us. Health—like education—is not easily regarded simply as a matter of individual preference and purchasing power. The failure to distribute it fairly and adequately raises fundamental questions about the quality of our communal life (see Campbell 1995). The moral issues raised are those of basic human rights and social justice. What is a person entitled to by virtue of his or her simple humanity? What are the obligations that every society has to its members in the sphere of health and welfare?

The 1948 United Nations Declaration of Human Rights includes a description of the right to health and welfare provision in Article 25(1): 'Everyone has the right to a standard of living adequate for the health and wellbeing of himself and his family, including food, clothing, housing, medical care and necessary social services.' But numerous problems are encountered in seeking to implement this right. The first arises from the problem of constantly increasing possibilities for the provision of improved health care. The more medical 'successes' we have, the higher the expectations are for what medicine should achieve. Thus supply constantly fails to meet demand, and the right to health care seems impossible to implement. A second—and more theoretical—problem relates to disagreement about the nature of the 'right' that is claimed, and about the theory of justice that underpins such a right. A third problem will remain, however, even if we can come to some resolution of the first two: how is 'adequate health care' to be defined, and what are the procedures that will ensure that such adequacy is achieved?

The Paradox of Health Care

In 1942 the Beveridge Report was presented to the British government. This formed the basis for the welfare state established by the Labour government in the immediate postwar era. Beveridge discussed arrangements for health care on the following assumption: 'A comprehensive health service will ensure that for every citizen there is available whatever medical treatment he requires, in whatever form he requires it.' This assumption now seems hopelessly ambitious because we are painfully aware that no country, however wealthy, can possibly afford all the possible treatments that might be beneficial to all its citizens. The reason for this is what Cochrane (1972) has called 'the nicest possible form of inflation'. As medical care has become more effective in providing cures for life-threatening conditions, the demands on health services have increased in line with people's enhanced expectations of what should be provided. This 'paradox of health care' has been well described by Maxwell (1974):

> The more infant lives are saved the more serious becomes the threat of handicap. The further life expectancy is extended the greater become the demands on geriatric services and long term facilities for the infirm and elderly. Each new advance which gives hope to another category of sufferers . . . converts a latent need into an immediate and continuing demand.

The resolution of this paradox depends upon a willingness to view health care provision in terms of its overall impact upon the health of a population, rather than as a series of individual interventions or responses to demand. Coordinated planning of this kind is notoriously difficult to achieve because of the numerous interests—professional, commercial and political—that operate in the health field. But an approach can be attempted in terms of the interrelationship of three things—efficiency, effectiveness, and equity.

The first two are assessed by health research and implemented by adequate resource management. In the United Kingdom the government has recently set up a National Institute for Clinical Excellence (NICE). The task of NICE is to analyse all the available evidence for the effectiveness of pharmaceuticals and other medical interventions and to advise on whether they achieve the outcomes claimed for them. Although such evidence is essential for an objective assessment of effectiveness, it cannot of itself provide the solutions to problems of rationing. The level of decision-making has to be decided: what types of decision should be a matter of national priority? And what types can be left to the discretion of local health institutions taking into account local circumstances? This is inevitably a political process. Goals and objectives have to be defined for different aspects of the health service, and ways devised to monitor the extent to which they are being achieved. Thus it might be decided that major causes of premature death should be reduced by a combination of preventive, health-educational, and curative measures. Priority would then be given to the financing of the measures selected, and the plan would be adjusted according to whether or not the desired outcomes were being achieved. Such planning solutions, although useful, depend upon a prior social agreement about which goals and objectives are to be selected out of a vast range of possibilities. Since not all health goals can be achieved, however efficient and effective our interventions become, we have to decide which are to be given favoured consideration. Therefore, we are faced with the problem of equity. How can we ensure that resources available to health care are allocated fairly? On which theory of justice do we base our judgments of equity in health care provision?

Equity and Theories of Justice

In one sense, equity is quite simply defined: it is ensured when people are treated in as fair a manner as possible by ignoring irrelevant differences between them but taking account of relevant differences. For example, it is inequitable to deny people the right to vote simply because of their gender or the colour of their skin. These differences are irrelevant to the issue being considered. On the other hand, it is equitable to deny the vote to those who are severely disturbed psychiatrically, or to persons below a certain age, if it can be shown that these factors are relevant to their capacity to make an informed choice. We have here what is sometimes called the 'formal principle of justice', which can be stated thus: 'treat equals equally and unequals unequally'. This formal principle is of some help in ensuring equity in health care, since it identifies the unfairness of the maldistribution of health care resources by, for example, social class or geographical region. However, it leaves unresolved the more difficult issue of deciding which differences are relevant in deciding health care priorities. Are some people's health care needs more deserving of attention than others? How are we to determine which?

To try to answer these questions we need to look more carefully at the theoretical debate underlying justice theory. Beauchamp and Walters (1989, p. 33) have described six different principles upon which a theory of distributive justice might be based:

1 To each person an equal share.
2 To each person according to individual need.
3 To each person according to acquisition in a free market.
4 To each person according to individual effort.
5 To each person according to societal contribution.
6 To each person according to merit.

If we consider how these might be applied to health care provision, we can see that some seem fairer than others. A stress on acquisition in a free market (Principle 3), for example, fails to allow for the vulnerability and disadvantage created by illness itself. The chronically ill or permanently disabled are certainly in no position to compete equally with their less disadvantaged fellow citizens. The same objection applies to the principle that rewards effort (Principle 4). This is based on the false assumption that there is a 'level playing field' on which all have an equal capacity to look after their own interests. The reality of ill health is that it removes the possibility of equal opportunity in a competitive situation. (This is not to deny that individual effort has a worthwhile contribution to make to the maintenance or the restoration of health, but fairness cannot be ensured by using effort as the sole criterion for the allocation of resources.)

A different kind of objection can be levelled against the last two principles. These assume that the health of some individuals is to be more highly valued than that of others, either because they have more to offer to society, or because they are more deserving of consideration and respect on account of their personal qualities. There are situations in which we use these principles to distribute benefits. Societal contribution may be recognised by appropriate income levels (though this is rarely the way things actually work in income distribution); and honours and distinctions are frequently used as a mark of excellence of character and achievement. However, to allocate health care according to these principles is to base matters of life and death on our highly fallible judgments of individual or social worth. Health is too vital an aspect of individual well-being for it to be dependent upon such potentially prejudiced judgments. In any case, to disregard a person's health care needs because we regard that person as being of lower value than others would commit us to a dangerous path of discrimination, in which only the worthy or the socially useful are to be accorded full rights.

We appear to be left, then, with a choice between either an equal distribution (Principle 1) or a distribution according to need (Principle 2). Each has some strong arguments in its favour. When there is a valued and scarce social benefit, an equal and impartial distribution would seem to be the fairest method of dealing with the scarcity. All would suffer equally from the scarcity and benefit equally from the benefits available. Although this appears to promote equality, the effect can often be the opposite, since the scarcity of resources can have a far more detrimental effect on some groups than on others. For example, a shortage of primary care facilities in a low-income area has much more serious effects than a similar shortage in more prosperous communities, which often have greater resources for self-help. Again, an equal distribution of resources across a range of types of service can have disproportionate effects on some particularly vulnerable groups, such as the intellectually handicapped, the very young or the elderly, who require a high concentration of health care resources.

Thus it seems essential to relate the distribution of resources to some criterion of need. Those with equal needs should get equal shares, but those with greater needs should get greater shares. By using need as a criterion we use equality of opportunity, or equality of *outcome* as a goal, rather than resting content with equality of distribution. It is the 'need theory' of distributive justice that has had the most influence on health care policy from Beveridge onwards. It does, however, raise some ferociously difficult practical problems.

Arbitrating Between Needs

An area health board has to make substantial cuts in services in order to balance its budget. A major saving would be obtained by closing down some smaller units in outlying areas and centralising these services in a major hospital. This is an unpopular move since it causes great inconvenience to these smaller communities. An alternative would be to allow waiting lists for elective surgical operations to lengthen, causing inconvenience and unnecessary disability to a smaller number of people, but at a more serious level.

Such hard choices are commonplace for health authorities at the present time, and innumerable other examples could be given. What criteria should be used to identify the least undesirable option? (There is no ideal option. Some group must suffer to some degree).

We begin by recognising that this decision is not one between individuals as such, but between relative funding of different types of service. This is a dilemma peculiar to countries that have some kind of integrated and nationally funded health service, and therefore already accept the basic premise that it is a national obligation to provide an adequate level of health care for all citizens. Thus, the debate about justice in health care provision is very different in countries like the United Kingdom, New Zealand, Australia, and the Scandinavian countries from that in the USA, for example, where this basic premise is still not accepted. Decisions about relative spending between types of service can be described as macro-allocation (to distinguish it from micro-allocation—choices between individuals as to who should receive a scarce resource, such as renal dialysis).

To make macro-allocation decisions we need to combine the three factors of efficiency, effectiveness, and equity with the overall aim of maximising the most efficient and effective form of health care delivery to those whose needs are greatest. Using this formula there seems, at first sight, no escape from the conclusion that services must be increasingly centralised in order to enable them to deliver effective and lower-cost intervention as equally as possible to a maximum number of people. An underutilised peripheral service uses up resources that could be put to effective use in a major centre.

Is this a fair conclusion? Why should people be penalised in terms of access to services simply because they live in a rural area? Moreover the effectiveness of health care services can be compromised if they are too inaccessible and located in larger, more impersonal institutions. A service based in a small community could achieve much earlier interventions for the people of that community, and thus be more cost-effective in the long run. These counter-arguments illustrate the uncertainty of decision-making in this area. There are bound to be compromises, and frequently the right balance of types of service and of efficient deployment of services will not be achieved. However, we might regard the isolated rural lifestyle as a 'package deal' that includes slightly, or significantly, worse access to certain services. This perspective regards it as reasonable to ask 'How much should society in general pay to mitigate the consequences of a chosen lifestyle?' Yet many people living in rural areas could fairly reply that, had they not chosen this rural isolation, society's agricultural needs would not be met.

So far we have been discussing problems of equitable distribution of services to meet roughly comparable medical needs. The criteria for just distribution become even more difficult to apply when we are attempting to compare widely disparate needs. For example, how are we to determine the relative weightings to be assigned to life-saving as opposed to life-*enhancing* interventions?

A health authority has to consider two competing claims for its strictly limited funds. The first comes from a group of senior cardiologists and cardio-thoracic surgeons who want to set up a heart transplant unit in the region. They have established that the necessary surgical and nursing skills are already available in a local hospital and that there would be a steady supply of appropriate recipients. The second claim for funds comes from a hospital catering for elderly and terminally ill patients. The wards are in a deplorable state and require extensive upgrading and greatly improved staffing levels. There are reports of neglect of patients, and a number of complaints from relatives about the state of the wards and the poor professional standards of the staff. Both schemes require capital expenditure plus ongoing revenue expenditure, and (given some funding from private sources for the transplant unit) the costs are roughly the same. Which project should the authority support, in the knowledge that due to budgetary restrictions the rejected project is likely to be indefinitely postponed?

This example forces us to consider how we might weigh survival for a few against increased quality of life, or more accurately, quality of care, for a larger group. As we have seen in Chapter 11, attempts have been made to provide a formula for such decisions in terms of Quality Adjusted Life Years (QALYs). A health care intervention is assessed in terms of both the *number* of years of life gained and the *quality of life* during those years of survival. However, although QALYs can be useful when we are considering two or more alternative interventions for the *same* group of people (for example, cardiac surgery versus medication for people with symptoms of heart disease), they do not provide a moral basis for arbitrating between interventions for *different* groups. Let us suppose that (a) the cardiac transplantation would gain for the recipients on average between five and ten years of high-quality survival; and (b) the upgrading of the geriatric wards would gain on average three to five years of improved quality of life for the patients on these wards before their deaths. These numbers do not tell us that the heart transplantation proposal is the preferred option for the health authority, unless they are always going to favour those who have longer survival prospects (with the necessary intervention) over those who are closer to death. Such an approach would be morally intolerable since it would create a huge bias in the health service against the old and terminally ill, in favour of those who are younger and can benefit from acute interventions. We would end up with a health care system that was seriously 'agist' (see Harris 1987).

Although QALYs are inevitably agist for between-person comparisons and difficult to calculate and apply to between-treatment comparisons, there is one licit use from an ethical perspective. Consider a person contemplating two modes of treatment for, say, a tumour of the bowel. On the one hand the patient is offered a resection with colostomy and five years of remaining life and on the other a conservative approach with a shorter survival but no colostomy. The actual QALY figures here may not be important, but the principle of a trade-off between longevity and quality and the need to take a careful look at this is important and useful for the person concerned. An even more compelling case for a QALY comparison is that of a person with an abdominal cancer, who is offered a chance of life for eight months severely constrained by dietary restrictions, with a major requirement for in-hospital care and chemotherapy.

Compare this with another case having a shorter survival time, say four months untreated, with palliative care only, and a relatively normal range of activity during that time. In such cases we can endorse the principle of comparing outcomes, and the probabilities of certain outcomes, in relation to quality and longevity as a means of assessing the relative economic and clinical merits of different health interventions.

Maximising the Minimum

When we contemplate the possibility that a group of elderly people could remain in deplorable conditions indefinitely in order to allow for an initiative saving the lives of others, we realise that something fundamental is at stake morally. This was expressed by Kant (1785) in the principle that we should never treat people as 'mere means to an end', which implies that we honour certain undertakings to them. However worthy the goal of the heart transplantation program, a more pressing demand for our attention is the dependency of elderly people, for whom society has already taken responsibility and for whom it has a continuing obligation for adequate care. There is thus a prior obligation to meet their needs adequately before launching new initiatives in life-saving medicine. Here we may perceive a special place for the value of personal freedom as a human quality, which all societies should seek to both protect and enhance. The less an individual is able to safeguard his or her own freedom, the more responsibility we have to ensure that there is no abuse of the dependency, and that freedom is fostered as far as possible.

These intuitions about the essential aspects of justice have been incorporated in a celebrated theory of justice formulated by the philosopher John Rawls (1971). According to Rawls, if we were to consider the basic constituents of justice under a 'veil of ignorance' (i.e. when we could not know our own particular social situation), we would support two basic principles of justice. The first principle (the 'Liberty Principle') would require that each person be accorded the maximum amount of equal personal liberty compatible with the same amount for all other persons. This combination is designed to ensure a degree of equalisation by social arrangements of those deficits in personal liberty that might be created by the fortuitous circumstances of such things as birth, disability, and childhood environment. Thus the first principle already has a definite bias towards the weak and disadvantaged in a society who, by reason of their disadvantage, might have significantly curtailed liberty unless special measures are taken.

However, Rawls's second principle prevents his theory from being a simplistic egalitarian one, in which no differences between individuals in terms of possession of property or other social goods would be permitted. Rather, Rawls believes that it is just to permit, or even promote, such differences, provided that the resultant inequalities enhance the position of the most disadvantaged in society. This 'Difference Principle' once more underlines the need to recognise the plight of those often disregarded by society and afforded inadequate care because they do not have a power base from which to actively promote their interests.

To what extent does Rawls's account of justice help in the complex issue of the fair distribution of health care resources? Certainly it prevents any over-simplified emphasis on life-saving at any cost. Clearly a health service that always gives life-saving measures priority will seriously inhibit the possibility of a fair distribution of resources that defend the freedom of the disregarded and the underprivileged. An outcome of this in health care provision could be that acute services would use up even more of the budget than they do at present, and services that provide basic care and support at a simple level on a long-term basis (community-based geriatric services, for example) would lose out badly. This does appear to be the case when a 'free market' is allowed to operate in health care. The health services then most favoured are those that appeal to the members of society with the income to purchase them and the information needed for consumers to decide which is the 'best buy', while the poor and dis-advantaged are more and more dependent on an inadequately funded public service, grudgingly supported by taxation.

On the other hand, the Rawlsian Difference Principle serves as a reminder that we need to pay attention to the overall social and economic impact of health care interventions. A service that allows for a healthy and productive younger group can rebound to the advantage of the more vulnerable groups, if the resources generated by their productivity are then devoted to effective pro-grams of long-term care. If the imbalance moves too far in favour of funding for the disadvantaged, then—paradoxically—it is the disadvantaged who them-selves suffer most in the long run.

A Basic Minimum?

Does this mean then that there is no right to a minimum level of health care, but only a juggling of resources to ensure that disadvantage is not too great? This could be the outcome of using the Difference Principle as the measure of whether a health care system is just. In our current situation of ever-expanding demands on the health services, combined with severe fiscal constraints, this can mean a rapidly sinking floor of health status, especially for the chronically ill. But this seems incompatible with some of the values implicit in a 'caring society'.

Improvements in screening for breast cancer and for cancer of the prostate have resulted in a dramatic increase in the number of cases referred for surgery, chemotherapy, and radiotherapy in a region that has already been exceeding its government-allocated health budget. The inability of the service to meet the escalating demand from its existing resources has resulted in longer and longer delays in the provision of relevant therapy. These delays have resulted in preventable deaths and in painful and disabling conditions caused by the spread of the cancer during the waiting period. Without increased funding, the prospects for cancer patients in these categories will rapidly worsen, but the government claims that increasing funds in this sector will cause equally serious problems in another, since there is only a finite amount in the total health budget. Since the medical staff have been warning these patients of their worsening prospects, those who can afford it are opting for private treatment. However, many patients have no such financial resources and have no choice but to wait.

The only answer to this difficulty is to seek a social consensus on what is a basic minimum of health care provision that all members of a given society must receive, whatever the financial cost. If governments cannot supply the minimum, they have a duty to increase the total funding to health care until it is met. In New Zealand this approach to justice in health care was attempted by the formation of a government committee to advise on 'core health services', which were defined as services to which all those needing them should have access without undue delay or cost. This attempt to define a core has failed to produce any definition of a minimum entitlement, despite nearly ten years of work. Instead it has had to confine itself to determining criteria for defining the urgency of cases, and assessing the relative effectiveness of different interventions for a given condition. Although these are useful tasks, they do not bind the government to any specific level of provision: the more urgent may be treated first, but (as the cancer example above illustrates) resource constraints may prevent large numbers of treatable conditions being high enough up the list to be treated in time. How low the floor sinks is defined by economics, not by ethics.

A more sophisticated version of Rawlsian theory than the one we used in the previous section provides an explanation of why defining a minimum is so difficult. In *Just Health Care*, the philosopher Norman Daniels has put forward an account of health care entitlement based on Rawls's first principle of justice— the Liberty Principle. One aspect of genuine liberty is ensuring an equality of opportunity for all members of a society, since without such opportunity the concept of freedom is empty. Since disability and ill health are potent barriers to equal opportunity, the principle of liberty requires that they be removed, to equalise everyone's chances in life. But what does this mean in practical terms? Daniels argues that we should use as a criterion 'species typical normal functioning'. He believes that we know enough about normal human functioning at various ages for us to establish a relatively objective 'normal opportunity range' for any given individual at any given point in life (Daniels 1985). This criterion will help us to determine how much entitlement to health care is a basic minimum for any given person. If people do not receive this minimum then their right to health care has not been respected and the health care system is not just.

Daniels's theory is an attractive and politically challenging one. It offers the potential for us to describe any given society's health care system as in breach of human rights, just as we currently do about social or legal systems that breach civil or democratic rights. But unfortunately, any attempt to apply his criterion to the actual dilemmas of health care provision runs into huge practical and theoretical difficulties, as he himself has subsequently admitted. The main problem is that the criterion specifies an unattainable goal: some people are so damaged by illness or disability that no amount of resources can restore to them the normal opportunity range, and any attempt to do so will swallow up all available resources for health care. But if we aim lower than Daniels suggests, how do we decide a minimum entitlement? How close to 'normal' is acceptable?

A second difficulty is whether we are going for aggregate or individual improvement. For example, a good immunisation program will keep millions of children within a normal opportunity range: but the same resource might be devoted to just a few individuals who had a rare condition requiring very expensive treatment. Does the aggregate benefit count for more ethically? Does it matter once rights to health care are not met whether this is for a few people or for a large number? The theory Daniels offers provides no answer to this question. A final difficulty is whether we should target the worse off (medically), in the hope of improving their condition to a point approaching the normal range, or whether our focus should be on those who are close enough to the normal range to make our interventions achieve a wholly satisfactory outcome. There is the problem of triage, when applied to emergency medicine, but should triage operate in our prioritising of non-acute conditions also?

Regretfully we have to conclude that a basic minimum standard of health status, which can clearly define a right to health care, is a will o' the wisp. In the world outside the philosopher's study, what happens is a political balancing act. One set of claims constantly competes with another set. Often it takes a media scandal to get resources reallocated or (rarely) increased. A pragmatist will try to keep the whole system functioning as effectively as possible, seeking to avoid gross disadvantage to any one group. But the idealism of medicine and of the professions involved in it requires that we do not give in to political expediency and cynically accept the sinking floor in health care. Rather, the debate about how we can define a basic minimum for any society that values justice must continue.

State-funded Care Versus Private Practice

The issue of private practice, and the differential access to health care created by it, is also a subject of ethical debate, particularly in countries like the United Kingdom and New Zealand, in which a state-funded service finds itself under ever-increasing pressure. There are those who opt for some kind of entitlement theory of justice corresponding to the principle 'to each according to acquisition in a free market'. We have argued that this disadvantages those who, through no fault of their own, may already be disadvantaged, and therefore it is incompatible with the idea of a caring society. Many will agree with this basic stand, but argue that a modified mutual health care system according to the principle 'to each according to individual need' is compatible with a limited private sector. In this sector, they argue, those who can provide service over and above what is required of them to serve our mutual need arrangements can contract with those who wish to pay over and above what they already contribute to our mutual system and provide extra health care services. On this basis, the existence of private medical care is thought to be no threat to a shared-care system that provides services according to need (and availability of resources). It seems hard to argue that once people have contributed to a public system through taxation they should be prevented from spending their disposable income as they choose. It seems ludicrous to allow people to spend their spare resources on holidays or other non-essential items but to try to prevent them purchasing an operation that will ease their discomfort or make their daily activities less burdensome.

The defenders of private practice would go so far as to say that it offers advantages to all to have such a system. They would say that it reduces competition for the limited resources in the public, needs-based system; that it gives the professionals greater earning power, which reduces pressure on the public system salary structure (and thus on costs); that it provides a carefully costed system that can streamline care in ways that might be copied where appropriate by the public system; and that it provides more choices and greater individual freedom within the society. These arguments have gained increasing force with evidence that countries with a private health care element spend a higher proportion of their national wealth on health care than countries like the United Kingdom in which the state sector predominates.

However, it should be noted that higher spending by no means always equates with a better or fairer service, and that the main beneficiaries of a mixed system are those who can afford private health care. Where the two systems co-exist, there is often pressure on the professionals concerned to shift a disproportionate amount of time and effort into the highly paid system. There is also pressure not to reduce the waiting lists in the public system because having to wait for care is an incentive to pay for private care. The best one can say is that where the professionals are highly motivated and acting in accordance with the standards of professional practice that we have outlined, there may be no harm in a two-tier system. However, there is great potential for abuse, and definite pressures to devalue one's involvement in public health care. It is to the credit of most professionals working in both, that the standards in their public health practice are so high. Equally, pressure mounts on patients, as resource constraints affect the public sector, to shift to private care or to seek a 'double indemnity' by having health insurance but using the public system as a safety net.

What is rarely perceived by the public is that if this shift into private care becomes a major component of the health system, then quickly the public service will be eroded, to everyone's detriment. Private medicine can work reasonably well with a public system so long as it is focused on extras and is used by a few. As soon as it becomes the major provider, costs begin to escalate. This happens because health care providers define the needs of their patients, and thus can easily create their own market by being generous in their estimate of requisite tests and so on. In the private sector there are few controls on this tendency to escalate costs: they are defined by what the market can bear, the only constraint being controls instituted by health insurers. All this has the effect of attracting professional staff more and more into the higher paid, private work, thus forcing the public sector to pay more to retain their services. These increased costs on the limited budget of the public sector cause a further reduction in the services available or an increase in the waiting times, thus pushing more health consumers into the private sector. As the spiral continues, the public health system becomes less and less sustainable and the overall costs of health care rise exponentially. The widely acknowledged crisis in US health care provides a clear example of this danger. Health care delivery is not a self-limiting market, and governments that want to provide an adequate health service to all of their citizens must avoid the fatal attraction of trying to save costs by encouraging a growth of the private sector.

Conclusion

Given the complexity of the debate about health care priorities, it is understandable that many doctors feel a sense of hopelessness in this area of medical ethics. What is the use of getting involved in such social or political matters? Isn't it best just to do what one can for one's own patients, within whatever resources are available, and, when it comes to cuts, to 'defend one's own corner' as well as possible?

To take up such a position ignores the possibility that a profession can play a prophetic role within the society that authorises it to practise (Campbell 1984, Chapter 2; 1995, Chapter 5). Doctors who refuse to see past the immediate illnesses or accidents dealt with by their speciality are depriving society of an important source of insight and critical demand for change. Of course, no one practitioner and no one group of specialists can see the whole picture in health care. However, if sufficient numbers of health professionals are willing to enter the debate about priorities, an impressively wide picture of the crisis areas in health care provision can be gained.

The purpose of this chapter has been to suggest some of the concepts doctors and other health professionals should use to improve the quality of the debate about justice in health care, a debate that should be everybody's concern, but to which the health care provider can contribute a great deal of detailed description of the inequities in the system. We may summarise the basic framework for a just system of health care provision as follows:

1 Justice in health care provision demands that every person be treated fairly, without regard to their social status, gender, ethnic group, or political views.
2 Since illness and accident strike people in arbitrary and unequal ways, the only fair basis for discrimination is the degree of need for health care.
3 When a society has decided that a health care need should be met, all those with that need should be treated equally, without discrimination according to age, gender, place of residence, ability to pay, or alleged merit as a citizen.
4 In trying to put different needs for health care into some order of priority, we should pay particular attention to the disadvantaged in the society, since their liberty to improve their own health is likely to be most severely curtailed.
5 A minimum entitlement to health care has to be defined and applied without discrimination to each person in the society. This minimum should be defined according to what is required to give each person an equal opportunity to exercise his or her personal liberty. However, it has to be admitted that an economically achievable minimum entitlement is very hard to define.

This attempt to ensure justice by equalising the opportunity to maintain one's own health reminds us that no one can ensure the health of another. Professionals do not 'give' people health; they make the achievement and maintenance of health a possibility by removing the barriers to it in the lives of individuals. Ivan Illich makes the point about the difference between health and medical intervention succinctly and well in his book *Limits to Medicine*: 'A world of optimal and widespread health is obviously a world of minimal and only occasional medical intervention' (Illich 1977).

16
Law, Ethics, and Medicine

Introduction

Medical law is complex in that health care professionals are affected by a number of areas of law in relation to their professional duties. In general, these fall into three major divisions:

1   the law as it relates to medical or health care practice through such things as Medical Practitioners Acts, Hospitals Acts, Mental Health Acts and so on;
2   the criminal law, which describes certain roles for doctors in relation to criminal behaviour but might also consider certain acts to be criminal in themselves even if performed by a health care professional;
3   the civil law, which may adjudicate in disputes between doctors and patients.

The first of these three areas of law defines what a society expects of a person who is to be regarded as a 'registered medical practitioner' or a 'registered nurse' and imposes certain duties and conditions of practice on such people. It also gives such people certain special roles in relation to those considered mentally ill, the use and disposal of bodies, public health and so on. For instance, a doctor designated by the coroner might be permitted to dissect a corpse for the sake of determining a cause of death, but a person who is not a registered practitioner could not do such a thing.

The second of these relates to certain crimes to do with death or injury and usually involves health care workers only where they are guilty of some serious breach of their professional role tantamount to criminal behaviour. For instance, a male doctor who acted inappropriately towards a woman attending him for a medical problem might be charged with sexual violation. This could happen even though doctors are entitled to do things that others are not, as part of their professional practice. The court would have to decide that either the woman did not consent to what was done or that what was done was not part of what a doctor would do in that clinical situation, in which case what he did would be treated exactly as if it were performed by others. The criminal or general law also outlines certain provisions about expert testimony, and the role of doctors in gathering certain kinds of evidence. For instance, a specialist pathologist may be asked in a criminal case whether he or she believes that certain wounds were caused by single or multiple blows.

The third area of law is invoked where a doctor has caused certain kinds of harm to a patient and the patient sues for damages. This area of litigation is limited in some countries such as New Zealand and Sweden where compensation arrangements are in place (Wall 1992) but is widespread in other countries such as Australia and the United Kingdom.

We should also notice the problems that arise when non-lawyers fail to appreciate the difference between statute law and common law. Statute law is what is written into acts of parliament or government statutes. For instance, in most Commonwealth countries, the law states that no person should withhold the necessaries of life from a person for whom he or she is responsible (Skegg 1988a). Taken one way this may mean that a doctor should provide all possible means to keep a person alive where there is any chance at all of doing that. But it is not usually interpreted that way and, in fact, doctors often do not administer every possible life-prolonging treatment to a person who is dying. The common law, or the law as it has been interpreted and applied by the courts, is an area that grows as cases are heard and judgments made. It is the common law or the decisions of courts that tell us that the giving of pain relief to a dying patient is most unlikely to be construed as culpable homicide even if the doses used are large enough to constitute a risk of hastening death (Skegg 1995). It is the common law that tells us that withdrawal of life support under approved conditions will not be treated as murder.

Before we consider these three areas further we will discuss the general considerations relating to ethics and the law.

Ethics and the Law

It is obvious that some of the behaviour and many of the cases described in this book involve actions that are on the borderline between the unethical and the illegal. The relationship between medical ethics and medical law is subtle and mirrors the general relationship between the moral intuitions of a community and the laws regulating that community (Honore 1993).

Our moral intuitions cause us to enact certain laws so as to safeguard what we consider important. For instance, we believe that one should be able to live without fear of violence, and so we have laws against murder, wilfully causing injury, and assault. We also believe that one should have a certain security of private property, and so we have laws against fraud and theft. On the other hand, we believe that each citizen should assume some responsibility for the welfare of all, leading to tax laws and social welfare laws. Each of these examples illustrates the fact that our laws are shaped by what we believe to be right conduct. What we accept as right conduct changes from age to age, as is witnessed by our current widespread relaxation of mores concerning marriage and the family. It must be accepted, however, that much law also depends upon unexamined assumptions or conventions, often inherited from the social arrangements of a previous age. Thus the law requires continuous revision and reform.

In medicine, we have a set of laws that dictates what a medical practitioner can and cannot do. And so, we have laws that proscribe assisting a person to die, we have constraints on the termination of pregnancy, and we demand of doctors that they show due care and skill. These laws encode the standards we have already discussed. But some health care professionals worry about the letter of the law, and whether they will be held guilty of a crime for doing what they believe to be correct according to ethical considerations.

> Dr D was caring for a 46-year-old man, Mr E, who had suffered a devastating brain haemorrhage. She spoke to the relatives and was told that he would never have wanted to live in the mute, dependent, bedridden and paralysed state to which he had been reduced. One night Mr E developed a high temperature, and over the next day or so it was clear that he had severe pneumonia and would die if this were not treated. She felt inclined not to treat it but to give him morphine for his respiratory distress. However, a colleague, Dr F, said she was obliged to because the law stated that a doctor could in no way withhold the necessaries of life, which included medical treatment required to save the life of the patient [this refers to the New Zealand Crimes Act, section 151].

Where should we turn in such a situation? Laws generally have qualifying phrases that allow one to exercise judgment: terms like 'reasonable', 'lawful excuse', 'sufficient', 'disproportionate' and 'unwarranted'. These phrases are applied by the courts in an effort to give substance to the moral convictions of reasonable or commonsense people, in relation to issues that require the judgment of sensible people. Therefore, there are often mitigating provisions that make the 'strict letter of the law' more of a myth than a reality in dealing with clinical practice.

In relation to the case of Mr E, Dr F declined to mention that the section he quoted qualifies 'omitting to provide' the 'necessaries of life' by inserting the words 'without lawful excuse'. Thus, one is not bound to give such 'necessaries' to the patient (Collins 1992, pp. 192 ff.). Judging by recent case law, it is likely that this would be interpreted to include those situations where, in the opinion of the doctor, the family, and the other health care professionals involved and in accordance with any known wishes of the patient, no 'substantial benefit' (see Chapter 1) was to be gained by giving the life-saving treatment in question (Gillett et al. 1995; Skegg 1988b).

Therefore, ethics influences not only the formulation of the laws governing medical practice, but also their interpretation in a given clinical situation. Most of the time the courts can be expected to take the view that the ethical standards that govern conduct between doctor and patient will be taken as a guide as to what can reasonably be expected of a competent practitioner.

We ought also to note that the law influences our common morality in that it tends to signal, especially in complex moral issues, what those who should know regard as a reasonable stand in a given area. For instance, most countries now have laws permitting abortion. We all realise that this is a difficult and contentious moral issue and, in most countries, the introduction of the law has signalled that abortion is a reasonable step only in certain circumstances where a greater evil must be avoided. Thus, even though the original provisions in any legislature allow abortion only under strictly limited conditions, there is gradual acceptance that it is a thing that can be done, and the conditions are gradually loosened to allow a wider and wider range of cases to qualify. Whatever our view on this particular matter, it provides a graphic illustration of the persuasive effect of law, in that the legalisation of a given practice signals to a community that that practice is reasonable (albeit under certain limited conditions), whereas its occurrence might previously have been considered to be a matter of grave moral concern.

Professional Requirements on Doctors and Others

In every country there are standards defining the properly qualified doctor, dentist, nurse, psychologist, and so on. These standards are generally administered by a licensing body that keeps a register of those who qualify. This body of registered practitioners then has a mechanism, usually defined by statute, that gives it certain powers to regulate and discipline members of the profession.

The reason for the profession having such power is that it is reckoned to know best what counts as good practice in its own area of expertise. In order to promote and make clear the standards it requires, each profession usually devises a code of ethics. Such codes define a set of duties for doctors, or the relevant professionals, with the appropriate moderating or qualifying conditions that apply to them. In addition to this, the profession works to a standard of competence according to which any practitioner is expected to act with a certain degree of skill and care in the way he or she cares for patients. Two cases will illustrate this.

> Dr A is treating Mr C for a chronic back problem, which he believes to be in part a method of malingering on Mr C's part. He has a brief note from a previous doctor in another town that indicates that there seems to be no physical problem that

can be detected as the cause of the back condition. While playing golf with a friend, who is one of the directors of a local manufacturing concern, he hears that his friend is about to employ Mr C. He mentions back trouble and the fact that it seems to be related to an aversion towards hard work. The facts about the conversation on the golf course emerge when Mr C is refused work and starts to ask why it might have happened, and Dr A is subjected to a complaint to the Medical Council on two counts:

  1 Dr A shared Mr C's confidential medical information without consent;
  2 Dr A had not taken the trouble to make a proper diagnosis of Mr C's back condition.

Dr A is in trouble. The profession has, as we have seen, adopted a standard of confidentiality that precludes the kind of information-sharing that Dr A indulged in. What is more, Dr A has not taken adequate steps to ensure that he knows what Mr C's back condition is. To do this Dr A would almost certainly have had to obtain previous records about Mr C and possibly to arrange for a specialist opinion. In this case Dr A has been both unethical and incompetent and will face disciplinary charges from the profession. These can include a fine and a limitation of practice.

Dr S does sterilisation procedures in her local, rural hospital. She has done a training period in gynaecology and has performed many successful operations, although not formally registered as a gynaecologist. She has also, in the past, done tonsillectomy and adenoidectomy (T&A) procedures on the basis of a time during which she worked in the ENT department of a district hospital. She undertakes a T&A on Jon, a child of seven with recurrent ear infections and chronically inflamed tonsils. Jon haemorrhages badly after the operation and, after a torrid time and having been transfused with two units of blood, survives. Jon recovers fully but his parents lay a complaint that Dr S was not qualified to perform the procedure.

Here the question is one of competence, and it is debatable whether a generally qualified medical practitioner is equipped to carry out such a procedure. In the case of surgery, all is well if things go smoothly and without complications, but complications require a level of skill hard to maintain with only intermittent or occasional practice. To decide whether Dr S has acted properly it is necessary to determine her skill level in this area, and the conditions required to make such a procedure fall within acceptable limits for safe practice.

Such matters as these are within the jurisdiction of the profession and its regulatory and disciplinary mechanism. The judgments of the professional regulation and disciplinary systems impact directly on the professionals involved. They may involve fines, which are not usually large, or limitations on practice. These may be radical or more moderate. The worst that can happen is that a doctor can be struck off the list of registered practitioners and therefore unable to practise. For a less serious matter a doctor may be temporarily suspended and unable to practise, and this would usually be conjoined with some sort of corrective training. Less serious again might be the case in which the doctor is fined but allowed to continue in practice provided that certain supervision or retraining conditions are met. For instance, if the parents' complaint about Jon were upheld, Dr S might be instructed either to stop performing minor ENT procedures such as tonsillectomy or to undertake an approved course of supervised retraining in that area. A doctor may also be fined and censured, which is mainly serious because of the criticism it would attract from fellow members of the profession; the fine would probably be met by the doctor's malpractice insurance. In each of these cases the penalties are far more effective than a damages settlement because they directly affect the income and practice of the offender.

Problems arising in clinical practice may, however, be linked with more serious charges and pass into the jurisdiction of a criminal court. This could, for instance, happen if a doctor was judged to have been guilty of professional misconduct because of sexual activity in a doctor–patient relationship, and then also had to face a criminal charge of indecent assault.

Health Care Workers and Criminal Law

Dr W is an anaesthetist. While anaesthetising one of his patients, Mr X, he leaves the operating room to get a cup of coffee as he is under pressure to get through a large number of operative cases and realises he will not have time for morning tea. He returns to find that Mr X's oxygen levels are dangerously low and falling. He asks what is happening and is told that an alarm on the machine went off but the staff were instructed by the surgeon, Mr Y, to 'Turn that blasted racket off!' as Mr Y was having trouble with a tricky bit of the operation. As Dr W tries to investigate what is happening Mr X's heart stops and, despite attempts to resuscitate him, he dies. After the event the relatives of Mr X make enquiries but cannot arrange a time to see either Dr W or Mr Y and discuss the situation with them. The family not only lays a complaint with the Medical Council but also asks the police to investigate. The coroner's report suggests that the anaesthetic tube slipped and that the equipment used gave fair warning of the serious hypoxia that ensued. Criminal charges to the effect that gross professional negligence led to culpable homicide are laid against both Dr W and Mr Y.

Here a matter of professional competence and care has crossed a boundary and becomes of concern to the criminal law. In the past, cases of this type in some countries (such as New Zealand) led to convictions for manslaughter against the doctors involved. This situation has now been changed so that only serious breaches of professional conduct (involving criminal negligence, sexual moles-tation, rape, or fraud) are subject to criminal prosecution.

The most worrying area for doctors is where a statute exists, for instance concerning the hastening of death, and the doctor becomes concerned about whether certain actions, such as prescribing large doses of pain-relieving drugs for a dying person, might be seen in a criminal light. In general, there are several ethical tests the doctor can apply to his or her actions, and they tend to reflect what a court would decide.

1   Is what is being contemplated a decision that falls within reasonable clinical practice? The best way of determining this is to consult another doctor for an independent opinion.
2   Does the decision, for instance, about withdrawing life-sustaining treatment, reflect, as far as can be ascertained, what the patient wants or would have wanted? This is best determined either directly through consultation with the patient or by discussing the patient's attitudes, values, and opinions rele-vant to such matters with his or her obvious 'kin' (these are the people who would be regarded as most closely in touch with the patient's wishes and are not necessarily legal relations).
3   Is the decision being made one that would probably be in accordance with the wishes of a reasonable person placed in the patient's situation?

Practitioners who can satisfy themselves on these points are likely to make decisions that would now be upheld in most jurisdictions, provided the act is not one that falls under a specific legal or professional prohibition, such as active voluntary euthanasia. In each case, as we have suggested in the section concern-ing ethics and the law, a course of action that meets with agreement from both the professionals concerned and patients or their representatives is not likely to be challenged by the courts. If the practitioner is genuinely concerned, he or she should consult a criminal lawyer well versed in the common law that has emerged in the relevant jurisdictions.

Civil Disputes

In a number of jurisdictions, disputes between doctors and patients are the sub-ject of civil damages cases. In others, New Zealand and Sweden for instance, there is a separate arrangement to compensate patients for the results of medical misadventure. The ethical comparison between these two systems is interesting.

It is clear that there are two requirements in the general area of harm to a patient caused by a health care professional. First, there is the requirement to compensate the sufferer for the injury he or she has suffered. Second, there is the requirement to guard against bad practice. Civil damages suits are supposed to do both; in fact, they do neither. Consider the following cases.

Mr Q was admitted for an operation to correct a disc prolapse in his neck causing pain in his arm and headaches. During the operation there was a serious complication, which caused damage to his spinal cord. He emerged partially paralysed down one side of his body and incontinent of urine. He made a complaint against his surgeon not because of the complication but because of the fact that he had not been warned that such a thing might happen, and would not have agreed had he known of the risk.

Ms R was admitted for bilateral tubal ligations as a means of sterilisation. After the operation she began to experience severe aching pain in her back and side. On investigation she was found to have a seriously swollen kidney on the right due to the ureter, the draining tube of the kidney, having been tied off during the procedure. Another operation was done but the kidney damage could not be reversed and caused ongoing health problems, whereas she had previously been healthy and active. Ms R also took legal action against her surgeon.

If a person is seriously or even slightly harmed by a procedure performed by a doctor, there are two possibilities: the doctor was, or was not, at fault. In the first case you may or may not be able to prove the fault and the fact that it was this (rather than an unfortunate combination of events) that caused the harm. In the case of Mr Q, a successful suit would depend on a court deciding that the doctor had indeed omitted the relevant information when Mr Q's consent was obtained, and that the omission had led to Mr Q's agreeing to the procedure when he would not have exposed himself to the risk had he known of it. In the case of Ms R, the consent may also be at fault and form part of her claim, but she is also claiming that the operation was done badly or negligently and caused her kidney damage and subsequent problems. This sounds good and fair but we should look carefully at the consequences of the possible findings in such cases.

If a patient does prove that a doctor is at fault, the claim will be settled by the doctor's professional insurance. If fault is not proven, the patient gets nothing. In either case, a great deal of strife for both doctor and patient is caused by the worry and strain of what are often protracted court proceedings with a highly adversarial atmosphere. Thus, the patient and the doctor must both go through a stressful process, the patient may or may not be compensated for his or her injury, and the doctor will not be punished either way because the burden of payment will be shared by all doctors.

But the rising costs of awards will increase the amount paid by all doctors for their professional practice insurance. They will, of course, pass this cost on to their patients. Thus, it is ultimately patients, and the health care system in general, that gets punished by civil damages claims against doctors. The only winners are those who are paid to keep the system going.

The alternative is to pay sufferers damages based on their injury and its severity rather than on the fault of the doctor concerned. This satisfies one of the two aims of the system, but by itself does nothing to address the other. Thus, there must be some just and impartial way to punish bad doctors. One way is to have the compensating body refer any claims they believe to involve negligence or incompetence to a separate body competent to make a judgment about the doctor's practice. If the judgment is unfavourable, direct punishments in terms of limitations on the doctor's practice might be imposed. These may involve any of the penalties mentioned in our discussion of professional discipline and regulation. The important point here is that these are real punishments on the individual practitioner concerned and not ones that can be diffused across the system and passed on to patients.

Both systems have their advocates, and the way in which the problems in this area are resolved is going to have far-reaching implications for the ethics of the profession and health system costs in the future.

Conclusion

The relationship between ethics and law is complex in two ways. First, there are various mechanisms according to which doctors may be dealt with by the law. These include professional regulation and discipline, criminal law, and civil law. The first of these is a kind of in-house or intraprofessional law. Where this is strongly and impartially administered, it has the capacity to impose real penalties on bad practitioners. There is also criminal justice, which is reserved for behaviour that amounts to gross negligence or outrageously bad practice. Alternatively, there is civil litigation, which is limited in some countries by no-fault compensation provisions. This system is expensive and ultimately ineffective in imposing real penalties on bad practitioners. In countries where there is a publicly funded compensation scheme the same considerations apply to exemplary damages as to other suits for damages.

The second complication arises from the intricate relationship between statute law or legislation and common law. Statutes consist of written laws that are interpreted by courts, which determine their applicability and significance in a range of circumstances. This means that a literal reading of a statute can be misleading about the legality or illegality of a given clinical decision.

It emerges from this chapter that the statement to or by a health care professional that this or that practice is 'illegal' is quite unclear and often hopelessly confused. It should always be carefully considered in terms of the type of law involved and with due regard to the qualifications and exemptions that may or may not make the law in question applicable to the situation under discussion.

References

Almond, B. (1990) 'Personal issues and personal dilemmas' in B. Almond (ed.), *AIDS: A Moral Issue*, 2nd edn, Macmillan, London.

American Psychiatric Association (1994) *Diagnostic and Statistical Manual of Mental Disorders*, Washington, DC.

Andersen, J. (1994) 'A time to remember: annual convocation of thanks' *Mayo Today* June/July, p. 13.

Angell, M. (1997) 'The ethics of clinical research in the third world' *New England Journal of Medicine* 337, pp. 847–9.

Annas, G. J. (1993) *Standard of Care: the Law of American Bioethics*, Oxford University Press, New York.

—— (1998) 'The Prospect of Human Cloning' in J. M. Humber & R. F. Almeder (eds), *Human Cloning*, Humana Press, pp. 53–63.

Anscombe, E. (1981) *Ethics, Religion and Politics*, Blackwells, Oxford.

Australian Academy of Science (1999) *A Position Statement on Human Cloning*, Canberra.

Bagasao, M. (1995) 'HIV/AIDS in Asia: editorial comment' *Venereology* 8, pp. 136–40.

Bahro, M., Silber, E. & Sunderland, T. (1995) 'How do patients with Alzheimer's disease cope with their illness? A clinical experience report' *Journal of the American Geriatrics Society* 43, pp. 41–6.

Bailey, L. L., Nehlsen-Cannarella, S. L., Concepcion, W. & Jolley, W. B. (1985) 'Baboon-to-human cardiac xenotransplantation in a neonate' *Journal of the American Medical Association* 254, pp. 3321–9.

Bancroft, J. (1981) 'Ethical aspects of sexuality and sex therapy' in S. Bloch, P. Chodoff & S. Green (eds), *Psychiatric Ethics*, Oxford University Press, Oxford, pp. 160–84.

Barraclough, B., Bunch, L., Nelson, B. & Sainsbury, P. (1974) 'A hundred cases of suicide: clinical aspects' *British Journal of Psychiatry* 125, pp. 355–73.

Bartlett, E. T. & Youngner, S. J. (1988) 'Human death and the destruction of the neo-cortex' in R. M. Zaner (ed.), *Death: Beyond Whole-Brain Criteria*, Reidel Publishing Company, Dordrecht, pp. 199–215.

Bauby, J.-D. (1997) *The Diving Bell and the Butterfly*, Fourth Estate Limited, London.

Bayley, A. (2000) 'Commentary: narrowing the gap' *Journal of Medical Ethics* 26, pp. 51–3.

Bayley, J. (1998) *Iris: a Memoir of Iris Murdoch*, Duckworth, London.

Beauchamp, T. & Childress, J. (1989) *Principles of Biomedical Ethics*, Oxford University Press, New York, pp. 141–7.

Beauchamp, T. & Walters, L. (1989) *Contemporary Bioethics*, Wadsworth Publishing Company, Belmont, California.

Beecher, H. K. (1970) *Research and the Individual*, Little, Brown, Boston.

Benfield, D. G., Flaksman, R. J., Lin, T-H., Kantak, A. D., Kokomoor, F. W. & Vollman, J. H. (1991) 'Teaching intubation skills using newly deceased infants' *Journal of the American Medical Association* 265, pp. 2360–3.

Berkowitz, J. (1995) 'Mummy was a fetus: motherhood and fetal ovarian transplantation' *Journal of Medical Ethics* 21, pp. 298–304.

Bernat, J. L. (1998) 'A defense of the whole-brain concept of death' *Hastings Center Report* 28, pp. 14–23.

Bertman, S. L. & Marks, S. C. (1989) 'Experiences with learning about death and dying in the undergraduate anatomy curriculum' *Journal of Medical Education* 55, pp. 48–52.

Bluml, S., Kopyov, O., Jacques, S. & Ross, B. D. (1999) 'Activation of neurotransplants in humans' *Experimental Neurology* 158, pp. 121–5.

Boddington, P. (1996) 'Organ donation and ethics—could Australia accept the Spanish model of organ donation?' *Monash Bioethics Review* 15, pp. 33–43.

Bok, S. (1980) *Lying: Moral Choice in Public and Private Life*, Quartet, London.

Boklage, C. E. (1990) 'Survival probability of human conceptions from fertilization to term' *International Journal of Fertilization* 35, pp. 75–94.

Boone, A. K. (1988) 'Bad axioms in genetic engineering' *Hastings Center Report* 18, pp. 9–13.

Boozang, K. (1998) 'Western medicine opens the door to alternative medicine' *American Journal of Law and Medicine* XXIV, pp. 185–212.

Botega, N. J., Metze, K., Marques, E., Cruvinel, A., Moraes, Z. V., Augusto, L. & Costa, L. A. (1997) 'Attitudes of medical students to necropsy' *Journal of Clinical Pathology* 50, pp. 64–6.

Brams, M. (1977) 'Transplantable human organs: should their sales be authorized by state statutes?' *American Journal of Law and Medicine* 3, pp. 183–95.

Bray, T. L. & Killion, T. W. (1994) *Reckoning with the Dead: The Larsen Bay Repatriation and the Smithsonian Institute*, Smithsonian Institution, Washington, DC.

British Medical Association (1988) *Euthanasia*, BMA, London.

—— (1999) *Euthanasia*, BMA, London.

Brown, H. G. (1984) 'Lay perceptions of autopsy' *Archives of Pathology and Laboratory Medicine* 108, pp. 446–8.

Brown, J., Henteleff, P., Rarakat, S. & Rowe, C. (1986) 'Is it normal for terminally ill patients to desire death?' *American Journal of Psychiatry* 143, pp. 208–11.

Burns, J. P., Reardon, F. E. & Truog, R. D. (1994) 'Using newly deceased patients to teach resucitation procedures' *New England Journal of Medicine* 331, pp. 1652–5.

Butler, D. & Gershon, D. (1994) 'Breast cancer discovery sparks new debate on patenting human genes' *Nature* 371, pp. 271–2.

California Supreme Court (1976) *Tarasoff versus Regents of the University of California* Report 14, 551 P 2d 347.

Callahan, D. (1987) *Setting Limits: Medical Goals in an Aging Society*, Touchstone, New York, pp. 141–52.

—— (1992) 'Dementia and appropriate care: allocating scarce resources' in R. H. Binstock, S. G. Post & P. J. Whitehouse (eds), *Dementia and Aging: Ethics, Values and Policy Choices*, The John Hopkins University Press, Baltimore, pp. 141–52.

Campbell, A. (1984) *Moderated Love: A Theology of Professional Care*, SPCK, London.

—— (1987) 'The hospital ethics committee' *Hospital Therapeutics* August, pp. 5–7.

—— (1995) *Health as Liberation*, Pilgrim Press, Philadelphia.

—— (1998) 'The "ethics of care" as virtue ethics' in M. Evans (ed.), *Advances in Bioethics* vol. 4, Jai Press, Stamford.

Caplan, A. L. (1984) 'Organ procurement: it's not on the cards' *Hastings Center Report* 14 (5), pp. 9–12.

—— (1987) 'Should fetuses or infants be utilized as organ donors?' *Bioethics* 1, pp. 119–40.

—— (1992) 'Is xenografting morally wrong?' *Transplantation Proceedings* 24, pp. 722–7.

Carter, A. H. (1997) *First Cut: A Season in the Human Anatomy Lab*, Picador, New York.

Central Office of Information (2000) *Bristol Royal Infirmary Enquiry*, London.

Charlesworth, M. (1993) *Bioethics in a Liberal Society*, Cambridge University Press, Melbourne.

Charlton, R., Dovey, S. M., Jones, D. G. & Blunt, A. (1994) 'The effects of cadaver dissection on the social attitudes of medical undergraduates' *Medical Education* 28, pp. 290–5.

Clark, M. (1999) 'This little piggy went to market: the xenotransplantation and xeno-zoonose debate' *Journal of Law Medicine and Ethics* 27, pp. 137–52.

Cochrane, A. (1972) *Effectiveness and Efficacy*, Nuffield Provincial Trusts Hospital, London.

Cochrane, J. (2000) 'Narrowing the gap: access to HIV treatments in developing countries' *Journal of Medical Ethics* 26, pp. 47–50.

Cole, D. (1987) *Medical Practice and Professional Conduct in New Zealand*, Roydhouse, Carterton.

Collins, D. (1992) *Medical Law in New Zealand*, Brooker & Friend, Wellington.

Cooper, Dame Whina (27 April 1987) Deposition in the Court of Appeal of New Zealand, Court of Appeal, Auckland.

Coulehan, J. L., Williams, P. C., Landis, D. & Naser, C. (1995) 'The first patient: reflections and stories about the anatomy cadaver' *Teaching and Learning in Medicine* 7, pp. 61–6.

Council for Ethical and Judicial Affairs (1994) 'Strategies for cadaveric organ procurement: mandated choice and presumed consent' *Journal of the American Medical Association* 10, pp. 809–12.

Council of Europe (1995) 'Recommendation No. R (94) 11 of the Committee of Ministers to Member States on Screening as a Tool of Preventive Medicine' *International Digest of Health Legislation* 46, pp. 13–18.

Council of Europe (1996) 'Convention for the Protection of Human Rights and Dignity with regard to the Application of Biology and Medicine', Strasbourg.

Coxon, A. (1990) 'Coping with the threat of death' in B. Almond (ed.), *AIDS: A Moral Issue*, 2nd edn, Macmillan, London.

Culver, K. W. (1993) 'Splice of life: genetic therapy comes of age' *The Sciences* January/February, pp. 18–24.

Daniels, N. (1985) *Just Health Care*, Cambridge University Press, Cambridge.

Dansey, H. (1975) 'A view of death' in M. King (ed.), *Te Ao Huruhuri: The World Moves On: Aspects of Maoritanga*, Hicks Smith, Wellington.

Davis, R. (1989) *My Journey into Alzheimer's Disease*, Tyndale House, Illinois.

Department of Health (1999) *Clinical Governance: Quality in the New NHS* (Health Circular HSC 1999/065), Department of Health, London.

—— (2000) *Stem Cell Research: Medical Progress with Responsibility*, Department of Health, London.

Deuchar, N. (1984) 'AIDS in New York City' *British Journal of Psychiatry* 145, pp. 612–19.

Dracopoulou, S. & Doxiadis, S. (1988) 'In Greece, lament for the dead, denial for the dying' *Hastings Center Report* 18 (4), pp. 15–16.

Editorial (1999) 'Xenotransplantation; time to leave the laboratory' *Lancet* 354, p. 1657.

ELSI Task Force on Genetic Testing (1997) 'Proposed recommendations of the task force on genetic testing' *Federal Register* 62, pp. 4539–47.

Emson, H. E. (1992) 'Notes on necropsy' *Journal of Clinical Pathology* 45, pp. 85–6.

Engelhardt, H. T. (1986) *The Foundations of Bioethics*, Oxford University Press, New York.

Evans, E. J. & Fitzgibbon, G. H. (1992) 'The dissecting room: reactions of first year medical students' *Clinical Anatomy* 5, pp. 311–20.

Evans, R. W. & Manninen, D. L. (1988) 'US public opinion concerning the procurement and distribution of donor organs' *Transplantation Proceedings* 20, pp. 781–5.

Ewing, T. (1990) 'Emphasis on "Aborigine rights"' *Nature* 344, p. 697.

Feinberg, J. (1985) 'The mistreatment of dead bodies' *Hastings Center Report* 15 (2), pp. 31–7.

Finkelstein, P. & Mathers, L. (1990) 'Post-traumatic stress among medical students in the anatomy dissection laboratory' *Clinical Anatomy* 3, pp. 219–26.

Formenty, P., Hatz, C., Le Guenno, B., Stoll, A., Rogenmoser, P. & Widmer, A. (1999) 'Human infection due to Ebola virus, subtype Côte d'Ivoire: clinical and biologic presentation' *Journal of Infectious Diseases* 179, pp. S. 48–53.

Foucault, M. (1981) *Power/Knowledge: Selected Interviews and Other Writings, 1972–1977*, Harvester, Brighton.

—— (1987) *Mental Illness and Psychology*, University of California Press, Berkeley.

Frame, J. (1982) *Faces in the Water*, Braziller, USA.

Gabbard, G. (1999) 'Boundary violations' in *Psychiatric Ethics*, S. Bloch, P. Chodoff & S. Green (eds), Oxford University Press, Oxford, pp. 141–60.

Gaylin, W. (1974) 'Harvesting the dead' *Harper's Magazine* September, pp. 23–30.

Gbadgesun, S. (1994) 'An African concept of health and disease' in J. McMillan (ed.), *Proceedings of the International Seminar on Bioethics*, Otago Bioethics Centre, Dunedin, pp. 64–8.

Gearhart, J. (1999) 'New Potential for Human Embryonic Stem Cells' *Science* 282, pp. 1061–2.

General Medical Council of Britain (1988) 'Advice on testing for HIV infection' *Lancet* 20 August, p. 465.

—— (1993) *HIV Infection and AIDS: The Ethical Considerations*, GMC, London.

—— (1999) *Seeking Patients' Consent: The Ethical Considerations*, GMC, London.

—— (2000) *Confidentiality: Protecting and Providing Information*, GMC, London.

Gethin Morgan, H., Burns-Cox, C., Pocock, H. & Pottle, S. (1975) 'Deliberate self-harm: clinical and socio-economic characteristics of 368 patients' *British Journal of Psychiatry* 127, pp. 564–74.

Gillam, L. (1989) 'Fetal tissue transplantation: a philosophical approach' in L. Gillam (ed.), *Proceedings of the Conference: The Fetus as Tissue Donor: Use or Abuse?*, Monash University Press, Melbourne, pp. 60–9.

Gillett, G. (1986) 'Why let people die?' *Journal of Medical Ethics* 12, pp. 83–6.

—— (1987) 'Reply to J. M. Stanley: fiddling and clarity' *Journal of Medical Ethics* 13, pp. 23–5.

—— (1989) 'HIV and the epidemiologist' *Lancet* 19 November, pp. 1228.

—— (1990) 'Consciousness, the brain and what matters' *Bioethics* 4, pp. 181–98.

—— (1996) 'AIDS and confidentialty: the doctor's dilemma in AIDS' in B. Almond (ed.), *AIDS: A Moral Issue*, 2nd edn, Macmillan, London.

—— (1999) *The Mind and its Discontents*, Oxford University Press, Oxford.

—— (2000) 'Ethics and images in organ transplantation' in A. Trzepacz & A. Dimartini (eds), *The Transplant Patient*, Cambridge University Press, Cambridge, pp. 239–54.

Gillett, G., Goddard, L. & Webb, M. (1995) 'The case of Mr L: a legal and ethical response to the court sanctioned withdrawal of life support' *Journal of Law and Medicine* 3, pp. 49–59.

Gillon, R. (1995) 'On giving preference to prior volunteers when allocating organs for transplantation' *Journal of Medical Ethics* 21, pp. 195–6.

Ginifer, C. & Kelly, A-M. (1996) 'Teaching resuscitation skills using the newly deceased' *Medical Journal of Australia* 165, pp. 445–7.

Glover, J. (1977) *Causing Death and Saving Lives*, Penguin, Harmondsworth.

Gormally, L. (1994) 'Against voluntary euthanasia' in R. Gillon (ed.), *Principles of Health Care Ehics*, Wiley, Chichester, pp. 763–73.

Griffiths, J. (1995) 'Assisted suicide in the Netherlands: the Chabot case' *Modern Law Review* March, pp. 232–48.

Grigg, M. M., Kelly, M. K., Celesia, G. G., Ghobrial, M. W. & Ross, E. R. (1987) 'Electroencephalographic activity after brain death' *Archives of Neurology* 44, pp. 948–54.

Gustavson, N. (1988) 'The effect of human dissection on first-year students and implications for the doctor–patient relationship' *Journal of Medical Education* 63, pp. 62–4.

Hacking, I. (1995) *Rewriting the Soul: Multiple Personality and the Sciences of Memory*, Princeton University Press, Princeton.

Hafferty, F. W. (1991) *Into the Valley: Death and the Socialization of Medical Students*, Yale University Press, New Haven.

Hahnemann, S. (1993) *Organon of Medicine* (tr. W. Boericke), B. Jain, New Delhi.

Hamblin, J. (1994) 'HIV in the developing world: lessons for health care in Australia' *National Bioethics Conference Proceedings*, Christian Centre for Bioethics, Sydney.

Hampton, J. (1983) 'The end of clinical freedom' *British Medical Journal: Clinical Research Edition* 287, pp. 1237–8.

Hare, R. (1991) 'The philosophical basis of psychiatric ethics' in S. Bloch, P. Chodoff & S. Green (eds), *Psychiatric Ethics*, Oxford University Press, Oxford, pp. 34–46.

Harris, J. (1987) 'QALYfing the value of life' *Journal of Medical Ethics* 13, pp. 117–23.

Harrison, M. R. (1986a) 'Organ procurement for children: the anencephalic fetus as donor' *Lancet* 2, pp. 1383–6.

—— (1986b) 'The anencephalic newborn as organ donor' *Hastings Center Report* 16 (2), pp. 21–3.

Heyd, D. & Bloch, S. (1991) 'The ethics of suicide' in S. Bloch, P. Chodoff & S. Green (eds), *Psychiatric Ethics*, Oxford University Press, Oxford, pp. 243–64.

Higgs, R. (1985) 'On telling patients the truth' in M. Lockwood (ed.), *Moral Dilemmas in Modern Medicine*, Oxford University Press, Oxford, pp. 187–202.

Hoffmaster, B. (1994) 'The forms and limits of medical ethics' *Social Science and Medicine* 39, pp. 1155–64.

Holden, W. (1994) *Unlawful Carnal Knowledge: The True Story of the Irish 'X' Case*, Harper Collins, London.

Holland, A. (1990) 'A fortnight of my life is missing: a discussion of the status of the pre-embryo' *Journal of Applied Philosophy* 7, pp. 25–37.

Holtug, N. (1995) 'Patents on human genes: is there a moral problem?' *Monash Bioethics Review* 14, pp. 26–35.

Honore, T. (1993) 'The dependence of morality on law' *Oxford Journal of Legal Studies* 13, pp. 1–16.

Human Fertilisation and Embryology Authority (1995) *Fourth Annual Report*, HFEA, London.

—— (1999) *Eighth Annual Report and Accounts*, HFEA, London.

Human Fertilisation and Embryology Authority & The Human Genetics Advisory Committee (1998) *Cloning Issues in Reproduction, Science and Medicine*, Her Majesty's Stationery Office, London.

Huxtable, R. (2000) 'Re M (medical treatment: consent) time to remove the "flak jacket"?' *Child and Family Law Quarterly* 12, pp. 83–8.

Iglesias, T. (1984) '*In vitro* fertilization: the major issues' *Journal of Medical Ethics* 10, pp. 32–7.

Illich, I. (1977 edn) *Limits to Medicine*, Penguin, Harmondsworth.

Iserson, K. V. (1993) 'Postmortem procedures in the emergency department: using the recently dead to practise and teach' *Journal of Medical Ethics* 19, pp. 92–8.

James, P. D. (1992) *The Children of Men*, Faber & Faber, London.

Jonas, H. (1992) 'The burden and blessing of mortality' *Hastings Center Report* 22 (1), pp. 34–40.

Jones, D. G. (1987) *Manufacturing Humans*, Inter-Varsity Press, Leicester.

—— (1989) 'Brain birth and personal identity' *Journal of Medical Ethics* 15, pp. 173–8.

—— (1994) 'Use of bequeathed and unclaimed bodies in the dissecting room' *Clinical Anatomy* 7, pp. 102–7.

—— (2000) *Speaking for the Dead: Cadavers in Biology and Medicine*, Ashgate Publishing Limited, Aldershot.

Jones, D. G. & Fennell, S. (1991) 'Bequests, cadavers and dissections: sketches from New Zealand history' *New Zealand Medical Journal* 104, pp. 210–12.

Jones, D. G. & Harris, R. J. (1998) 'Archeological human remains: scientific, cultural and ethical considerations' *Current Anthropology* 39, pp. 253–64.

Jones, D. & Sagee, S. (2001) 'Xenotransplantation: hope or delusion? *Biologist*, 48, pp. 129–32.

Jones, D. G. & Telfer, B. (1995) 'Before I was an embryo, I was a pre-embryo: or was I?' *Bioethics* 9, pp. 32–49.

Kant, I. (1785) *Fundamental Principles of the Metaphysic of Morals*, Liberal Arts Press, New York, 1949.

—— (1963 edn) *Lectures on Ethics*, trans. L. Infield, Harper & Row, New York.

Karasu, Y. (1981) 'Ethical aspects of psychotherapy' in S. Bloch, P. Chodoff & S. Green (eds), *Psychiatric Ethics*, Oxford University Press, Oxford, pp. 135–66.

Kass, L. R. (1985a) 'Thinking about the body' *Hastings Center Report* 15, pp. 20–30.

—— (1985b) *Toward a More Natural Science: Biology and Human Affairs*, Free Press, New York.

Kawashima, H. (1988) 'Commentary' *Hastings Center Report* 18 (4), pp. 27–8.

Kennedy, I. (1988) *Treat Me Right*, Clarendon Press, Oxford.

Keown, J. (1992) 'The law and practice of euthanasia in the Netherlands' *Law Quarterly Review* 108, pp. 51–78.

Kesey, K. (1962) *One Flew Over the Cuckoo's Nest*, Viking Penguin, New York.

Kirby, M. (1989) 'Legal implications of AIDS' in R. Paterson (ed.), *Legal Implications of AIDS*, Legal Research Foundation, Auckland.

Kleinig, J. (1985) *Ethical Issues in Psychosurgery*, George Allen & Unwin, London.

Kocan, P. (1980) *The Treatment and the Cure*, Angus & Robertson, North Ryde, NSW.

Kopelman, L. (1994) 'Female circumcision/genital mutilation and ethical relativism' *Second Opinion* 20, pp. 55–71.

Kubler-Ross, E. (1969) *On Death and Dying*, Macmillan, New York.

Laing, R. (1965) *The Divided Self*, Penguin, Harmondsworth.

Lamb, D. (1985) *Death, Brain Death and Ethics*, Croom Helm, London.

Langarek, E. A. (1979) 'Abortion: listening to the middle' *Hastings Center Report* 9 (5), pp. 24–8.

Leenen, H. (1987) 'Euthanasia, assistance to suicide and the law: developments in the Netherlands' *Health Policy* 8, pp. 197–206.

Levitt, M. (1995) 'Ethics of genetic screening: a new report on genetic screening in the Netherlands' *Euroscreen* 3, pp. 1–5.

Llano-Escobar, A. (1988) 'In Colombia, dealing with death and technology' *Hastings Center Report* 18 (4), pp. 23–4.

Lloyd, G. E. R. (ed.) (1978) *Hippocratic Writings*, Penguin, Harmondsworth.

Lundberg, G. D. (1984) 'Medicine without the autopsy' *Archives of Pathology and Laboratory Medicine* 108, pp. 449–54.

Lurie, P. & Wolfe, S. (1997) 'Unethical trials of interventions to reduce perinatal transmission of the human immunodeficiency virus in developing countries' *New England Journal of Medicine* 337, pp. 853–6.

Marcus, R. & the CDC Cooperative Needlestick Surveillance Group (1988) 'Surveillance of health care workers exposed to blood from patients with the human immunodeficiency virus' *New England Journal of Medicine* 319, pp. 1118–23.

Martin, R. J. & Post, S. G. (1992) 'Human dignity, dementia, and the moral basis of caregiving' in R. H. Binstock, S. G. Post & P. J. Whitehouse (eds), *Dementia and Aging: Ethics, Values, and Policy Choices*, The Johns Hopkins University Press, Baltimore, pp. 55–68.

Marwick, C. (1995) 'Pathologists request autopsy revival' *Journal of the American Medical Association* 273, pp. 1889–91.

Maxwell, R. (1974) *Health Care: The Growing Dilemma*, McKinsey & Co., New York.

May, W. F. (1983) *Physician's Covenant: Images of the Healer in Medical Ethics*, Westminster Press, Philadelphia.

—— (1985) 'Religious justification for donating body parts' *Hastings Center Report* 15 (2), pp. 38–42.

McCullagh, P. (1993) *Brain Dead, Brain Absent, Brain Donors: Human Subjects or Human Objects?*, John Wiley & Sons, Chichester.

McGarry, L. & Chodoff, P. (1981) 'The ethics of involuntary hospitalisation' in S. Bloch, P. Chodoff & S. Green (eds), *Psychiatric Ethics*, Oxford University Press, Oxford, p. 217.

McLaren, A. (1984) 'Where to draw the line?' *Proceedings of the Royal Institution of Great Britain* 56, pp. 101–21.

—— (1986) 'Embryo research' *Nature* 320, p. 570.

McMahan, J. (1995) 'The metaphysics of brain death' *Bioethics*, 9, pp. 91–126.

McNeill, P. (1993) *The Ethics and Politics of Human Experimentation*, Cambridge University Press, Cambridge.

Meighan, C. W. (1993) 'The burial of American archeology' *Academic Questions* 6, pp. 9–19.

Micale, M. & Porter, R. (1994) *Discovering the History of Psychiatry*, Oxford University Press, Oxford.

Mirkin, B. (1995) 'AIDS clinical trials: why they have recruiting problems' *AIDS Treatment News* 217, pp. 1–4.

Monaghan, D. (1991) 'The body-snatchers' *Bulletin* 12 November, pp. 30–8.

Moody, H. R. (1992) 'A critical view of ethical dilemmas in dementia' in R. H. Binstock, S. G. Post & P. J. Whitehouse (eds), *Dementia and Aging: Ethics, Values, and Policy Choices*, The Johns Hopkins University Press, Baltimore, pp. 86–100.

Moussa, M. & Shannon, T. A. (1992) 'The search for the new pineal gland: brain life and personhood' *Hastings Center Report* 22 (2), pp. 30–7.

Mulhern, S. (1994) 'Satanism, ritual abuse, and multiple personality disorder: a sociohistorical perspective' *International Journal of Clinical and Experimental Hypnosis* 42, pp. 265–88.

Multi-Society Task Force on PVS (1994) 'Medical aspects of the persistent vegetative state I' *New England Journal of Medicine* 330, pp. 1499–508.

Murphy, G. (1973) 'Suicide and the right to die' *American Journal of Psychiatry* 130, pp. 472–3.

Nairne, P. (1996) *Animal to Human Transplants: The Ethics of Xenotransplantation*, Nuffield Council on Bioethics, London.

National Commission for the Protection of Human Subjects of Biomedical and Behavioral Research (1975) *Research on the Fetus*, Department of Health, Education and Welfare, Washington, DC.

National Health and Medical Research Council (1984) 'Ethics in medical research involving the human fetus and human fetal tissue' *Medical Journal of Australia* 140, pp. 610–20.

—— (1991) *Guidelines on Ethical Matters in Aboriginal and Torres Straits Islander Health Research*, Canberra.

National Institute of Health (1985) 'Recombinant DNA research: request for public comment on 'Points to Consider in the Design and Submission of Somatic Cell Gene Therapy Protocols' *Federal Regulation* 50, pp. 2940–5.

National Medical Council of New Zealand (1990) '*A Statement for the Medical Profession on Information and Consent*', Wellington.

Nelson, J. (1992) *The Rights and Responsibilities of Potential Organ Donors: A Communitarian Approach*, The Communitarian Network, Washington, DC.

Newkirk, I. (1986) 'Who will live, who will die?' Quoted in K. McCabe *Washingtonian Magazine* August, p. 115.

Newton-Smith, W. (1981) *The Rationality of Science*, Routledge, London.

Nnodim, J. O. (1996) 'Preclinical student reactions to dissection, death and dying' *Clinical Anatomy* 9, pp. 175–82.

Nowell Smith, P. (1989) 'Euthanasia and the doctors' *Journal of Medical Ethics* 15, pp. 124–8.

Nuffield Council on Bioethics (1993) *Genetic Screening: Ethical Issues*, Nuffield Council, London.

—— (1995) *Human Tissue: Ethical and Legal Issues*, Nuffield Council, London.

—— (1996) *Animal to Human Transplants: The Ethics of Xenotransplantation*, Nuffield Council, London.

—— (2000) *Stem Cell Therapy: The Ethical Issues*, Nuffield Council, London.

Nussbaum, M. (1993) 'Non-relative virtues: an Aristotelian approach' in M. Nussbaum & A. Sen (eds), *The Quality of Life*, Clarendon Press, Oxford, pp. 243–76.

Oakley, J. (1992) 'Basic ethical principles in aged care' in L. Gillam (ed), *Frail, Elderly— Fairly Treated? Meeting the Ethical Challenges of Aged Care*, Monash University Centre for Human Bioethics, Clayton, Victoria, pp. 19–27.

Ofosu-Amaah, S. (1982) 'Ethical aspects of externally sponsored research in developing countries: an African viewpoint' *Human Experimentation and Medical Ethics*, CIOMS.

Omine, A. (1991) 'Right and wrong in the brain-death debate' *Japan Echo* 18, pp. 68–71.

Orlowski, J. P., Kanoti, G. A. & Mehlman, M. J. (1990) 'The ethical dilemma of permitting the teaching and perfecting of resuscitation techniques on recently expired patients' *Journal of Clinical Ethics* 1, pp. 201–5.

Otago Bioethics Research Centre (1991) *Biotechnology Revisited: Report to the Medical Council of New Zealand*, Wellington.

Pallis, C. (1983) *ABC of Brain Stem Death*, The Devonshire Press, Torquay.

Pappworth, M. H. (1967) *Human Guinea Pigs: Experimentation on Man*, Routledge & Kegan Paul, London.

Paradis, K., Langford, G., Long, Z., Heneine, W., Sandstrom, P., Switzer, W., Chapman, L., Lockey, C., Onions, D. & Otto, E. (1999) 'No evidence of pig DNA or retroviral infection in patients with short-term extracorporeal connection to pig kidneys' *Lancet* 352, pp. 699–701.

Peart, N. & Gillett, G. (1998) 'A life worth living' *Journal of Law and Medicine* 5, pp. 239–51.

Peel Committee Report (1972) *The Use of Fetuses and Fetal Material in Research*, Her Majesty's Stationery Office, London.

Pellegrino, E. D. (1991) 'Families self-interest and the cadaver's organs: what price consent?' *Journal of the American Medical Association* 265, pp. 1305–6.

Pellegrino, E. D. & Thomasma, D. (1981) *A Philosophical Basis of Medical Practice*, Oxford University Press, Oxford.

—— (1988) *For the Patient's Good*, Oxford University Press, Oxford.

Peters, T. G. (1991) 'Life or death: the issue of payment in cadaveric organ donation' *Journal of the American Medical Association* 265, pp. 1302–5.

Pewhairangi, N. (1992) 'Learning and tapu' in M. King (ed.), *Te Ao Hurhuri: the world moves on: aspects of Maoritanga*, Reed, Auckland, pp. 10–11.

Pietroni, P. (1992) 'Beyond the boundaries: relationships between general practice and complementary therapy' *British Medical Journal* 305, pp. 564–6.

Pinching, A. (1990) 'AIDS: clinical and scientific background' in B. Almond (ed.), *AIDS: A Moral Issue*, 2nd edn, Macmillan, London.

Pinching, A., Higgs, R. & Boyd, K. (2000) 'The impact of AIDS on medical ethics' *Journal of Medical Ethics* 26, pp. 3–8.

Poplawski, N. & Gillett, G. (1991) 'Ethics and embryos' *Journal of Medical Ethics* 17, pp. 62–9.

Popper, K. (1959) *The Logic of Scientific Discovery*, Hutchinson, London.

Post, S. G. (1990) 'Severely demented elderly people: a case against senicide' *Journal of the American Geriatrics Society* 38, pp. 715–18.

—— (1994) 'Genetics, ethics, and Alzheimer's disease' *Journal of the American Geriatrics Society* 42, pp. 782–6.

President's Commission for the Study of Ethical Problems in Medicine and Biomedical and Behavioral Research (1981) *Defining Death: Medical, Legal and Ethical Issues in the Determination of Death*, United States Government Printing Office, Washington, DC.

—— (1983) *Deciding to Forego Life-Sustaining Treatment*, United States Government Printing Office, Washington, DC.

Privacy Commissioner (1994) *Health Information Privacy Code 1994*, Privacy Commissioner, Auckland.

Putnam, F. (1991) 'The satanic ritual abuse controversy' *Child Abuse and Neglect* 15, pp. 95–111.

Rachels, J. (1975) 'Active and passive euthanasia' *New England Journal of Medicine* 292, pp. 78–80.

Rawls, J. (1971) *A Theory of Justice*, Oxford University Press, Oxford.

Reich, W. (1999) 'Psychiatric diagnosis as an ethical problem' in S. Bloch, P. Chodoff & S. Green (eds), *Psychiatric Ethics*, Oxford University Press, Oxford, pp. 193–224.

Resnick, D. (1998) 'The ethics of HIV research in developing nations' *Bioethics* 12, pp. 286–306.

Richardson, R. (1988) *Death, Dissection and the Destitute*, Penguin Books, Harmondsworth.

Rimene, C., Hassan, C. & Broughton, J. (1998) *Ukaipo Te Roopu Rangahau Hauora Maori o Ngai Tahu*, Department of Preventive and Social Medicine, University of Otago, Dunedin.

Rollin, B. (1989) *The Unheeded Cry*, Oxford University Press, Oxford.

Royal College of Paediatrics and Child Health (1997) *Withholding or Withdrawing Life Saving Treatment in Children: A Framework for Practice*, RCPCH, London.

Royal Commission on Social Policy (1988) 'The Treaty of Waitangi and Social Policy', Government Printing Office, Wellington.

Royal Society (1990) *The Case for Human Embryological Research*, Royal Society, London.

Sanner, M. (1994a) 'A comparison of public attitudes toward autopsy, organ donation, and anatomic dissection: a Swedish survey' *Journal of the American Medical Association* 271, pp. 284–8.

—— (1994b) 'Attitudes towards organ donation and transplantation: a model for understanding reactions to medical procedures after death' *Social Science and Medicine* 38, pp. 1141–52.

Saunders, J. (1996) 'Alternative, complementary, holistic . . .' in D. Greaves & H. Upton (eds), *Philosophical Problems in Health Care*, Avebury Press, Aldershot, pp. 103–25.

Schüklenk, U. & Ashcroft, R. (2000) 'International Research Ethics' *Bioethics* 14, pp. 158–72.

Seneca (1920 edn) *Epistua Morales*, Harvard University Press, Cambridge, Massachusetts.

Serour, G. (1994) 'Islam and the four principles' in R. Gillon (ed.), *Principles of Health Care*, Wiley, Chichester, pp. 75–92.

Shamblott, M. J., Axelman, J., Wang, S., Bugg, E. M., Littlefield, J. W., Donovan, P. J., Blumenthal, P. D., Huggins, G. R. & Gearhart, J. D. (1998) 'Derivation of pluripotent stem cells from cultured human primordial germ cells' *Proceedings of the National Academy of Sciences USA* 95, pp. 13726–31.

Sherwin, S. (1996) 'Feminism and bioethics' in S. Wolf (ed.), *Feminism and Bioethics: Beyond Reproduction*, Oxford University Press, New York, pp. 47–66.

Singer, P. (1975) *Animal Liberation*, New York Review/Random House, New York.

—— (1983) 'Sanctity of Life or Quality of Life? *Paediatrics* 72, pp. 272–8.

—— (1992) 'Xenotransplantation and speciesism' *Transplantation Proceedings* 24, pp. 728–32.

Singer, P. & Kuhse, H. (1985) *Should the Baby Live?*, Oxford University Press, Oxford.

Singer, P. & Wells, D. (1984) *The Reproductive Revolution: New Ways of Making Babies*, Oxford University Press, Oxford.

Skegg, P. (1988a) 'The edges of life' *Otago Law Review* 6, pp. 517–32.

—— (1988b) *Law, Ethics and Medicine*, Clarendon Press, Oxford.

—— (1989) 'Heterosexually acquired HIV infection' *British Medical Journal* 298, pp. 401–2.

—— (1995) 'Pain killing drugs and the law of suicide' *Otago Bioethics Report* 4, pp. 8–10.

Skene, L. (1991) 'Mapping the human genome: some thoughts for those who say "there should be a law on it"' *Bioethics* 5, pp. 233–49.

Smith, D. H. (1992) 'Seeing and knowing dementia' in R. H. Binstock, S. G. Post & P. J. Whitehouse (eds), *Dementia and Aging: Ethics, Values, and Policy Choices*, The Johns Hopkins University Press, Baltimore, pp. 44–54.

Smith, T. (1983) 'Alternative medicine' *British Medical Journal* 287, p. 307.

Smithurst, M. (1990) 'AIDS: risk and discrimination' in B. Almond (ed.), *AIDS: A Moral Issue*, 2nd edn, Macmillan, London.

Sommers, C. H. (1985) 'Tooley's immodest proposal' *Hastings Center Report* 15 (3), pp. 39–42.

Steinberg, A. (1994) 'Jewish perspective on the four principles' in R. Gillon (ed.), *Principles of Health Care*, Wiley, Chichester, pp. 65–74.

Stierman, E. D. (1987) 'Emotional aspects of perinatal death' *Clinical Obstetrics and Gynecology* 30, pp. 352–61.

Storr, A. (1970) *Human Aggression*, Penguin Books, Harmondsworth.

Suokas, J. & Lonnqvist, J. (1991) 'Outcome of attempted suicide and psychiatric consultation: risk factors and suicide mortality during a five year follow-up' *Acta Psychiatrica Scandinavica* 84, pp. 545–9.

Szasz, T. (1983) 'Objections to psychiatry' in J. Miller (ed.), *States of Mind*, BBC, London.

Tackaberry, E. & Ganz, P. (1998) 'Xenotransplantation: assessing the unknowns' *Christian Medical Journal Association* 159, pp. 43–5.

Teo, B. (1991) 'Organs for transplantation: the Singapore experience' *Hastings Center Report* 21 (6), pp. 10–13.

—— (1992) 'Is the adoption of more efficient strategies of organ procurement the answer to persistent organ shortage in transplantation?' *Bioethics* 6, pp. 113–29.

Tew, M. (1990) *Safer Childbirth: A Critical History of Maternity Care*, Chapman & Hall, London.

Thomasma, D. C. (1992) 'Mercy killing of elderly people with dementia: a counter-proposal' in R. H. Binstock, S. G. Post & P. J. Whitehouse (eds), *Dementia and Aging: Ethics, Values, and Policy Choices*, The Johns Hopkins University Press, Baltimore, pp. 101–17.

Thomson, J., Itslovitz-Eldor, J., Shapiro, S., Waknitz, M., Swiergiel, J., Marshall, V. & Jones, J. (1998) 'Embryonic stem cell lines derived from human blastocysts' *Science* 282 pp. 1145–7.

Tolstoy, L. (1960 edn) *The Death of Ivan Ilyich*, Penguin Books, Harmondsworth.

Tooley, M. (1983) *Abortion and Infanticide*, Clarendon Press, Oxford.

UNESCO (1997) 'Universal Declaration on the Human Genome and Human Rights'.

Van Tongeren, P. J. M. (1991) 'Ethical manipulations: an ethical evaluation of the debate surrounding genetic engineering' *Human Gene Therapy* 2, pp. 71–5.

Vawter, D. E., Kearney, W., Gervais, K. G., Caplan, A. L., Garry, D. & Tauer, C. (1990) *The Use of Human Fetal Tissue: Scientific, Ethical and Policy Concerns*, University of Minnesota, Minneapolis, Minnesota.

Veatch, R. M. (1981) *A Theory of Medical Ethics*, Basic Books, New York.

—— (1988) 'Whole-brain, neocortical, and higher brain related concepts' in R. M. Zaner (ed.), *Death: Beyond Whole-Brain Criteria*, Reidel Publishing Company, Dordrecht, pp. 171–86.

—— (1993) 'The impending collapse of the whole-brain definition of death' *Hastings Center Report*, 23 (6), pp. 18–24.

Walker, A. (1992) *Possessing the Secret of Joy*, Random House, New York.

Wall, J. (1992) *Compensation and Accountability: Keeping the Balance*, Medical Defence Union, London.

Warren, V. (1992) 'Feminist directions in medical ethics' in H. Bequaert Holmes & L. Purdey (eds), *Feminist Perspectives in Medical Ethics*, Indiana University Press, Bloomington, pp. 32–45.

Weiss, R. A. (1998) 'Xenotransplantation' *British Medical Journal* 317, pp. 931–4.

Wennberg, R. (1985) *Life in the Balance*, Eerdmans, Grand Rapids.

Wertz, D. C., Fanos, J. H. & Reilly, P. R. (1994) 'Genetic testing for children and adolescents: who decides?' *Journal of the American Medical Association* 272, pp. 875–81.

Wilmut, I., Campbell, K. & Tudge, C. (2000) *The Second Creation: the Age of Biological Control by the Scientists Who Cloned Dolly*, Headline Book Publishers, London.

Winch, P. (1958) *The Idea of Social Science and its Relation to Philosophy*, Routledge, London.

Wittgenstein, L. (1922) *Tractatus Logico-Philosophicus*, Routledge, London.

Wolterstorff, N. (1978) *Lament for a Son*, Eerdmans, Grand Rapids.

Wright, S. (1999) 'Human embryonic stem-cell research: science and ethics' *American Scientist*, 87, pp. 352–61.

Appendix

The Hippocratic Oath

I swear by Apollo the healer, invoking all the gods and goddesses to be my witnesses, that I will fulfil this Oath and this written Covenant to the best of my ability and judgment.

I will look upon him who shall have taught me this Art even as one of my parents. I will share my substance with him, and I will supply his necessities, if he be in need. I will regard his offspring even as my own brethren, and I will teach them this Art, if they would learn it, without fee or covenant. I will impart this Art by precept, by lecture and by every mode of teaching, not only to my own sons but to the sons of him who taught me, and to disciples bound by covenant and Oath, according to the Law of Medicine.

The regimen I adopt shall be for the benefit of the patients according to my ability and judgment, and not for their hurt or for any wrong. I will give no deadly drug to any, though it be asked of me, nor will I counsel such, and especially I will not aid a woman to procure abortion. Whatsoever house I enter, there will I go for the benefit of the sick, refraining from all wrongdoing or corruption, and especially from any act of seduction, of male or female, of bond or free. Whatsoever things I see or hear concerning the life of men, in my attendance on the sick or even apart therefrom, which ought not to be noised abroad, I will keep silence thereon, counting such things to be as sacred secrets. Pure and holy will I keep my Life and my Art.

If I fulfil this Oath and confound it not, be it mine to enjoy Life and Art alike, with good repute among all men at all times. If I transgress and violate my oath, may the reverse be my lot.

The Geneva Convention Code of Medical Ethics

This was adopted by the World Medical Association in 1949.

I solemnly pledge myself to consecrate my life to the service of humanity;
I will give to my teachers the respect and gratitude which is their due;
I will practise my profession with conscience and dignity;
The health of my patient will be my first consideration;
I will respect the secrets which are confided in me;
I will maintain by all the means in my power, the honour and the noble traditions of the medical profession;
My colleagues will be my brothers;
I will not permit considerations of religion, nationality, race, party politics or social standing to intervene between my duty and my patient;
I will maintain the utmost respect for human life from the time of conception, even under threat. I will not use my medical knowledge contrary to the laws of humanity;
I make these promises solemnly, freely and upon my honour.

Council for International Organizations of Medical Sciences (CIOMS)

International Guiding Principles for Biomedical Research Involving Animals, June 1984

This is an extract from the document.

1. Basic Principles

I The advancement of biological knowledge and the development of improved means for the protection of the health and well-being both of man and of animals require recourse to experimentation on intact live animals of a wide variety of species.

II Methods such as mathematical models, computer simulation and in vitro biological systems should be used wherever appropriate.

III Animal experiments should be undertaken only after due consideration of their relevance for human or animal health and the advancement of biological knowledge.

IV The animals selected for an experiment should be of an appropriate species and quality, and the minimum number required, to obtain scientifically valid results.

V Investigators and other personnel should never fail to treat animals as sentient, and should regard their proper care and use and the avoidance or minimization of discomfort, distress, or pain as ethical imperatives.

VI Investigators should assume that procedures that would cause pain in human beings cause pain in other vertebrate species although more needs to be known about the perception of pain in animals.

VII Procedures with animals that may cause more than momentary or minimal pain or distress should be performed with appropriate sedation, analgesia, or anaesthesia in accordance with accepted veterinary practice. Surgical or other painful procedures should not be performed on unanesthetized animals paralysed by chemical agents.

VIII Where waivers are required in relation to the provisions of article VII, the decisions should not rest solely with the investigators directly concerned but should be made, with due regard to the provisions of articles IV, V, and VI, by a suitably constituted review body. Such waivers should not be made solely for the purposes of teaching or demonstration.

IX At the end of, or, when appropriate, during an experiment, animals that would otherwise suffer severe or chronic pain, distress, discomfort, or disablement that cannot be relieved should be painlessly killed.

X The best possible living conditions should be maintained for animals kept for biomedical purposes. Normally the care of animals should be under the supervision of veterinarians having experience in laboratory animal science. In any case, veterinary care should be available as required.

XI It is the responsibility of the director of an institute or department using animals to ensure that investigators and personnel have appropriate qualifications or experience for conducting procedures on animals. Adequate opportunities shall be provided for in-service training, including the proper and humane concern for the animals under their care.

World Medical Association Declaration of Helsinki

Ethical principles for medical research involving human subjects. Adopted by the 18th World Medical Assembly, Helsinki, Finland, June 1964 and amended by the 29th World Medical Assembly, Tokyo, Japan, October 1975, 35th World Medical Assembly, Venice, Italy, October 1983, the 41st World Medical Assembly, Hong Kong, September 1989, 48th World Medical Assembly, Somerset West, Republic of South Africa, October 1996, and 52nd World Medical Assembly, Edinburgh, Scotland, October 2000.

A. Introduction

1 The World Medical Association has developed the Declaration of Helsinki as a statement of ethical principles to provide guidance to physicians and other participants in medical research involving human subjects. Material research involving human subjects includes research on identifiable human material or identifiable data.

2 It is the duty of the physician to promote and safeguard the health of the people. The physician's knowledge and conscience are dedicated to the fulfilment of this duty.

3 The Declaration of Geneva of the World Medical Association binds the physician with the words, 'The health of my patient will be my first consideration', and the International Code of Medical Ethics declares that, 'A physician shall act only in the patient's interest when providing medical care which might have the effect of weakening the physical and mental condition of the patient'.

4 Medical progress is based on research which ultimately must rest in part on experimentation involving human subjects.

5 In medical research on human subjects, considerations related to the well-being of the human subject should take precedence over the interests of society.

6 The primary purpose of medical research involving human subjects is to improve prophylactic, diagnostic, and therapeutic procedures and the understanding of the aetiology and pathogenesis of disease. Even the best proven prophylactic, diagnostic, and therapeutic methods must continuously be challenged through research for their effectiveness, efficiency, accessibility and quality.

7 In current medical practice and in medical research, most prophylactic, diagnostic and therapeutic procedures involve risks and burdens.

8 Medical research is subject to ethical standards that promote respect for all beings and protect their health and rights. Some research populations

are vulnerable and need special protection. The particular needs of the economically and medically disadvantaged must be recognised. Special attention is also required for those who cannot give or refuse consent for themselves, for those who may be subject to giving consent under duress, for those who will not benefit personally from the research and for those for whom the research is combined with care.

9   Research investigators should be aware of the ethical, legal and regulatory requirements for research on human subjects in their own countries as well as applicable international requirements. No national ethical, legal or regulatory requirement should be allowed to reduce or eliminate any of the protections for human subjects set forth in this Declaration.

B. Basic Principles for all Medical Research

10 It is the duty of the physician in medical research to protect the life, health, privacy, and dignity of the human subject.

11 Medical research involving human subjects must conform to generally accepted scientific principles, be based on a thorough knowledge of the scientific literature, other relevant sources of information, and on adequate laboratory and, where appropriate, animal experimentation.

12 Appropriate caution must be exercised in the conduct of research which may affect the environment, and the welfare of animals used for research must be respected.

13 The design and performance of each experimental procedure involving human subjects should be clearly formulated in an experimental protocol. The protocol should be submitted for consideration, comment and guidance and where appropriate, approval by a specially appointed ethical review committee, which must be independent of the investigator, the sponsor or any other kind of undue influence. This independent committee should be in conformity with the laws and regulations of the country in which the research experiment is performed. The committee has the right to monitor ongoing trials. The researcher has the obligation to provide monitoring information to the committee, especially any serious adverse events. The researcher should also submit to the committee, for review, information regarding funding, sponsors, institutional affiliations, other potential conflicts of interest and incentives for subjects.

14 The research protocol should always contain a statement of the ethical considerations involved and should indicate that there is compliance with the principles enunciated in this Declaration.

15 Medical research involving human subjects should be conducted only by scientifically qualified persons and under the supervision of a clinically competent medical person. The responsibility for the human subject must always

rest with a medically qualified person and never rest on the subject of the research, even though the subject has given consent.

16 Every medical research project involving human subjects should be preceded by careful assessment of predictable risks and burdens in comparison with foreseeable benefits to the subject or to others. This does not preclude the participation of healthy volunteers in medical research. The design of all studies should be publicly available.

17 Physicians should abstain from engaging in research projects involving human subjects unless they are confident that the hazards involved have been adequately assessed and can be satisfactorily managed. Physicians should cease any investigation if the risks are found to outweigh the potential benefits, or if there is conclusive proof of positive and beneficial results.

18 Medical research involving human subjects should only be conducted if the importance of the objective outweighs the inherent risks and burdens to the subject. This is especially important when the human subjects are healthy volunteers.

19 Medical research is only justified if there is a reasonable likelihood that the populations in which the research is carried out stand to benefit from the results of the research.

20 The subjects must be volunteers and informed participants in the research project.

21 The right of research subjects to safeguard their integrity must always be respected. Every precaution should be taken to respect the privacy of the subject and to minimise the impact of the study on the subject's physical and mental integrity and on the personality of the subject.

22 In any research on human beings, each potential subject must be adequately informed of the aims, methods, sources of funding, any possible conflicts of interest, institutional affiliations of the researcher, anticipated benefits and potential risks of the study and the discomfort it may entail. The subject should be informed of the right to abstain from participation in the study or to withdraw consent to participate at any time without reprisal. After ensuring that the subject has understood the information, the physician should then obtain the subject's freely-given informed consent, preferably in writing. If the consent cannot be obtained in writing, the non-written consent must be formally documented and witnessed.

23 When obtaining informed consent for the research project the physician should be particularly cautious if the subject is in a dependent relationship to him or her or may consent under duress. In that case the informed consent should be obtained by a well-informed physician who is not engaged in the investigation and who is completely independent of this relationship.

24 For a research subject who is legally incompetent, physically, or mentally incapable of giving consent, or is a legally incompetent minor, the

investigator must obtain informed consent from their legally authorised representative in accordance with applicable law. These groups should not be included in research unless the research is necessary to promote the health of the population represented and this research cannot be instead performed on legally competent persons.

25 When a subject deemed legally incompetent, such as a minor child, is able to give assent to decisions about participation in research the investigator must obtain that assent in addition to the consent of the legally authorised representative.

26 Research on individuals from whom it is not possible to obtain consent, including proxy or advance consent, should be done only if the physical/mental condition that prevents obtaining informed consent is a necessary characteristic of the research population. The specific reasons for involving research subjects with a condition that renders them unable to give informed consent should be stated in the experimental protocol for consideration and approval of the review committee. The protocol should state that consent to remain in the research should be obtained as soon as possible from the individual or a legally authorised surrogate.

27 Both authors and publishers have ethical obligations. In publication of the results of research, the investigators are obliged to preserve the accuracy of the results. Negative as well as positive results should be published or otherwise publicly available. Sources of funding, institutional affiliations and any possible conflicts of interest should be declared in the publication. Reports of experimentation not in accordance with the principles laid down in this Declaration should not be accepted for publication.

C. Additional Principles for Medical Research Combined with Medical Care

28 The physician may combine medical research with medical care, only to the extent that the research is justified by its potential prophylactic, diagnostic or therapeutic value. When medical research is combined with medical care, additional standards apply to protect the patients who are research subjects.

29 The benefits, risks, burdens and effectiveness of a new method should be tested against those of the best current prophylactic, diagnostic or therapeutic methods. This does not exclude the use of a placebo, or no treatment, in studies where no proven prophylactic, diagnostic or therapeutic method exists.

30 At the conclusion of the study, every patient entered into the study should be assured of access to the best proven prophylactic, diagnostic or therapeutic methods identified by the study.

31 The physician should fully inform the patient which aspects of the care are related to the research. The refusal of a patient to participate in a study must never interfere with the patient–physician relationship.

32 In the treatment of a patient, where proven prophylactic, diagnostic or therapeutic methods do not exist or have been ineffective, the physician, with informed consent from the patient, must be free to use unproven or new prophylactic, diagnostic or therapeutic measures, if in the physician's judgement it offers hope of saving life, re-establishing health or alleviating suffering. Where possible, these measures should be made the object of research, designed to evaluate their safety and efficacy. In all cases, new information should be recorded and, where appropriate, published. The other relevant guidelines of this Declaration should be followed.

Index